PLANETARY HERBOLOGY

PLANETARY
HERBOLOGY

An Integration Of Western Herbs
Into The Traditional Chinese
And Ayurvedic Systems

DR. MICHAEL TIERRA, C.A., N.D., O.M.D.

Edited and Supplemented
By DR. DAVID FRAWLEY, O.M.D.

Supplemented By Christopher Hobbs

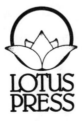

LOTUS
PRESS

Twin Lakes, Wisconsin

DISCLAIMER

This book is a reference work not intended to treat,
diagnose or prescribe. The information contained herein
is in no way to be considered as a substitute for consultation
with a duly licensed health-care professional.

FIRST EDITION, 1988
Printed in the United States of America

Library of Congress Cataloging-in-Publication Data

Tierra, Michael, 1939–
    Planetary herbology: an integration of Western
herbs into the traditional Chinese and Ayurvedic sys-
tems/Michael Tierra: edited and supplemented by
David Frawley.
        p.   cm.
    Bibliography: p.
    Includes Index.
    ISBN 0-941524/27/2: $16.95
    1. Herbs—Therapeutic use. 2. Medicine, Chi-
nese. 3. Medicine, Ayurvedic. I. Frawley, David.
II. Title.
RM666.H33T52 1988
615′.321—dc19   88-15901
                                    CIP

Published in 1992 by Lotus Press/P O Box 325/Twin Lakes/Wi/53181

DEDICATION

To all green, growing, flowering ones

of this beautiful planet,

who embody the universal creative healing

energy,

and with each moment,

humbly assume

the grand task

of transforming light into life,

and who patiently bear

the crude assaults and insults of our

misguided ignorance,

all in the dream of awakening.

Without their conscious, living presence,

nothing,

no breath nor food,

no life,

no delight,

none of our earthly endeavors would be possible.

TABLE OF CONTENTS

PART TWO
Planetary Materia Medica

PART THREE
Appendices

Publisher's Acknowledgement

This book greatly benefitted from the input of Harriet Slavitz who edited for style and clarity, as well as attending to the related minutiae of copy editing. Her labors were very ably supplemented by the sharp eye and boundless patience of Lavon Alt, a fine herbalist, who single handedly managed the inputting and indexing of this substantial manuscript through its several incarnations. Mina Yamashita designed the book and coordinated art production. The Publisher is indebted to them for the unusually devoted exercise of their skills.

FOREWORD

Herbs are a natural and primary therapeutic remedy for human ailments. Therefore, human beings have relied upon plants for healing for many thousands of years.

Drugs are poor substitutes for plants. They may be helpful for short-term or acute conditions, but their long-term action often depletes the primary life-force because of their inorganic nature. I believe that the reliance on chemical medicine contributes to a culture that is destroying our innate love of nature. Herbal medicine, therefore, relates to larger spiritual and political issues. If we do not reestablish our connection with the universe and natural healing, we may not be likely to survive as a species. We must replace our present medicines of death with those of life. Our concern as herbalists is not merely technical or medical, but planetary and humanistic.

An organic herbalism is, above all, an energetic herbalism. Yin and yang, the elements and humors, are part of the language of nature, a language of life. It is the appropriate language for understanding plants, their properties and their uses. Unfortunately, much of modern medicine and Western herbalism has become too focused on the chemical analysis of herbs as a basis for understanding them. This knowledge is useful but cannot substitute for the language of nature which is alchemical more than chemical. The value of this book is that it attempts to systematize Western herbs in a wholistic planetary manner.

I first came in contact with Michael Tierra when he wrote the forward to my book on the Ayurvedic method of herbal healing, *The Yoga of Herbs*. In this book, my co-author Dr. Vasant Lad and I attempted to discuss Western herbs according to the energetic principles of Ayurvedic medicine. Michael relates this project to his endeavor to classify Western herbs according to the energetic system of Chinese medicine.

Over the years, as a practitioner and teacher of Chinese as well as Ayurvedic medicine, I too have attempted to classify Western herbs according to the Chinese system. Since Michael also works in Ayurveda, and we found our work had other parallels, we began to share ideas and insights concerning herbs. Michael later suggested that I help him with this book.

As editor of the book, I rewrote some portions, particularly in the explanatory material relative to the different herbal categories. I also added some additional information on some of the individual herbs and contributed to the appendices.

We went over the materia medica together and Michael incorporated a number of my suggestions into the final text. Working together, I think we have brought harmony to a topic which should finally reach the audience it deserves. At the same time, I hope we have brought an equal share of clarity to those two traditional natural healing systems, the Ayurvedic and the Chinese. It is time to help bring into being a global culture, not merely a brief association with one culture or another, but a true synthesis. Healing systems which may appear cumbersome or "artificial" (and may be rejected by those who wish to stay with only one tradition) need to be examined in the light of others that are different. It is the fruit of such creative application which makes knowledge our own and enables it to work for us.

Herbs transcend their usage in any particular system. This is because they have such a wide variety of potential uses. In a basic state of nature, any given herb may be useful in treating almost any condition. The concept here is similar to a "primitive" state of society in which any given person plays different roles according to a variety of needs. As a culture evolves it becomes more specific in terms of specialization. The same thing is true of herbal medicine. Herbs can become very specific in terms of what they are used for. This is both a gain and a loss. The gain is that the specific therapeutic properties of individual herbs may be more efficiently utilized. The loss is that herbs may become artificially limited by specific classification.

Specialization has happened to a greater extent in Chinese and Ayurvedic herbalism as part of the long-term development of these great and enduring cultures. In Western herbalism, owing to a break down of natural healing traditions, this specialization has not occurred in the same way. Herbs may be presented as the tonic that is good for all that ails you—the same herb may, therefore, be classified as diaphoretic, diuretic, carminative, tonic and emmenagogue. We must always remember that herbs are a means of linking with the cosmic life-force. This is what matters ultimately—not the technicality, or complexity, or generality of the remedy

In comparing herb usage in different systems, we should discriminate between those uses which are primary in a specific herb and those which are secondary; between those which are intrinsic to an herb and those which it can fulfill only by special adaptation or preparation. We should note further that almost every single plant has some valid herbal usage, of which only a limited number can ever be used in a major way. In examining an herb we should also consider the role it plays in a particular system. Naturally, we should always consider the particular bias of this system.

Classification of herbs is not a fixed thing, but part of an overall strategy. Different traditions within the same tradition may classify or use the same herb in different ways. However, the uses of herbs are remarkably similar worldwide. (Examples are the use of gentian in Europe, America, India and China for detoxifying the liver. Conversely, hawthorn berries are used for treating food stagnation in Traditional Chinese Medicine and as a heart tonic in Western herbalism).

Sometimes an herb may be used centrally in one tradition and only peripherally in another. The usage of an herb should not be gauged by a tradition in which it is only of secondary use. Haritaki (*Terminalia chebula,*) a prime rejuvenative herb in Ayurvedic medicine, for example, is a minor astringent in Chinese medicine. We must not assume, therefore, that the Chinese terminalia is a different or inferior herb than the Indian. Similarly, such herbs as dandelion or nettles (used more widely in Western herbalism than in the oriental systems) may possess more significant therapeutic effects in the area of their wider use.

Traditional Chinese Medicine (T.C.M.), like other systems, has developed around the use of certain key herbs, mainly those used in classical formulas. In China there is also traditional folk medicine which uses a much larger number of herbs, owing to many localities. The herbs in the T.C.M. system are not necessarily better than those of their folk medicine, though they are among the better ones. Some folk medicines are entering into T.C.M. today, as they have through the passage of time, particularly in the treatment of modern problems for which we may not have specific classical formulas. Many commonly used anti-cancer herbs in China have been derived in this way.

Western herbal medicine is primarily a folk medicine. It has been unable to maintain a system of herbal practice along with diagnosis and formula development. Though originally it did have such system—through the Greeks and during the middle ages in Europe—today it lacks the sophistication of the oriental systems. The energetics of the East can be used to help us restore the energetics of our older Western tradition. They are not as alien as we would think, but in the fabric of the intuitive side of our own older culture, the values are all there to be rediscovered.

While Chinese and Ayurvedic medical systems have many advantages, they sometimes can become too focused on disease as a physical process. In both Eastern and Western systems, there is the need to emphasize the more spiritual, naturalistic approach to herbalism. This practice brings the plant into communion with the healer. The right healers, therefore, can do more with limited remedies and intuitive understanding than certain widely- based herbal medical professionals. Healing is through the life-force, and works in direct connection with the individual. Herbal medicine can be used mechanically, but this cannot do justice to its real power. So while systematic knowledge is important in approaching healing with herbs, it is necessary for us as individuals to take responsibility for our own health.

I would also like to make the following qualification: Traditional Chinese Medicine therapeutically uses certain animal and insect products which require the killing of living creatures. Ayurveda uses some of these as well, but it states that when we do so, we incur the negative karma of harming life. According to Ayurveda, these substances can only be rightfully used when our own life is in danger.

Otherwise, the negative karma of using them will, in the long run, outweigh the temporary good they do us. Hence, the use of these substances in this work is referential—not to encourage their use.

In conclusion, I would like to express my hope that this book becomes a tool in the ongoing renaissance of herbal medicine and natural healing. It may serve as the first modern planetary materia medica—a point of dialogue and synthesis for the future. I hope it further encourages those working along similar lines to have faith in what they are doing and persist in their work. Much more needs to be done to bring love and healing into the world

David Frawley
Santa Fe, New Mexico, March 1988

INTRODUCTION

This work is conceived out of a need to integrate Western herbalism into the more developed diagnostic and therapeutic systems of traditional Chinese and East Indian herbalism. It is apparent to anyone trained in the rigors of traditional Chinese and Ayurvedic herbalism that these systems are superior to ours. They better integrate differential diagnosis and treatment and demonstrate a more profound understanding of the actions and applications of herbs, and on these important counts have much to teach us. Our Western herbal tradition, on the other hand, hardly has progressed from the Galenic traditions of the ancient Greeks and Romans.

The contemporary practitioners of Western medical science disregard the traditional herbal systems. While there is a growing interest in looking for medicinal plants throughout the threatened forests and jungles of the world, it is focused on discovering genetic models for the development of new synthetic drugs rather than on the fullest uses of the whole herb legacies of wisdom that were systematized in the herbalism of traditional peoples.

Traditional Chinese and Ayurvedic herbal medicine are complete and thorough alternative medical systems developed, respectively, more than 3,000 and 5,000 years ago. Their pharmacopoeia and their methods of diagnosis and treatment are, not surprisingly, far superior to those of Western herbalism. Let us consider some of the serious shortcomings of the latter.

To begin with basics, quality commercial herbal material is very difficult to find. Most of these herbs are grown, harvested and prepared for sale according to less than optimum standards. While this situation is changing gradually as more people become more experienced in recognizing and using herbs, laymen (including not only the consumer, but the merchant and the distributor) may have good reason to doubt whether the herb they purchase is genuinely as represented by the seller.

There is also a serious need for the cultivation of certain valuable wild species such as lady's slipper *(Cypripedium)*, which is one of the most valuable nervines in North America. Although it is an endangered species, its harvesting from the wild is not prohibited in some areas. Such herbs will become even more gravely threatened as interest in herbalism grows and they are illegally harvested for monetary gain.

Many herbs essential to an effective, complete clinical practice are unavailable. One reason is that they are banned by governmental agencies because of alleged toxicity. This is unproven in such cases, for example, as sassafras and comfrey, but the ban persists. Many common spices such as nutmeg are useful as condiments and medicines in certain dosages and poisonous in higher amounts. Through a system of processing and assessment of dosage, extremely valuable yet somewhat toxic herbs like pokeroot *(Phytolacca)*, mandrake *(Mandragora)*, skunk cabbage *(Symplocarpus)*, blood root *(Sanguinaria)*, wild ginger *(Asarum)*, baptisia, wild indigo *(Isatis)*, bryonia, aconite *(Aconitum)*, datura and belladonna can be reinstated into the clinical armamentarium of the practicing herbalist.

Further, there is a need for Western herbalists to seek out adaptogenic tonics similar to certain Chinese herbs like ginseng and astragalus. These may not have been recognized in the traditions of the Native Americans and early settlers but may have a value comparative with that of herbs that are well known in oriental cultures.

Traditional systems of differential diagnosis employ a truly holistic assessment of the individual. This involves observation of the patient's over-all appearance and complexion, examination of the tongue and pulse, and palpation of certain areas of the body. The person's emotional attitude is observed, and details of the family history are gathered. Using all this accumulated data, the practitioner then makes a differential evaluation of symptoms, keying the prescription of specific herbs and formulas to these findings.

Although both can be extremely useful to the herbalist for a balanced understanding of specific herbs, the traditional energetic classification of herbs allows one to practically and efficiently encompass a greater range of therapeutic actions than the scientific biochemical model. To date, it has been the tendency in the West to consider herbs as substitutes for drugs, but, generally, Western medicine ignores the over-all effect of drugs on the individual. Because of the numerous side effects of doctor-prescribed drugs, resulting in iatrogenic (doctor-caused) dis-orders, there is a growing dissatisfaction with these and other practices of contemporary Western medicine.

Since traditional Chinese and Ayurvedic medicine are the most artic-ulated alternative herbal systems extant, it would be much to our advan-tage to be able to integrate Western herbs into the Oriental diagnostic and therapeutic models. When I was in China in 1980, I spoke with my teachers there about classifying our native North American herbs into the energetic system of Chinese medicine. They said that what I pro-posed could not be done, that it had taken the efforts of countless her-balists over many centuries to evolve such a complete system and phar-macopoeia. After many years of pondering this problem, I agree that this process cannot be satisfactorily accomplished by a single individual. All I may hope to achieve is a modest beginning which, over the coming years, will be enriched by my own practice and evolution in understand-ing, and that of many other herbalists as well.

This book represents my study of the nature and properties of Chi-nese, Indian and Western herbs. I compared the Chinese categories of *surface-relieving herbs* or *herbs to relieve wind and dampness*, for instance, to the similarly-acting and commonly known Western herbs such as the diaphoretics or antirheumatics. In the same way, I studied the common characteristics of Ayurvedic herbs whose energetics were determined by their taste, and by their action on broad physiological processes classified under the three humoral categories of air, fire and water. Fortunately, a sufficient number of models of classifications by the Chinese and Indians were already available and very well known in the West.

I then took note of therapeutic characteristics, properties and flavors in common among the herbs already classified by the Chinese. Chinese herbs classified as *chi tonics*, for example, were mostly regarded as sweet in taste with a neutral energy and as acting on the spleen and lung meridians. According to Western classifications, many of these have demulcent, carminative and nutritive actions. I particularly took note of common factors found in the majority of herbs classified as chi or yang, blood or yin tonics, for instance, and also noted seemingly irrational inconsistencies in the classification of many herbs that could easily fit into several categories. The Chinese herb bupleurum classified as a *cool surface-relieving* diaphoretic is mostly used as a *chi-regulating* carminative. Hawthorn berry, a Western herb used for its cardiac and circulating properties is classified by the Chinese as an herb for removing food congestion, but in practice they too use it for heart and circulatory problems.

Through comparing all of these factors, I arrived at the classifications presented here, offering them with the understanding that they must be considered to be to some extent arbitrary until they have been verified through further practical testing—not only my own but that of other herbalists as well. Since I have been able to make this pharmacopiea available on computer data base,[1] it will be possible for individuals to use this book as a model, revising classifications and dosages as their experience informs them.

In my book *The Way of Herbs* (New York: Washington Square Press, 1980), I presented a popular herbal, with suggestions for self-treatment, useful for the general public. The present volume, to which I have devoted six years of effort, continues and builds upon that earlier work, and is addressed principally to the serious herbal practitioner as well as to other therapists such as the acupuncturist, naturopath, chiropractor, medical doctor and lay practitioner.

This work was written to further a lively tradition of energetic usage and classification of herbs, and to incorporate into those systems Western herbs that may be used in conjunction with Chinese and Ayurvedic herbalism. It is my fervent hope that it will prove useful to its readers.

Michael Tierra
Santa Cruz, California

[1]see pg 485

PART ONE

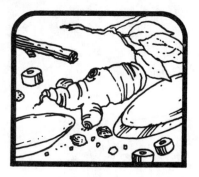

The Art and
Science of
Planetary Herbalism

THE ROOTS OF PLANETARY HERBALISM

Healing herbs are everywhere. A hike in the country or a brief stroll through the garden may reveal a pharmacopoeia of medicines for body, mind and spirit. If we have some knowledge of the herbal arts, our finds may then inspire us to envision some of their countless healing possibilities. For herbalism is a religion of nature, representing a balance of head and heart, that relies more on artful intuition than precise scientific reasoning.

Since all substances possess energies and qualities, all plants must have potential therapeutic application. What remains is for us to discover and understand what these uses might be. This may include exploring the uses of exotic plants from distant lands, as well as of the common vegetables and weeds growing in our yards and gardens.

The energetic description of herbs based upon their heating and cooling energies, the five flavors (bitter, sweet, spicy, salty and sour), along with their more specific therapeutic actions, is probably the oldest way of classifying herbs. It makes possible a system of medicine whose integration of the physical and psychological aspects of disease and holistic approach to diagnosis and treatment is unrivaled by contemporary Western scientific medicine.

Contemporary Western scientists are critical of traditional herbal medical systems for their tendency to be too general, inviting inconsistencies and subjective ambiguities that are difficult to measure with current medical technologies. This accounts for the period of eclipse of traditional herbal medicine. Its reliance on subjective evaluations and diagnoses, based upon observation of the pulse, tongue and appearance of the patient, has been replaced by a mechanistic evaluation. Mainstream medicine involves more technology, with much less time spent by doctor with patient. There is a risk involved in ignoring or not sufficiently considering those immeasurable factors of emotions and lifestyle, that always will be part factors in the complete symptomology of the patient.

Traditional systems of herbalism also include the patient's reaction to treatment in the diagnosis. The reaction to a particular remedy is a further indication of the patient's over-all condition, and care must be taken so that the possible negative reactions to food or herbal remedies do not prove too extreme. With Western drugs and therapies, the allowable margin of error is much narrower; and with them there is a far greater possibility of harmful side effects.

Herbs, as "special foods", tend to be absorbed as a complete food with active therapeutic properties. In order to understand the over-all effect of a particular substance on an individual, one must take into account its total "personality" or energetic nature as well as its specific therapeutic action. This is more possible with herbs than with drugs because of their greater resemblance to whole foods. Drugs may possess specific therapeutic actions that are helpful in the short term or in acute conditions but energetically in the longer term their inorganic or non-food nature makes them deranging.

The knowledge of the energetic classification of herbs has largely been lost in the West, but remains intact in the traditional herbal systems of India and China. The vitality of these systems continues to be maintained, evolving beyond the simple theoretical principles of the bipolar energies of yin and yang, the elements and humors, that were a common legacy to East and West in the ancient world. Properly understood, their depth of understanding and wisdom about their plant remedies can connect us all with what Dr. Paul Lee has called "the vital roots of existence."

Herbs, used as "special foods" in accordance with energetic principles, have proved effective in treating the majority of diseases, both acute and chronic, including some that may not respond to standard Western medicines. They are further useful offsetting the possible harmful side effects of Western drugs when used in conjunction with them.

The tendency of Western technological medicine has been to focus on the eradication of symptoms rather than on removing the underlying conditions and causes from which disease arises. This approach allows the disease to progress to a chronic condition, while the symptoms are masked by technological drug medicines and therapies. The herbalist, on the other hand, using mild therapeutic agents, is committed to a proc-

ess of eliminating and adjusting those factors that are likely to perpetu-
ate the disease process.

The primary focus of holistic herbalism is to support the body's
inherent healing capacity. The primary action of herbs is less to provide
substantive nourishment, as in the case of vitamin supplements, than to
stimulate and increase the body's inherent ability to synthesize, extract
and utilize the special nutrients that are available only in whole foods.
The food-like quality of herbs also, in many cases, supply nutritional
needs as well, from their content of essential vitamin, mineral and trace
elements. It is exactly their food-like quality that makes it easier for the
body to organically process and eliminate herbs; while synthetic drugs
may have a much longer and often devastating effect upon the body.

Traditional systems of herbal diagnosis use four main methods:

1. interrogation (symptoms, case history)
2. observation (manner, facial appearance, tongue)
3. palpation (trigger points on the body, pulse)
4. listening (tone of voice, breathing, heart)

These methods provide a simple and profound understanding of the
patient and of the nature of the disease.

The unified theoretical basis of yin-yang theory in Chinese herbalism and the humoral theory of Ayurveda provide a similarly balanced
approach to the understanding of health, disease and treatment. They
agree closely, too, in their understanding of herbs and other natural substances obtained from the vegetable, animal and mineral kingdoms.
These are used as directly harvested, or in special preparations and formulas, to encourage the metabolic processes of the body and to reinstate
homeostasis. Their use is based on classification in terms of over-all
effects, and specifically, according to their therapeutic properties and
innate biochemistry.

Up to the seventeenth century, with the advent of the rational phi-
losophy of Descartes, Western medicine classified herbs according to
their bipolar heating or cooling nature much as they were classified in
other cultures throughout the world. Astrological symbolism, now
popularly understood in the the West as a kind of fortune telling, once

was used here as a way of describing an integration of humankind with the cosmos. Herbs and diseases were classified and described energetically in terms of astrological symbolism, from the times of the ancient Egyptians and of Hippocrates until a few centuries ago. In fact, an understanding of the principles of diagnosis and treatment according to the occult science of astrology was considered an essential part of the study of the art of medicine.

The seventeenth century herbalist, Nicolas Culpeper, 1616-1654, (whose *Complete Herbal* is still in print in England,) states that "physic (study of medicine) without astrology is like a lamp without oil." European herbals and materia medica designated not only the physical therapeutic effects of herbs but also their astrological indications.

While the herbal-astrological system was never standardized in the West (as it was in the *Vedic* astrology of India), certain principles of energetic classification indicated how the herbalist might apply certain herbs for certain types of individuals and diseases. Thus, herbs ruled by the Sun (cayenne, calendula) are warming and drying, while those ruled by the Moon (spinach, chickweed) are cooling and soothing. Herbs and foods ruled by Jupiter (seeds and nuts) are nourishing, while those ruled by Mars (prickly ash, garlic) have more active, circulating properties. Herbs ruled by Saturn (ginseng, comfrey root) have a slower, moistening action. Those ruled by Mercury (lady's slipper root, dill) affect the nervous system, whereas those ruled by Venus (sage, uva ursi), promote purification of the blood and genito-urinary tract.

The early twentieth century visionary, Dr. Rudolf Steiner, inspired by the scientific writings of the poet Goethe (*The Metamorphosis of Plants*), taught and wrote about the therapeutic energetics of botanical medicine. Steiner began where the poet Goethe left off, with the understanding that the innate healing potential of plants is revealed more in their unique patterns of growth and development than in their biochemical constituents. A system of Anthroposophical herbal medicine, inspired by Steiner's teachings and lectures, continues to exert a profound influence among its adherents.

Homeopathic medicine is a purely energetic system of healing that uses many herbs and other substances. Many of these in crude form are deadly poisons; but in the infinitesimal dilutions of homeopathy they are safe and effective remedies. The theoretical basis of homeopathic medicine is "like cures like" and the use of the minimal dose. Medicines are selected which when taken in substantial amounts precipitate a variety of reactions and symptoms that mirror the disease to be treated. Diluted to a minute dose, this is the homeopathic remedy prescribed. In this way, substances relieve, in subtle amounts, the conditions they would cause if taken in gross amounts

First developed by the eighteenth century German scientist Hahnemann, homeopathy has had and continues to have many thousands of adherents and practitioners around the world. Because of its low cost (one drop of a tincture can be diluted and prepared to effectively treat hundreds of patients) and negligible toxicity, it is very popular in economically depressed countries such as India, but also in more affluent ones as well. When the correct remedy is used in accordance with the physiological and emotional patterns of the patient, homeopathic medicine can be astoundingly effective for the treatment of both acute and chronic diseases.

The energetic basis of herbalism is represented in Chinese and East Indian Ayurvedic medicine. Aspects of this approach to medicine were known in ancient times throughout the Mediterranean, among the Babylonians, Egyptians, Greeks and Romans. Though this older European counterpart passed away, an Islamic form survives in the Unani system of medicine. Curiously enough, it is most widely practiced and studied today in India, where it has become reintegrated into Ayurveda.

If one looks deeply into the mythic symbolisms of traditional peoples, archetypal counterparts to the traditional healing systems of India and China may be seen. In the Native American's use of the medicine wheel, for example, there is a relationship to the fire-element systems of Chinese and Ayurvedic medicine.

The medicine wheel assigns animal totems to each of the four directions. These symbolically represent various personality types and spiritual energies and qualities, as well as diseases and plant medicines. Symbol-systems vary among tribes. According to one tribal system, the energy of the West, symbolized by the elk or grizzly bear, represents the powers of introspection, strength and responsibility; the South, symbolized by the mouse or coyote, represents the energies of maturing, growth and compassion; the East, symbolized by the hawk or eagle, represents the powers of wisdom, mental clarity and enlightenment; the North, symbolized by the white buffalo, represents the energies of renewal, purity, balance and patience.

The nineteenth and early twentieth century Eclectic herbalists of North America evolved a less esoteric system of differential diagnosis that stressed the treatment of the whole person rather than only of specific diseases. They integrated the medicine and science of their day with the use of hundreds of herbs, mainly from the Native American tradition.

It is unfortunate that the contribution made by the American Eclectic herbalists, homeopathic medicine and lay midwifery has been devalued by the medical monopoly of the allopathically-supported American Medical Association. In 1907, Andrew Carnegie and John D. Rockefeller commissioned a man named Flexnor to investigate hospitals and schools in order to advise them on investments in American medicine. Flexnor's report found that the "heroic" doctors, whose heroism consisted in the free use of surgery, would best represent the development of industrial technology and would provide the greatest profit to his sponsors. With this financial support, allopathic medicine began to flourish.

Within a few years, well established Eclectic medicinal schools, herbal pharmaceutical companies, homeopathic schools, schools for midwifery, medical schools for black doctors disappeared owing to lack of funding. Herbalism was so denigrated that medical doctors of the 1930s were ashamed to admit their knowledge and use of traditional herbal remedies. Powerful opponents of herbalism were the financially booming chemical drug companies. They had discovered how lucrative exclusive patent rights on synthetic drug medicines could be. Herbalists, on the other hand, employed substances that could be found and used by anyone.

While it should be acknowledged that mainstream medicine literally has saved millions of lives, perhaps its greatest contribution has been in disease prevention through introduction of the principles of urban sanitation and personal hygiene. Perhaps the ideal system of the future would incorporate the best of Western scientific medicine with traditional medical systems and herbs.

Today, more than three-quarters of the world's population still rely on the use of medicinal herbs for their primary health care. The recent popularity of alternative medicine and of health foods in the urbanized West is an encouraging sign. As environmental pollution increases, as health care provided by the medical establishment becomes increasingly unaffordable and dangerous, as denatured foods fail to support our immune systems, surely the holistic alternatives of diet and therapy will gain in importance.

Planetary Herbalism is a term that denotes the integration of the world's most developed systems of traditional herbal medicine. It integrates the traditional differential classification of diseases with the energetic classification of herbal medicines, and includes all useful contributions, past or present, including scientific knowledge. It embraces not only plant medicines but remedies derived from the animal and mineral kingdoms as well.

To achieve a planetary system first we must examine the principles of diagnosis and classification of the two great systems of holistic herbal medicine, traditional Chinese herbalism and East Indian Ayurvedic medicine. Using these systems as models, we can begin to develop standards and principles of classification and treatment that will have practical value both to the clinical practitioner and the interested layperson. This will include the classification of herbs according to their energies, flavors, organs and meridians affected, humoral designation according to the Ayurvedic *Tridosha* theory, as well as their therapeutic properties and biochemical components.

THE NATURE OF HERBS
IN THE CHINESE, AYURVEDIC AND
WESTERN SYSTEMS

Herbs have both broad food-like qualities as well as specific medicinal effects. The traditional herbalist recognizes the value of integrating both their general and specific properties by using the whole herb in its natural state, in special preparations, or combined with other herbs in formulas.

The broad effects of foods and herbs will be described energetically, using systems that classify them according to their heating or cooling qualities. This approach is integral to nearly all traditional wholistic systems of herbal healing, but was most highly developed and evolved by the traditional systems of Chinese herbalism and East Indian Ayurvedic medicine. It also was used by the ancient Greeks and Romans, and by herbalists throughout Europe until the 17th century.

TRADITIONAL CHINESE CLASSIFICATION OF FOOD AND HERBS

The Chinese have developed their understanding of food and herbs through centuries of observation and use under many different conditions. Their classification is based upon four categories:

1. Four Natures
2. Five Flavors
3. Four Directions
4. Organs and Meridians Affected.

Four Natures

Herbs are classified as cold, cool, warm and hot and their curative properties are related in this way to the general nature of various diseases. Thus one uses cold or cool herbs for diseases of a hyper-metabolic, hot or yang nature and, conversely, hot or warm herbs for diseases of a hypo-metabolic, cold or yin nature.[1] Contraindicated, therefore, would be the use of hot or warm-natured herbs for hot diseases, or cool or cool-natured herbs for cold diseases.

Despite the fact that they may actually have a slightly cool or warm energy, many herbs are classified as mild or neutral which means that they may be used either for hot or cold diseases.

Five Flavors

The five flavors are sour, bitter, sweet, spicy and salty. In addition there is a bland taste which usually is classified as mildly sweet.

Each of the flavors relates to a general physiological effect. The sour flavor tends to contract flaccid tissues and stop abnormal secretions. It is yin, cooling and refreshing, and promotes digestion, enzyme secretion and liver function. Sour-flavored herbs and foods include lemon, rose hips, hawthorn berries and Chinese dogwood berries.

The bitter flavor is yin, cooling, clearing, detoxifying, antibiotic, anti-inflammatory, antiviral and antiparasitical. When taken in a normal dosage it stimulates the release of antibodies and enhances the production and secretion of bile through the liver, thus aiding this important organ in its function of detoxification. In small amounts it possesses a tonic or digestion-promoting action. Bitters are taken daily as a tea in many Oriental and European countries to help protect the body against disease and parasites and to cleanse the blood. Taken as a wine (in half to full teaspoonful doses) before meals, alcoholic bitters are used as a tonic to promote the secretion of hydrochloric acid, improving stomach function. Because bitter-tasting herbs also clear the veins and arteries of cholesterol, they ease circulation and benefit the heart. Bitter herbs include golden seal, gentian, centaury and mugwort.

The sweet flavor is yang, warming, soothing, tonic, building and nourishing. All herbs that are considered nourishing and most foods are classifed as sweet. Most common foodstuffs, including whole grains, beans, dairy and meat, are classified as "full" sweet. Foods that possess an abundance of simple sugars (such as sweet fruits, juices, honey and sugar) lack a balance of complex carbohydrates and proteins and are considered "empty" sweet: rather than satisfying they intensify the craving for sweet taste. Tonic, nutritive herbs and foods with a sweet flavor include ginseng, rehmannia, dates and barley malt sugar.

The spicy or pungent flavor is yang, warming, dispersing and drying. It distributes energy from the interior to the surface of the body and is used to counteract feelings of coldness, poor circulation, poor digestion and as a natural stimulant. It is useful for the treatment of hypometabolic conditions, mucous congestion, arthritic and rheumatic complaints, delayed menstruation, colds and flu. To relieve pain from bruises and injuries it is applied topically. Some spicy-tasting herbs are peppers, cinnamon, ginger and prickly ash.

The salty flavor is classified as yin, cooling and moistening because of its ability to help maintain fluid balance. Besides sodium chloride (common salt), there are many other salts such as sodium sulphate which is purging. The Ayurvedic classification of salt as being heating or "pitta" (fire) predominant is a matter of perspective. Salt in itself is cold, while its ultimate effect on the body can be irritating, fluid-retaining, and thus heating. Sources include the various seaweeds.

The bland flavor is mild and classified in the sweet category. It generally is regarded as being diuretic. Mushrooms are in this category.

Macrobiotics seems to reverse the traditional yin-yang classification of the flavors. Thus foods and herbs that are spicy, sweet and sour are considered yin while foods and herbs that are bitter and salty are considered yang. This may be a special adjustment of George Ohsawa who first introduced macrobiotics in the West. Again, the difference is probably one of perspective. The traditional Chinese approach evaluates the flavor and nature of the substance itself and its relatively immediate physiological reaction as opposed to the reaction that Ohsawa observed as a result of excess and long-term use.

Four Directions

All substances are said to be floating, descending, rising or sinking in relation to the body. These directions relate closely to the five flavors and they agree with the four seasons: summer is floating, fall is descending, winter is sinking and spring is ascending. The direction of yang is upwards while that of yin is downwards. Thus, lighter herbs, like leaves and flowers, tend to float and ascend, making them useful for more acute and surface diseases such as colds, flu and inflammations. Heavier herbs such as barks, seeds and roots descend and sink, and are more effective in treating deeper, more chronic diseases.

Organs and Meridians Affected

Historically, since this system of the Chinese is a comparatively recent one, having originated only a few hundred years ago, it is not yet as fully developed as the more ancient classification of herbs. Nevertheless, it is very useful, connecting herbs and foods with specific organic effects as well as with their influence on the acupuncture meridian pathways.

The principal way of discerning what organs and meridians an herb affects is by defining its predominant properties. In order to do this, one needs to understand how the Chinese evaluate the specific organs and meridians. Chinese physiology is based upon the dynamic interaction of the 12 vital organs, and not simply on their separate, local, and specialized functions. This is best expressed in the Five Phases of Transformation, which will be explained below.

THE YIN ORGANS OF TRANSFORMATION

The lungs rule the skin and are involved with the production of mucus. Most colds, flu and skin diseases, for instance, are considered superficial diseases. Sweating or diaphoretic herbs are said to affect the energy of the lungs because they open the surface of the skin, helping to clear skin blemishes and in treating the initial stages of simple acute colds and flu. The lungs are considered to partake of the energy of metal and are associated with paleness and whiteness. Thus, herbs that are white and mucilaginous are often used to moisten and tonify the lungs.

The kidney-adrenals dominate the urinary and hormonal systems of the body. They are characterized by the water element according to the Chinese and are associated with the color black. Herbs that are diuretic, aphrodisiac, tonic and nourishing, and are heavy and black in color, are regarded as working on the kidney organ and meridian.

The liver is classified as wood element and is represented by the color green. Most green, leafy vegetables, herbs that release bile or possess the green-yellow color of bile and calm hypertension are believed to affect the liver organ and meridian.

The heart partakes of the fire element and is represented by the color red. It is said to dominate the blood and circulation. Most herbs that are red and bitter and that clear cholesterol from the veins and arteries are said to affect the heart organ and meridian.

The spleen-pancreas is of the earth element and is represented by the golden-yellow color of the sun. It rules the processes of digestion and assimilation. Herbs that are tonic, nutritive, warming and beneficial to digestion are said to affect the spleen organ and meridian.

THE YANG ORGANS OF TRANSPORTATION

The colon is the yang of metal and counterbalances the lungs. It is affected by herbs that have a laxative action.

The bladder is the yang of water and counterbalances the kidneys. It is affected by herbs that have a lighter, superficial diuretic action as opposed to the heavier, deeper tonic effects of herbs associated with the kidneys.

The gall bladder is the yang of wood and counterbalances the liver. It is usually affected by lighter herbs which promote the secretion of bile.

The small intestine is yang of fire and counterbalances the heart. It is associated with digestion, and its disorders may produce blood in the urine. Herbs that arrest this symptom are said to affect the small intestine organ and meridian.

The stomach is the yang of earth and counterbalances the spleen. It is affected by herbs that are more carminative and digestive rather than sweet-flavored tonics.

Finally, the Chinese assign the organ functions including the triple warmer and pericardium meridians to the fire element. The triple warmer is affected by herbs that have a combined action of aiding digestion and regulating the circulation of fluids. The pericardium meridian is the emotional companion of the heart and is affected by these herbs that act on the heart.

THE AYURVEDIC CLASSIFICATION OF HERBS AND FOODS

Ayurvedic medicine is based upon constitutional analysis and evaluation of disease according to the three humors (or *tridosha*) and the seven vital tissues of the body (*dhatus*). There are many herbs used in common by Ayurveda and Chinese herbalism. Several of these may be found also in the West. The therapeutics of the Ayurvedic, like the Chinese system is based upon energy,(*virya*), and taste, (*rasa*). Ayurveda, however, adds two other categories: post-digestive effect, *vipaka,* and special potency, *prabhava.*

Before describing the four methods of classification used in Ayurvedic herbalism it is important to offer a brief description of the three-humor system.

Ayurveda recognizes five elements, two of which differ from two of the Chinese five elements. The Chinese elements are earth, water, fire, wood and metal. As in the older European system, the Ayurvedic elements are earth, water, fire, air and ether. In Ayurveda the humors describe three constitutional types based upon qualities of these elements.

Vata, the air humor, relates most directly to the nervous system and combines the air and ether elements. It is described as being dry, cold, light, mobile, subtle, rough, hard, irregular and clear. Because it embodies the very essence of the life energy, it is considered the most powerful of the three humors; and can carry and/or combine with either of the other two.

Vata governs respiration, movement, will, equilibrium, and acuity of the senses. In a deranged condition it will cause coldness, dryness, dark discolorations, tremors, abdominal distention, constipation, weakness, insomnia and other neurological problems, and lack of energy.

Herbs that reduce excess vata are demulcent, nutritive tonics with a sweet taste and warm energy. Herbs that aggravate vata are drying, diuretic, bitter and astringent.

Pitta, the fire humor, is hot, light, fluid, subtle, malodorous, soft and clear. It is catabolic and governs thermogenesis and all chemical reactions.

Pitta governs digestion, circulation, heat, visual acuity, hunger, thirst, skin luster, intelligence, courage, determination and pliability and softness of the body. In a deranged condition it will cause a jaundiced appearance or yellowish color of the urine, feces, eyes and skin. This may be accompanied by inflammatory and burning symptoms, insomnia, and greater hunger and thirst.

Herbs that increase pitta have a warm, moist nature with pungent, sour or salty flavors. Herbs that eliminate excess pitta are drying and cooling, with bitter, astringent and sweet flavors.

Kapha, the water or mucous humor, is cold, wet, heavy, slow, dull, smooth, and cloudy. It is anabolic or building.

Kapha governs bodily stability and strength, body fluids and lubrication of the joints and fosters peacefulness, love and patience. In a deranged state it will cause a diminution of digestive power, excessive phlegm and mucus, exhaustion, heaviness of the body and mind, pallor, coldness, difficult breathing and excessive desire for sleep. Herbs that increase kapha are moist, demulcent, nutritive, tonic, sweet and salty. Herbs that eliminate excess kapha are drying, warm and eliminative with spicy, bitter and astringent flavors.

Mental and spiritual qualities are attributed to the three biological humors, as has been indicated above. Temperament types may be classified from observing how the humors combine in an individual and which predominates.

The seven *dhatus* or vital tissues are plasma, blood, muscle, fat, bone, marrow and reproductive tissues. Herbs and foods of particular properties are used to counterbalance and remedy the diseases that affect them. The fundamental essence and strength of a given organism, however, is considered to derive from its healthy functioning as a whole, and the Ayurvedic term for this is *ojas*. This literally means 'to invigorate' and includes the functioning of the auto-immune system and the hormonal balance of the body. *Ojas* results from the refined functioning of all seven vital tissues, particularly the reproductive tissues or semen.

The difference between the traditional Chinese and Ayurvedic systems of diagnosis and treatment is primarily one of emphasis. Each system contains elements that are present in the other, but the heart of Ayurvedic medicine is its theory of *tridosha*. An understanding of *tridosha*, greatly contributes to recognition of a person's constitutional predisposition, assisting the practitioner in creating a therapeutic program that integrates all aspects of that individual's life. The prescription of diet and herbal therapy, counselling as to health-promoting lifestyle and exercise, understanding of emotional problems and recommendations of spiritual practices—all are based on diagnosis of the humoral balance. Like Ayurveda, traditional Chinese medicine, which is rooted in ancient Taoist tradition, is based on a mind-body unity. However, since the Communist revolution, Chinese medicine has tended to eliminate the psychological and spiritual components of healing, emphasizing the efficient and effective treatment of physical symptoms.

According to the Ayurvedic system, diseases which match the constitutional nature of a patient are much harder to cure than those that do not. For instance, a mucous type of disease that arises in a water-predominant (kapha) individual is harder to cure than if it arose in a fire (pitta) or air-predominant (vata) type. A neurological or vata disease that occurs in a vata person is harder to cure than it is in a pitta or kapha person. And, an inflammatory disease that develops in a pitta constitution is harder to cure than if it occurred in a kapha or vata person.

As with Traditional Chinese Medicine, the Ayurvedic system is designed to enable us to understand and to prevent disease. It also offers the tools for diagnosing and treating the many strange and seemingly intractable minor symptoms that are signs of minor humoral imbalances to the trained practitioner.

Energy
(Virya)

Both Ayurveda and Chinese herbalism classify herbs according to the heating or cooling properties. As one might expect, heating herbs promote warmth, circulation, digestion and motivation. In excess, they can create burning sensations, irritation, sweating, thirst, dizziness and exhaustion. They increase pitta (fire) and decrease vata (air) and kapha (water).

Cooling herbs create a sense of refreshment, a lifting of feelings of oppression. They promote detoxification and clarity. They tend to clear pitta and the blood but can also increase vata and kapha. When taken in excess, cooling substances produce an undesirable coldness, hypo-enervation, frailty, sadness, nervousness, poor memory and gradual degeneration.[2]

Agni and Soma

In Ayurveda, the life energy of the body is called *agni* or fire and cor-responds to the fiery essence of life included under the concepts of essen-tial yang and chi in Chinese medicine. The nature of *agni*, like that of yang, is warm, dry and motivating. It is this vital energy that provides the spark of life with which digestion of food begins.

In contrast, the material bodily essence which Ayurveda calls *soma* corresponds to all those cooling qualities which in Chinese medicine are classified as yin and blood. Like yin, *soma* is substantial, cool, and fluid. Herbs that are stimulants, carminatives, yang or chi tonics tend to pro-mote *agni;* while herbs that are anti-inflammatory, demulcent, blood and yin tonics tend to promote *soma*.

The Flavors
(Rasa)

Both Chinese herbalism and Ayurveda relate the flavors of herbs and foods to their therapeutic properties. Unlike Chinese medicine, Ayur-veda defines six tastes, counting sour and astringent as distinct from each other. This is because of their differing actions. Sour, acidic things like citrus and hawthorn berries possess stimulating and digestion-promoting properties and are thirst-relieving. Astringent taste, as in oak bark or alum, weakens digestion and promotes thirst. In this instance, Ayurveda is more refined in how the tastes function.

As stated, Ayurveda regards salt as heating because of its irritating and burning effect (for example, its effect when rubbed on an open wound). The Chinese regard salt as cooling because of its inert, heavy and sinking aspects. Both systems, however, agree that the therapeutic action of salt is moistening and water-retaining. Sweet and astringent are considered cooling in Ayurveda. Bitter is universally considered cooling in Eastern cultures (although alcoholic bitters are used as a digestive tonic in Western countries).

The important point of common understanding here lies in the therapeutic use of the flavors. Any differences are based upon the preferred strategies of healing and the approach to stimulating biological change. For example, cayenne pepper may be used in moderate amounts to warm up the body and even is classified in some Chinese herbals as a yang tonic. Used in substantial amounts however, cayenne (or chili peppers) disperses stagnation, moving the heat from the center of the body to its surface, ultimately causing coolness. It is commonly used in this way and for this purpose in hot, humid climates.

The sweet flavor is composed of the elements of earth and water. It is cooling, nutritive, pleasant and softening. It is commonly known that both sugar and honey are cooling and anti-inflammatory and that applying sugar or honey directly to a wound prevents infection.

The essence of nourishment, the sweet flavor is used for general debility, weakness, symptoms of aging, lack of semen and impotence. It is contraindicated for kapha (water) disorders, including obesity, mucous diseases like cough and asthma, diabetes, goiter and filaria. Some sources of sweet flavor are dates, licorice, marshmallow root, slippery elm and comfrey root.

The sour flavor is composed of the elements of earth and fire. It is heating, causes salivation, increases secretions, cleans the mouth, induces sweating and causes burning in the mouth and throat. It is used for loss of appetite, dyspepsia, and vata disorders or diseases of the nervous system. It is contraindicated for disorders of pitta (fire) and blood, gastritis, internal bleeding and jaundice.

Citrus fruits, rose hips and hawthorn berries are sources of sour flavor.

The salty flavor is composed of the elements of water and fire. It is heating, easily soluble, water-retaining, softening, and causes a burning sensation in the mouth and throat. It is used for loss of appetite and dyspepsia, as an expectorant for coughs, as a diuretic, and for neurological or vata disorders. It is contraindicated for disorders of pitta (fire) and blood, skin diseases, swelling, ascites, hypertension, hemorrhage and gastritis.

Salt, epsom salt (sodium sulphate) and seaweeds are salty flavor substances.

The spicy or pungent flavor is composed of the elements of fire and air. It is heating, counteracts congestion and stagnation, stimulates the nervous system, warms, stimulates digestion, causes tears, headaches and tingling sensations. Spicy taste is effective in treating loss of appetite and indigestion, and as an anthelmintic for dysentery. It also is helpful for coughs, colds, asthma, obesity, skin diseases and as a dentifrice. It reduces excess kapha (water) and vata (air). Hot, spicy-tasting herbs and foods are contraindicated in disorders of pitta (fire) and blood, eruptive skin diseases and semen disorders.

Some spicy or pungent flavor substances are peppers, cinnamon, asafoetida, garlic, aconite, and prickly ash.

The bitter flavor is composed of the elements of air and ether. It is cooling, overwhelms all the other flavors, and is clearing, drying and cleansing to the mouth. It is antipyretic, clears fevers, is detoxifying, removes pus, is anthelmintic, antiparasitical, inhibits bleeding, relieves burning sensations, treats skin diseases and also is useful in anorexia. Bitter taste in excess is contraindicated in nervous disorders, as it would further derange vata (air). It also is not recommended for semen disorders.

Golden seal, gentian, centaury, colombo, boldo and barberry or Oregon grape are bitter flavor.

The astringent flavor is composed of the elements of earth and air. It is cooling, contracting, clearing, drying, causes stiffness, mouth dryness, heart pains and feelings of heaviness. It also promotes healing, stops bleeding, is antidiuretic, stops diarrhea, is absorbent, and normalizes skin pigmentation. Astringent herbs are contraindicated in conditions of general debility and weakness, anorexia and loss of appetite, and disorders of vata (air) or neurological disorders.

Oak bark, cranesbill, alum, witch hazel and bayberry are astringent flavor.

Post-Digestive Effect
(Vipaka)

A special classification unique to Ayurveda reduces the six flavors to three in terms of their ultimate physiological effects after digestion. These correspond to three stages of digestion and assimilation.

The first stage is dominated by the alkaline secretions in the mouth and stomach characterized by the sweet and salty flavors (kapha). The second stage is the heating reaction characterized by the secretion of hydrocholoric acid and various digestive enzymes, and is represented by the sour stage (pitta). The third stage is the drying reaction when the intestines reabsorb fluid from the wastes and is represented by the spicy (or pungent), bitter and astringent flavors (vata).

Thus the sweet and salty flavors are said to have a sweet *vipaka* or post-digestive effect because they tend to increase bodily substance in accordance with the nutritive aspects of the sweet flavor. The sour flavor has a sour *vipaka,* while bitter, astringent and pungent flavors have a pungent *vipaka.* There are some exceptions. When the *vipaka* of certain herbs differs from their primary taste, this gives us special information about their action. Gotu kola, for example, though bitter in taste, has an exceptional sweet *vipaka,* indicating its special tonic properties for the brain and nervous system.

While in acute short-term application one may refer only to the primary flavor as an indicator of the primary therapeutic effects, in long-term use it is important to pay special attention to the secondary effects or *vipaka.* Thus sweet and salty because of their moist qualities will protect the body's essence, regulate elimination and strengthen sexual potency. An excess of them, however, will aggravate mucous conditions, arthritis and obesity. Because the sour flavor promotes bodily secretions it also can aggravate pitta, since the essence of pitta humor is oily (fire can exist in the body only in the form of oil). Thus sour, being fiery, will reduce sexual secretions in both men and women. Pungent *vipaka* in excess, or the long-term effect of taking too many; pungent, bitter or astringent things, will cause gas, constipation, high blood pressure, skin eruptions and dryness.

Special Potency
(Prabhava)

Energy, flavor and post-digestive effects account for most of the effects of herbs. In addition the biochemical constituents of plants may have unique effects and properties that are not necessarily accounted for in their broader energetic actions. These properties are classified as *prabhava* or "special potency".

For instance, an herb such as hawthorn berries has a sour, warm energy and is used by the Chinese as a digestive, but Western herbalism recognizes its special potency or *prabhava* in treating for the heart and circulation. Dandelion root is classified as a bitter, heat-clearing herb, but is potent in promoting and enriching breast milk and treating breast tumors.

The special potency of a particular herb may reside not only in physical properties, but in psychological or spiritual effects.

The concept of *prabhava* or special potency, by whatever name, is universal to all systems of herbalism, including the Chinese and Western. It explains the following aspects of exceptional herbs:

1. Specific biochemical constituents.
2. Specific effect upon a particular area of the body.
3. Specific psychological or spiritual actions.

THE SPIRITUAL QUALITIES OF HERBS

Both the Chinese and Ayurvedic doctors were often associated with a priest class of Taoists, Buddhists and yogis who, it was said, were able by processes of intuition to discern the psycho-spiritual qualities and energies of herbs.

They found that herbs that are light and bitter tend to lift depression, stimulate mental clarity and foster new directions and possibilities of being. Herbs and foods whose energies are heavier, salty and sweet are more stabilizing and grounding. Those whose energies are eliminative encourage one to release dependent tendencies. Herbs whose nature and strength are strong will foster personal growth and development. Herbs and foods whose natures are gentle and bland stimulate transformation and completion.

They further found that spicy and ascending herbs help overcome psycho-physical stagnation. Salty-tasting substances like salt and sea-weed will help one to store energy and feel more confident and secure. Sour herbs stimulate contraction and utilization of one's innate reserves. Bitter herbs generate purity, clarity and light. Sweet herbs generate strength, compassion and love. Rough, sharp, dry herbs stimulate inner clarity and motivation. Soft, demulcent, nutritive herbs stimulate feelings of love and compassion.

Using these findings, herbal combinations that promote various psycho-spiritual qualities may be formulated. This ultimately may be a more powerful means for creating health and harmony than the use of herbs to affect merely physical changes.

WESTERN EVOLUTION OF ENERGETIC HERBALISM

Europe

Until the seventeenth century, which was characterized by the mechanistic thinking of the philosopher, Descartes, European herbalism was dominated by the energetic system of classification and diagnosis associated with Galen and the medicine of ancient Rome and Greece. In this system, as in Ayurveda, people were classified according to the biological humors, of which four were recognized:

1. Sanguine (air), hot/moist.   3. Phlegmatic (water), cold/moist.
2. Melancholic (earth), cold/dry. 4. Choleric (fire), hot/dry.

The sanguine person was said to be hot and moist, with a ruddy complexion, cheerful, confident and optimistic, with a tendency towards inflammatory diseases.

The melancholic person is opposite in qualities, with a tendency to be cold and dry, pale in complexion, very sensitive; and, on the positive side, a visionary. They are more susceptible to mental and sexual disorders.

The phlegmatic person is cold and moist, but duller, slower and more indifferent than the sanguine individual. They have a tendency towards congestion, stagnation and rheumatic and mucous diseases.

The choleric person, the opposite of the phlegmatic, is hot and dry. They have a hot and fiery temperament and are easily angered. They have a tendency towards liver diseases, high blood pressure, rashes, burns, fevers without perspiration, and sunburn.

All herbals written in Western countries before the seventeenth century (and a few written later) classified herbs energetically. Two of the most famous were Macer's *Virtue of Herbs,* dating from the 11th century and considered the most popular herbal of the Middle ages; and Culpepper's *Complete Herbal,* published in the early part of the seventeenth century. They classified herbs as being, to various degrees, hot or cold and dry or moist.

This genuine system of holistic herbalism was practiced throughout most of European history. It is an approach that treats both the causes and the symptoms of disease. The modern medicine that succeeded it, on the other hand, focuses primarily on the symptoms.

Native American Herbalism

The Native American peoples, like traditional peoples throughout the world, also practiced an energetic approach to herbal healing. While ethnobotanists down through the ages have provided us with the names of many of the herbs they used, little is known how they used them, or of the systems of differential diagnosis practiced by the various North American tribes. Professor Richard I. Ford states that "the outside observer would expect general principles for organizing classes of folk medicines to have priority over the learning of specific cures."

The treasure of medicinal herbs that grows naturally throughout the wilderness areas of the North and South American continents is largely unknown. It is easy to forget that America was discovered because of the European quest for spices and herbs. American herbs were considered exotic botanicals much in demand in Europe and other parts of the world.

While we ignore our native botanicals in favor of the development of industrial, technological medicine, our herbs are being exported, grown, researched and made into preparations that are sold and appreciated throughout the European continent. Two of the most outstanding of the Native American herbal remedies are golden seal (*Hydrastis canadensis*) and echinacea. Another is American ginseng (*Panax quinquefolium*), of which the Chinese continue to import tons yearly. Many Chinese doctors even prefer the American species to their own.

There is such a diversity of plant life in the world's rain forests that undoubtedly some of the most powerfully effective herbs in those areas of South American and Africa have yet to be discovered. Argentina and Brazil have recently given us pau d' arco, or *taheebo* as it is called in Argentina. This herb has shown considerable effectiveness in the treatment of inflammatory diseases, cancers, tumors and candida yeast infections.

The traditional wisdom of native cultures can be of even greater value to us than the specific herbs they used. The greatest loss, surpassing that of the extermination of a particular medicinal plant, is the partial loss of these traditional systems of diagnosis and treatment.

The Eclectics

At one time there were more than 20,000 so-called Eclectics; herbalists of late nineteenth century North America who developed a profound understanding of medicinal plants. Eclectic medicine evolved from a combination of the earlier Thompsonian herbalism based on the work of the iconoclastic herbalist, Samuel Thompson, and other herbal doctors, and the medical practices of the "regulars". The latter were the mainstream practitioners of the day and the forerunners of modern scientific physicians.

Eclectic medicine was founded and named by Dr. Wooster Beech. It was an alternative to the "regular" medicine of the day, which was the object of increasing criticism for its abuse of such therapies as bloodletting and purging. Some of these excesses often left the patient in worse health than before undergoing treatment. Beech was trained in the orthodox medicine of the day but apprenticed himself to an herbalist and studied the methods of Dr. Samuel Thompson. Thompson's system of self-treatment recommended the use of such herbs as cayenne pepper, lobelia and bayberry bark and such natural therapies as the vapor bath.

Beech's system was founded on herbology (he used mainly North American herbs) as well as on the scientific principles of physiology and biochemistry.

By the middle of the nineteenth century the Eclectics had founded a college in Cincinnati, Ohio. Soon after, many trained Eclectic doctors were practicing throughout the United States. They published a medical journal as well as several books and monographs, mostly dealing with the use of particular North American herbs. Among the many outstanding and dedicated eclectic doctors was Dr. John M. King, who wrote the monumental *American Dispensatory,* a comprehensive two-volume work of more than two thousand pages, describing various herbs and various medicines and preparations in great detail.

Toward the end of the nineteenth century, the Eclectics began to define a system of differential diagnosis incorporating observation of the pulse, tongue, complexion and mental attitude of the patient as a means of accurately prescribing herbs and herbal formulas. In so doing, they came very close to creating an alternative system of herbal medicine strikingly similar to Ayurvedic and Chinese medicine. This system is probably best described in Dr. John M. Scudder's two volumes, *Study of Disease and Specific Medicine,* first published in 1874. Scudder begins his *Study of Diagnoses* with the following statement, "We wish to make a new study of diagnosis—one that will show us the relation between symptoms of disease and the curative action of drugs." Later he states that "We study disease, therefore, as a method of living; and we treat the diseased body as a living body, which has been placed in such position that its life has been enfeebled or deranged."

John Uri Lloyd was the outstanding herbal pharmacist for the Eclectics. His formulas and methods of preparation of herbal extracts were those most followed in his day (and probably also are in ours). He was regarded as an outstanding teacher and lecturer, with consummate knowledge of biochemistry using unique methods of extraction. Lloyd was a colorful personality with diverse interests that included metaphysics. He also wrote several novels, including his then famous visionary novel *Etidorpha or The End of the World.*

With the shift of popularity and funding to industrial technological medicine, which emphasized surgery and synthetic drugs, the Eclectics' college closed in the early 1930s. This signalled the end of Eclectic medicine as an active tradition.

The Eclectics left a profound legacy of accumulated herbal knowledge, which survives in the Lloyd Library and Museum in Cincinnati, Ohio. The library, maintained and funded by a grant from John Uri Lloyd's extinct pharmaceutical company, is a modern three-story building housing the library of the college and also many private collections bequeathed by doctors throughout the country. Some herbals in the library date back to the fifteenth century, and it maintains an international and up-to-date collection of books, monographs and periodicals on botanical medicine.[3]

SUMMARY

Despite local differences in terminology and in the herbs used, there is a common thread joining the systems of herbal medicine, all of which base their diagnosis and treatment upon a holistic, energetic model. Thus energetic herbal systems of classification—as seen in the Chinese, Ayurvedic and original Western systems—addresses considerations of diet and lifestyle and try to identify underlying emotional and spiritual causes for disease. A medicine that does not sufficiently take these factors into account is compelled to use ever stronger methods of treatment, such as drugs, surgery, radiation and chemotherapy. On the other hand, it will be seen that cures for most human ailments can be effected much more gently when the underlying causes of disease are attended to and adjustments made, simply through the use of mild herbs and foods.

---

[1]Please note, that in these traditional systems, the hot or cold nature of herbs is a quality inherent in the action of the herb and not an atmospheric temperature.

[2] The heating and cooling properties of herbs and foods are usually evaluated according to the flavors.

[3] The Lloyd Library and Museum, 917 Plum Street, Cincinnati, Ohio 45202, phone (513) 721-3707.

PREPARATION AND PROCESSING OF HERBS

The art of herbalism lies not only in selecting the most effective herbs for the condition being treated but also in determining how those herbs should best be prepared. In addition to treating internally, it is helpful to apply the herbs directly, and as close as possible to the site of the problem. This is done by means of medicated oils, poultices and suppositories.

In general, a greater variety of herbs will be used in a formula for chronic conditions. The purpose is to encourage healthy organic function and thus help the body heal itself. A rule of thumb is to use an appropriate herbal preparation for approximately one month for every year since the problem began. From two to six grams of a compound herbal formula may be taken two or three times a day. Children are given half this dose or less, according to age.

For acute conditions fewer herbs are used, or even just one: for example, echinacea alone may be given for infections and inflammatory conditions. The principle of administration in such cases is to keep the healing properties of the herbs continually available for the body to draw upon as needed. Thus a moderate dose of echinacea or another herb might be taken every two hours for acute conditions, and the dose then tapered off gradually as the symptoms abate. For especially acute conditions, herbs may be taken every fifteen minutes.

FORMULATIONS

The main principles of formulation are based upon four categories of herbal function:

Chief herbs: a single herb or herbs that address the main symptom complex. These will predominate in the prescription.

Supporting herbs: A single herb or group of herbs that support the primary function of the chief herbs. This group develops the effects of the chief herbs.

Assisting herbs: These herbs treat associated symptoms and also help to bring out the main effects of the chief herbs.

Conducting herbs: These direct the assimilation and maximum utilization of the other herbs in the formula.

The therapeutic function of a formula may be either to cool with alterative and anti-inflammatory herbs or to warm with stimulants or tonics. If the formula is strong, the heating or cooling activity, along with the primary therapeutic effects, is preserved by not adding herbs with opposite qualities. To modify, balance or lessen what may be an overly strong reaction to a particular herb or formula, varying amounts of herbs with opposing energies and actions may be added. Thus a small amount of ginger, cinnamon or pepper may be added to a cold formula or a small amount of a soothing and cooling herb, like marshmallow or chickweed, may be added to a hot formula. If the formula is a cold purgative, for instance, the patient will experience symptoms of metabolic coldness, such as abdominal cramping. For this reason a small amount of a warming, antispasmodic stimulant, such as ginger, is added for counterbalancing action.

Antispasmodic herbs, such as peony root in the Chinese tradition or lobelia in the Thompsonian Western tradition, are added to formulas in small amounts to relax the body for better utilization of the herbs. The common practice among Western herbalists of adding to formulas a small amount of a stimulant such as ginger and an antispasmodic such as lobelia assures the best absorption and utilization of the main herbs in the formula.

The Chinese also add small amounts of sweet herbs such as licorice or jujube dates to sweeten the generally bitter herbs which usually comprise the chief herbs in a formula. The mild tonic properties of these sweet-tasting substances also protects the stomach from the excess bitterness which the Chinese say can "injure the righteous chi". The bitter taste can overly stimulate the secretion of hydrochloric acid in the stomach and create chronic digestive weaknesses, especially when used over a long period of time. Perhaps many Western herbalists who say "sweeten with honey to taste" have the same protective purpose in mind.

The following simple classical Chinese formula illustrates the basic principles of formulation:

Decoction of Herba Ephedrae (*Ma Huang Tang*):

Ephedra (6-9 gm.):	Chief herb; primary property stimulating diaphoretic.
Cinnamon twigs (6-9 gm.):	Supporting herb; primary property warming diaphoretic.
Apricot seed (6-9 gm.):	Assisting herb; moistening and descending property, helps ameliorate the harsher effects of the two preceeding herbs.
Licorice root (3-6 gm.):	Conducting herb; sweet taste, harmonizes the other herbs in the formula, prevents unfavorable reactions, protects the stomach and digestion.

HERB QUALITY

How herbs are prepared is important to their efficacy. In the field, select the finest quality herbs with the most visible life force. They should be gathered in a place where they seem to be thriving in abundance and have good color and aroma. The same criteria should be applied to herbs that are purchased. As with anything that is of vital importance to your well being, be willing to pay the extra price for the superior quality of herbs that may have been picked and prepared under more ideal circumstances.

METHODS OF PREPARATION

The vessel in which herbal teas are prepared should be made of clay, glass or some insoluble metal, such as stainless steel. Soluble metals will somewhat alter the properties of herbs. Further, it always is preferable to cook herbs over an open flame rather than electrical heat.

There are various methods of herbal preparations, of which most are included in the five methods of Ayurvedic herbal preparations discussed by David Frawley and Dr. Vasant Lad in *The Yoga of Herbs* (Lotus Press). A comprehensive description of methods follows.

Herb Juice

This is usually made with fresh herbs by mashing and squeezing the pulp through a natural fiber cloth. Herb juices are commonly made with parsley, garlic and onions and fruits such as lemons and limes. Dry herbs are somewhat weaker in properties than the fresh. If dried herbs are used, they are soaked in twice their weight of water for 24 hours and then the fluid is pressed out.

Herb Paste

This is made by grinding and mashing the fresh herbs into a mass. A little water may then be added, which is necessary with dry herbs.

The paste may be taken as is or mixed with honey, ghee or oil, usually in double the quantity. Pastes will keep almost indefinitely if refrigerated. If only honey and no other moisture is added, they will keep indefinitely even without refrigeration. These pastes may be used as an electuary (powdered or mashed herbs mixed with honey or syrup) and eaten with a spoon, or stirred into a decoction. They also can be the basis for externally applied poultices and plasters.

Decoction

Heavier roots and barks and substances in which the volatile oils are not essential to the therapy are made in decoction. Thus, aromatic herbs such as mints are not decocted, as the volatile oils will evaporate. In Western herbalism, the average amount used of most herbs is an ounce decocted in a pint of water. A convenient method of approximating the amount needed is to fill the middle of the palm of the hand with heavier roots and barks. For lighter substances, such as red clover, a large handful may be required.

A decoction is made by bringing the water to a rolling boil, adding the herbs and covering. Let the mixture continue to simmer for twenty to thirty minutes over a low flame.

The methods of preparing Chinese decoctions vary according to the practitioner. However, the basic method is to simmer an ounce or more of herbs in three cups of water until the liquid reduces to two cups. The herbs may be double decocted by draining off and setting aside the two cups of the first decoction, adding two more cups of water, and simmering them down to one cup. This second decoction added to the two cups of the first yield a total of three cups of double decocted tea.

Ayurvedic medicine uses the basic formula of one part dry herbs simmered in sixteen parts water, or about a half ounce of herbs per eight ounce cup of water. The herbs are then slowly boiled over a low flame down to one-quarter of the original amount, so that four cups of water would reduce to one. A milder decoction is made by reducing the volume of water only to half.

Both the Oriental and Western Herbal traditions differentiate between single, double or more reduced decoctions. These indicate different levels of extraction. On the first level, the more sensitive volatile constituents are extracted. With each subsequent level of decoction, other biochemical constituents, and finally the minerals, are extracted. The problem is that without separating out the first decoction, longer cooking may tend to dissipate the previously extracted constituents.

One method of avoiding this is to use a ginseng cooker. This is a special ceramic container (available from most Chinese herb or grocery stores) which is a double boiler with two glass covers. The container is partially submerged in a pan of water which is then brought to a boil. It can be simmered for two to three hours, for maximum extraction of the valuable therapeutic properties. This method is expecially useful for cooking and fully extracting the valuable constitutents of ginseng. Both the delicate and sensitive volatile substances of the ginseng and its deeper constituents are extracted as fully as possible by this method.

Hot Infusion

This is made by steeping and covering about one ounce of herbs with a pint of boiling water, for from ten or twenty minutes up to several hours. In this method no fire is used, and the aromatic principles of the herbs are thereby kept intact.

Since many formulas combine aromatic herbs with heavier barks and roots, a compromise in such cases is to simmer the mixture on a low flame for from twenty minutes to an hour.

Cold infusion

This is made by allowing the herbs to stand in cool water for at least an hour. Some people prefer to place the infusion in the sun to make what is called "sun tea"; others allow the infusion to stand overnight. This method, too, is used for herbs with delicate volatile oils such as mints, hibiscus, lemon grass and sandalwood, which are chiefly cooling or refrigerant in nature. It is most commonly used with powders. Since powders are already partially broken down, stirring them into a cup of cool water and allowing them to stand will sufficiently extract their therapeutic substances.

Certain herbs, such as apricot seeds and wild cherry bark, are better extracted in cold water, since one of their active ingredients (amygdaline) is harmed by heat.

Powders

Powders are made from dried herbs by grinding, using a mortar and pestle or an electric herb grinder. Powders are the best way to achieve an even mix of ingredients from several herbs, in a form that is readily extracted and assimilated. Because powders are more efficiently utilized, less quantity is needed than when using whole herbs.

Powders may be taken in several ways. One is to put them into gelatin capsules. Another method is to stir them directly into a liquid, using from a teaspoonful to two tablespoonsful to an eight-ounce glass of warm water or milk. Thus, tonics can be taken by stirring the powders into warm milk, and this has a similar building effect to the use of tonic Chinese herbs taken with meat soups. Ayurvedic medicine combines herbal powders with ghee (clarified butter), oil, honey or raw sugar. These are considered carriers or *anupans* (see section on anupanas, pg. 69).

One of the problems in using herbal powders is that they will oxidize and lose their potency much more quickly than the whole dried herb. The period of effectiveness for herbal powders is from three months to a year.

Pills

Pills are taken for convenience and are more effectively utilized if taken with boiled warm water. Rather than make one large pill, Chinese pharmacies prepare several small grain-sized pills for quick, efficient utilization.

Pills are made in a variety of ways. One is to decoct the herbs down to a paste at the bottom of the vessel. This is then scraped off the bottom of the pan, rolled into small pellets and set out on a clean paper container to dry. Another is to mix a little water, syrup or honey with powdered herbs and then roll them into a pill mass of desired size.

Herbal Wines

Herbal wines are made by making 2-3 quarts of the herbal tea and dissolving about three to four pounds honey or whole sugar in it. When this mixture cools to around 68 degrees Fahrenheit, add a suitable live yeast culture. This is allowed to slowly ferment in a loosely covered container so that the carbon dioxide can freely escape. When the fermention is nearly complete, the brew is finely strained and bottled, with a vaporlock inserted so that no further fermentation can occur. Later do a final straining through a cloth. Then the herbal wine can be bottled for later use. The maintaining of cleanliness and a temperature of from 65 to 78 degrees are the most important factors in preparing herbal wines. In a sense they preserve themselves, making their own alcohol. They seem to be most effective as tonic beverages, but less effective than tinctures for acute conditions.

Some herbs lend themselves particularly to herbal wine preparations. These include Siberian ginseng (*Eleutherococcus senticosus*) and its Chinese near relative, called *Wu jia pi (Acanthopanax gracilistylus)*. Another excellent herbal wine is made with hawthorn berries.

Tinctures

Tinctures are made by combining 1-4 ounces of powdered or thoroughly crushed herb with 8-12 ounces of alcohol. Enough water is added to make a 50% solution or, alternatively, start with a 30% (60 proof) vodka poured over the herbs. The amount of liquid should be more than the herbs will absorb, so more should be added as needed. This is then shaken and allowed to stand in a warm place for two weeks, with daily stirring and shaking. Then the liquid is poured out through a muslin cloth and the herbal content squeezed until as much of the extract is removed as possible. The tincture is then kept in a dark bottle and taken by dropper, in amounts averaging from 1 to 30 drops according to the herb used. Most of the alcohol can be evaporated away from a tincture by placing the drops in boiling hot water for a few minutes.

Acetic tinctures are made in the same way, usually with apple cider vinegar, because of its healthful properties. However, acetic tinctures, while best for extracting alkaloids, are not as good for extracting the more acidic biochemical ingredients which often are of significant biological importance. Western herbalists usually make an acetic extract of lobelia, since the major active ingredient in lobelia is an alkaloid.

Glycerite tinctures are more soothing and milder on the digestive tract and are non-alcoholic. Their major disadvantage is that glycerine cannot dissolve resinous or oily materials as efficiently as alcohol. To make a glycerite tincture, mix one part vegetable glycerine with four parts warm water. Add the powdered herb and proceed as above, allowing to stand in a warm place for at least two weeks.

Tinctures are more successful when started on the new moon and strained on the full moon.

Liniments

Liniments are made in the same way as tinctures but, since they are intended for external use only, the cheaper isopropyl alcohol available in drug stores may be used. For external sprains, bruises and pains of the muscles and joints, warm circulating herbs such as cayenne, ginger, myrrh, angelica, wild ginger (*Asarum*), cloves, cumin seed or bay leaf are used. As with tinctures, they are macerated in alcohol for two weeks Then they are strained and used as an external rubbing oil.

Syrups

Syrups are especially useful for throat and lung problems, because of their ability to soothe and coat the throat. A basic syrup is made by boiling three pounds of raw or brown sugar in a pint of water until it reaches a syrupy consistency. To make an herb syrup, substitute the tea for the water; or add alcoholic extracts of the herbs to the syrup while it is cooking, to allow the alcohol to boil off. Honey may be substituted for sugar, although boiled honey is considered to have a mildly toxic residue. Herbal syrups are more easily taken by children.

An example of an herbal cough syrup is Old Indian Cough, Cold and Flu Syrup. This is made by decocting the following herbs:

Old Indian Cough, Cold and Flu Syrup

Loquat leaves (6 pts.)	Wild cherry bark (4 pts.)
Yerba santa leaves (6 pts.)	Elecampane root and flower (4 pts.)
Osha root (5 pts.)	Licorice root (3 pts.)
Gumweed (4 pts.)	Mullein (3 pts.)
Coltsfoot (4 pts.)	

Garlic-Lemon and Honey Syrup

Another simple and quick syrup helpful in treating mucous conditions, especially of the lungs, is garlic-lemon and honey syrup. This is made by blending a few cloves of fresh garlic into honey and adding freshly squeezed lemon juice. This is an excellent treatment for sore throat, lung and bronchiole affections.

Poultices and Fomentations

A poultice is made by crushing the fresh herbs and binding directly onto the affected part of the body. They relieve pain and promote local healing of injuries, cuts and fractures. A common poultice is made from comfrey root and plantain, with a sprinkle of cayenne pepper to activate its healing potential.

A plaster is made by spreading a thin coat of honey on a piece of cloth and sprinkling it with powdered stimulant herbs, such as cayenne, ginger or prickly ash. This is then taped directly over the painful area. It serves as a counterirritant to relieve pain and congestion.

A fomentation is made by making a decoction of an herb, soaking a cloth in it, and applying it as hot as possible to the affected area. A ginger fomentation, made by grating fresh ginger into hot water, is most commonly used. Turmeric also is good.

A drawing poultice, to pull out slivers and other matter embedded in the flesh, is made from a combination of comfrey root (fresh or powdered), plantain leaves and a small amount of cayenne pepper.

Medicated Oils

Medicated oils have a broad application in Ayurvedic medicine, since oil is considered an *anupan* or carrier into the vata humor or nervous system. Various oils may be used, such as olive, sesame, safflower, coconut and castor bean. Most Ayurvedic herbal oils are made either with the warming sesame oil or the cooling coconut oil. The basic Ayurvedic formula is one part herbs to sixteen parts water and four parts oil. This is then decocted until all the water has evaporated. For example, two ounces of herbs, one cup of oil and four cups of water make one cup of medicated oil. It is difficult to strain herbs that have been decocted in oil. A simpler method is to prepare the decoction, then strain the herbs out and proceed as above.

As mentioned above, herbs with volatile oils, such as mint, camphor and rose, lose their potency when over-heated. The best method of preparing them is to macerate the dried and powdered herbs directly in the oil. This mixture should then stand for one to two days before being strained through a cloth and bottled for use.

Still another method of making an oil is to crush and mash the whole herb, such as grated ginger, garlic or onions, and allow to stand overnight before squeezing the herbal oil through a cloth. Typically, garlic oil is made in this way, as is mullein flower oil, both of which are then used as drops to treat earaches in children.

Medicated oils are used chiefly for external massage, as ointments for the eyes and ears, as dressings for wounds, ulcers and burns, in enemas and douches, and as nasal applications. Some may be taken internally.

Brahmi Oil

A medicated oil made with gotu kola and calamus root, called *brahmi* oil, is ideal for the treatment of mental and central nervous system disorders. *Brahmi* oil is liberally applied to the scalp each day for individuals undergoing treatment for chronic emotional disorders, brain damage and related problems. It may be washed off after an hour or so.

Mullein Flower Ear Oil

Mullein flower oil is made by macerating mullein flowers in olive oil. This is then squeezed and strained through a muslin cloth and bottled for use. A drop or two is placed in each ear in the evening to relieve earache.

Garlic oil

Press several cloves of garlic and macerate in olive or sesame oil for a few days, then squeeze and strain through a muslin cloth. This may be taken hourly by the tablespoonful for colds and flu, for sore throats, and to prevent bacterial infections. The oil alleviates the sometimes harsh effect of the garlic. It also may be used for ear drops and to rub on bruises and injuries.

Chickweed Oil

This is made by grinding and macerating fresh chickweed (*Stellaria media*) in olive oil for a few days. This makes a soothing oil used for eczema and other itching.

According to Chinese medicine, oils have soothing, yin tonic properties which are strengthening to the nervous system.

Salves and Ointments

There are several methods of making ointments. Some use petroleum jelly and others oil and beeswax. The petroleum jelly base is best if a heating counterirritant, such as Vick's Vapo-Rub or Tiger Balm, is desired. Oil and beeswax are more absorbent and useful for promoting the healing of burns, bites and abrasions.

For the oil, one may use either leaf lard, ghee, sesame or olive oils. Boil the herbs in water until sufficiently extracted and then strain them out. Add the oil to the decoction and continue to simmer until all the water evaporates. Add sufficient beeswax until the desired consistency is achieved, or melt about 2 ounces of beeswax to 5 ounces of oil. To preserve, add a drop of tincture of benzoin (available at most drug stores) to each ounce of base.

Comfrey-Plantain Ointment

This is made with dried comfrey, plantain leaves, golden seal and echinacea.

Medicated Ghee

Though similar to medicated oils, medicated ghee is more specific as a carrier to the fire (pitta) humor making it useful for inflammatory conditions of the gastrointestinal tract, and for fevers and ulcers.

Ghee or clarified butter is made by heating one pound of raw unsalted butter on a medium flame until the white saturated fats condense and separate out from the pure unsaturated oil. Ghee is the best oil to use for cooking and is excellent for use in salves and ointments.

One preparation that is particularly good is made with gotu kola and calamus root. This is made like gotu kola oil but uses ghee instead. One teaspoon of the gotu kola ghee is stirred into a cup of warm water or mixed with food. It is taken internally two or three times a day to strengthen the mind and improve memory.

Ghee is cooling and therefore is excellent in preparations for treating chronic inflammatory conditions. It serves a similar function in Ayurveda to the yin tonics in Chinese medicine. Like yin tonics, it is thought to be building to the vital fluids of the body, including plasma, blood, muscle, fat, reproductive secretions and the all-important *ojas*, the essential vitality which dwells in the heart.

Alchemy and Spagyric Tinctures

Many herbalists believe that tinctures or alcoholic preparations do not necessarily represent the complete balance of all the herb's therapeutic components. This is recognized also in the tradition of alchemy, which dates back to the Middle Ages.

Alchemists have a unique way of separating out the respective components of an herb, then purifying and recombining them in the final alcoholic elixir. Simply expressed, a spagyric tincture, as it is called, is prepared by making a standard alcoholic extract in which the 'mark' or solid residue, which normally is discarded, is calcined to a fine white ash, ground into a powder, and returned to the strained liquid extract. The liquid is then carefully redistilled, leaving the residue of ash at the bottom. Such alchemical preparations represent a secret or lost art of herbal preparation that may contain keys to more direct means of extracting the life-force from plants.

Various principles are considered in deciding what kind of preparation is best for treating a given condition. Generally speaking, teas are good for most conditions; powders are best for digestive problems; pills for bitter-tasting substances and herbs which are to be taken in small amounts or for a long period of time; electuaries (herbal pastes) and soups as nutritive tonics, and medicated oils for neurological problems.

PROCESSING OF HERBS
Detoxifying and Altering the Properties of Herbs

Both Ayurvedic and traditional Chinese medicine have developed methods of processing herbs so as to reduce their toxicity, increase their therapeutic effectiveness, alter their properties, and remove any offending odors. Western herbalists can learn a great deal from these techniques.

Because Western herbalists have been unable to detoxify such deadly poisonous herbs as aconite, this otherwise valuable therapeutic agent is used in the West with extreme care, in miniscule or homeopathic doses. Because it is so deadly, this herb has been avoided altogether by most Western herbalists in recent years. The Chinese and the Hindus, on the other hand, have known for centuries how to use this herb in its prepared form (*Aconitum praeparatum*), detoxifying its poisonous principle and thus neutralizing most of its toxic potential.[1] (For further information, see aconite in the pharmacopoeia section, pg. 246).

Steaming and Drying

A glutinous and demulcent root such as *Rehmannia glutinosa,* which has a cool energy, is repeatedly steamed with wine and sun-dried by the Chinese. By these processes they literally add a little fire or circulatory energy to it. The same may be done with Western glutinous herbs such as marshmallow and comfrey.

Dry-Roasting and Stir-Frying

Dry-roasting certain herbs will enhance their fiery yang characteristics. Herbs such as Chinese bupleurum, which is used for the liver, are prepared in this way. By dry-roasting herbs in the oven or by frequently turning them in a wok until they are slightly brown, their ascending energy is enhanced and they may be used to raise the spirits, treat prolapse and elevate the yang. Herbs that are commerically dry-roasted for added flavor are dandelion, chicory and comfrey roots. We can expect them to have a similar property. In the raw state they have a cool energy, when roasted they should become a little warmer.

By adding a small amount of honey to an herb as it is stirred and dry-roasted in a wok, we add sweetness which gives the herb more of a tonic effect, especially on the spleen-pancreas. Licorice and astragalus often are dry-roasted with honey to increase the effectiveness of the digestive system (what the Chinese call *spleen chi).*

Soaking in Spirits or Wine

Herbs soaked in grain spirits are similar to western alcoholic tinctures or extracts. They enter the blood with maximum efficiency and have an ascending energy. The alcohol acts as a conductor as well as a stimulant to blood circulation. Such preparations are commonly used in Chinese medicine as tonics, treating circulatory disorders such as arthritic and rheumatic complaints. A common form is made by soaking Siberian ginseng in 40 to 50% grain spirits for from two weeks to six months. A teaspoon or so may be taken three or four times daily throughout the winter by the elderly to prevent circulatory problems and counteract rheumatic complaints. A good yang tonic to promote metabolic and hormonal strength is made by soaking a whole oriental ginseng root with some Chinese deer antler in a pint of cognac. This may be taken in doses of one teaspoon throughout the winter months only, as it is very warming. Tonifying the yin is more important for women, for whom grape wines are more beneficial. A root of angelica or Chinese dong quai macerated in brandy or good quality grape wine makes a blood tonic for women.

Processing with Salt

A pinch of salt usually is added to herbs intended as tonic for the urinary tract. Salt acts as a carrier for the other herbs in the formula, bringing their action to the kidneys. It enhances the descending action of a formula. If the urinary tract is intended to be cleansed rather than tonified, the salt is omitted. Processing herbs in salt, for example pickling them in salt, adds to their moistening effect because salt aids water retention.

Processing with Vinegar

The sour taste generally, and vinegar in particular, goes to the liver and has a descending and contracting energy. It causes astringency of tissues and thus enhances a certain kind of tonicity. Vinegar is used as a medium to extract alkaloids such as those found in lobelia, corydalis, golden seal and other antispasmodic and analgesic herbs. Water will not be as effective for this purpose.

Leaching with Water

This is done mainly to remove tannic acid and certain toxic substances. Acorns, a good yin tonic food, are prepared by shelling, grinding and then leaching them in running water for a few hours to remove the tannic acid.

Sand Heating

Certain herbs can be more evenly roasted by mixing them in sand and heating them in a wok while stirring frequently. This allows a much higher temperature than stir-frying without sand, and the roots will heat better. This method also can be used with roots such as burdock, dandelion and chicory.

Baking

Herbs can be baked with honey, ginger or other "carriers" to enhance certain effects. Honey makes herbs more tonic and moistening, while ginger makes them more warming and dispersing, promoting circulation and digestion.

DOSAGE

The dosage of individual herbs is expressed differently by the Chinese and by Western herbalists. Western herbalists tend to express the total effective dosage regardless of whether one or more herbs is used. Thus the standard effective Western dosage for mild non-toxic herbs is one ounce of herb to a pint of water and one cup taken three times daily. More active or toxic herbs are given special indications.

The Chinese give the range of standard dosage for each of their herbs as 3 to 9 grams on the average. Since Chinese herbalism is based upon formula compounds with considerations of balance and counterbalance, a single day's total dosage can range from 50 to 200 grams of herbs and there can be as many as 20 herbs in a single formula (consider that 28 grams equal one ounce).

Weights and Measures Chart

ENGLISH MEASURES

A few grains = less than 1⅛ teaspoon
60 drops = 1 teaspoon
1 teaspoon = ⅓ tablespoon
1 tablespoon = 3 teaspoons
2 tablespoons = 1 fluid ounce
4 tablespoons = cup
16 tablespoons = 1 cup or 8 ounces

METRIC EQUIVALENTS

1 teaspoon = 5 milliliters   1 grain = approx. .65 milligrams
1 tablespoon = 15 milliliters   1 ounce = approx. 28 grams
1 pint = .528 liters   1 pound = approx. 454 grams
1 quart = 1.056 liters   1 teaspoon cornstarch = 3 grams

Dosage Guidelines

Age	Fractional Adult dosage
one year and under	from $\frac{1}{10}$th to $\frac{1}{75}$
2 to 6 years	$\frac{1}{3}$ to $\frac{1}{10}$
6 to 12 years	$\frac{1}{3}$ to $\frac{1}{2}$
12 to 15 years	$\frac{1}{2}$ to $\frac{2}{3}$
15 years and up	full dose
over 70	$\frac{1}{2}$ dose

These guidelines apply to individuals of average weight, height and sensitivity. Dosage should be adjusted accordingly.

CONSIDERATIONS IN ADMINISTRATION OF HERBS

The way an herb is administered can lessen or optimize its effectiveness. Out of habit or for convenience, herbalists may exclusively use one form of herbs—such as teas, tinctures or pills—when another might be more effective. For example, in administering strong-tasting herbs to adult patients or sick children who are resistant to strange flavors and textures, one should, if possible, use a form of administration that does not have those qualities.

1. Use fresh herbs of the best quality available whenever possible.
2. Herbs with strong, active therapeutic actions (such as strong diaphoretics, febrifuges and purgatives) should be used with great care for individuals who are in a severely weakened state.
3. Strong blood-moving herbs or emmenagogues and purgatives with a strong downward action should not be used for pregnant women, as they can cause miscarriages and abortions.
4. Acute diseases should be treated more quickly, using strong herbs, and often using few herbs in a given formula. Chronic diseases are treated more slowly and gently, with a more balanced formulation given over a prolonged period of time.

5. In treating acute diseases, small frequent doses taken hourly or every two hours are best, tapering off the frequency as the symptoms subside. In such cases, a lower dose is continued for a few days after all symptoms have been alleviated.
   For chronic diseases, the herbs should be taken regularly three times daily, for one month to each year since the symptoms began.

6. Acute diseases should show improvement within one to three days at most. If they do not, the herbs used should be reevaluated and possibly changed.
   Chronic conditions should show some benefit within two weeks or so. If they do not, the approach may need to be reevaluated.

7. Excessive cooling and bitter herbs should not be taken too frequently over a prolonged period, since they can damage the digestive system (spleen-stomach).

8. Excessive heating herbs and yang tonics should be used rarely in summer. Cold-natured herbs with strong eliminative properties are used rarely in winter. Fasting and detoxification is best practiced during the spring and fall. (This should be adjusted according to geographical climatic conditions.)

9. For gastrointestinal diseases, the best method of administration is a powder.

10. To effect a more rapid recovery from skin diseases and disorders of internal surfaces such as the throat, vagina, rectum, eyes, ears and nose, one should consider, in addition to any internal treatment, the use of special preparations such as fomentations, gargles, douches, boluses, herbal enemas, suppositories and eye and ear drops.
    In addition to internal treatment, respiratory conditions may be treated with vapor inhalations through the lungs and syrups for sore throat and bronchial conditions.

12. Herbal tonics intended to have a nutritional action should be taken with food: the tonic teas used to cook rice porridges or meat soups, the powdered herbs or teas mixed with boiled warm milk.

13. Herbs used for the circulation of chi and blood are best taken as a wine or tincture, since alcohol acts as a carrier into the blood.

14. Infants and small children may be treated with herbal baths and fomentations. For the young, herbs can be powdered and mixed with honey to form a paste, and administered in teaspoonful doses followed by warm water.

15. There is some question about the use of herbs for people undergoing drug therapy. Generally, if the herb is prescribed according to the presenting symptoms, including any possible drug-induced symptoms and influences, herbal treatment will be very beneficial. The key is to treat the patient according to what is directly perceived, not according to Western systems of diagnosis.

16. The standard dosage indicated for mild herbs is approximate and represents a general effective minimum. When using mild herbs gathered in the wild or in the garden, use more if desired.

17. Anyone with sensitivity to alcohol (such as individuals who have been alcoholics or have suffered liver damage) should use alcoholic herbal extracts in the following way. Add the required dosage to a cup of boiling water so as to evaporate the alcohol, and then drink the water.

TIMES OF ADMINISTRATION

1. Empty Stomach: herbs taken on an empty stomach will have a stronger effect. This is the preferred time for those who have a watery condition with mucus and for detoxification.

2. Before Meals: herbs taken before meals will be more effective in treating nervous diseases, toning the intestines and reducing fat.

3. After Meals: herbs taken after meals will treat gas and indigestion and can also help prevent mucus.

4. Mixed With Food: herbs mixed with food are best as a tonic and for weak individuals.

5. Between Meals: herbs are best taken between meals by people with urinary and nervous disorders.

ANUPANS
(VEHICLES)

Anupana is a term used in Ayurveda that describes a particular substance used as a carrier. Chinese herbalism has a similar concept, adding certain herbs to a formula to carry the action of another herb to the area of the body to be treated. (*Anupans* in Ayurveda refers also to the particular tissues and humors to be treated.) Their use aids assimilation and efficacy of the herbs in the area being treated.

For vata or nervous conditions, herbs that are warm and mucilaginous are most effective. For pitta or fire conditions (like burns and ulcers), herbs that are sweet and cool-natured are most effective. For kapha or watery mucous conditions, herbs that are dry, rough textured and warm will be best. The primary vehicles used are cold and warm water, honey, butter, ghee, sugar, milk and other herbs that have a strong carrying property.

When treating a kapha or mucous condition it usually is best to mix the herbs with honey or to take honey with the tea. When treating a pitta or fire condition, it is best to mix the herbs with ghee or butter, following which one may drink warm water. When treating a vata or nervous condition, herbs are best mixed with sesame or other oils. These usually are rubbed on the skin, but they also may be taken internally.

Because of the anti-vata (pain relieving) properties of oil and because of its thick nature, castor oil is excellent to rub onto painful areas and joints. Ghee and honey combined in equal amounts can be toxic if taken over a prolonged time. They may be safely used in unequal proportions, however. They serve the purpose of making the combinations more food-like.

Often a particular formula, such as trikatu, triphala, or Herbal Uprising (Composition powder), which has well defined properties is added to a combination of ingredients as if it were one herb.

SIDE EFFECTS AND CONTRAINDICATIONS

Unless specifically indicated, most mild herbs are more or less equivalent in toxicity to most common foods. Just as certain individuals may have adverse reactions to certain foods, so some will react adversely to some herbs. Usually this can be prevented by using a carefully balanced formulation. If the formula is not properly balanced, a cleansing reaction or a downright aggravation can occur.

How is a cleansing or healing crisis distinguished from an aggravation? Generally a healing reaction is a recurrence of an illness that was previously suppressed. It also usually is of short duration, lasting from a few hours to a day or so. If the reaction is severe, discontinue the herbs until it subsides and then resume them gradually in smaller doses.

A reaction to herbs can help the diagnostic evaluation. If one at first misjudges a condition, as can happen to the most experienced practioner, a reaction to a formula can help define the condition more accurately. Mild herbs have the virtue of creating virtually no side effects. The practitioner can use them not only as a treatment but as an element to help the over-all diagnosis and analysis.

Anything taken to excess can cause reactions and side effects, but usually there are indications and symptoms that anyone with common sense and a little experience easily can recognize. Some herbs, indeed, are very toxic. Chinese and Ayurvedic herbalists have devised ingenious methods of preparing them to destroy or lessen their toxicity. Dosage requirements must be strictly studied and followed when using these substances.

These warnings are not intended to deter anyone from using herbal therapies. With care and intelligence, anyone should be able to utilize mild herbs both for food and medicine. Of course, there are advantages on occasion in consulting with an expert, although even so-called experts are not always right.

GATHERING AND DRYING HERBS FOR USE

The experience of gathering herbs is one of the most rewarding to an herbalist. We may choose to grow medicinal herbs, find them as common weeds in our surrounding garden or waste areas, or go into the forest, deserts and mountains to harvest them. This experience, like others, should be integrated both with our external needs and desires and with our internal ideals and longings.

The gathering of herbs either from our garden or from the wild should be practiced with spiritual awareness and prayerful thankfulness. Plants have a consciousness and are part of the same dynamic life energy of which we all are made. Essentially, it is that energy in its most gross form that manifests as specific therapeutic properties, in its less gross form as heating and cooling effects, and in an invisible form beyond our external consciousness.

To capture the subtlest, divine energy of herbs they should be handled with reverence and respect. A simple prayer, a moment of silence, or some token of offering made before picking herbs will assure that the subtle divine essence of the plant does not recede from our touch. Our inner state of mind is communicated to the plant. The words or token offering are more for ourselves. We need select only a single representative plant in a stand to which to make our silent offering before freely gathering its many nearby relatives.

I recommend leaving the grandparent plant undisturbed. Be careful to take not more than a tenth of what is growing, taking reasonable measures to assure the continued growth of the plant in the area.

It is important to harvest only in areas where the desired herbs grow most abundantly and to allow solitary specimens to proliferate and grow. If roots are dug out, cover the hole in respect for Mother Earth. In some cases, this will assure that any piece of the root left will grow another plant. Take the attitude of a wildcrafter, in which you are only pruning the plants in the area and assisting their growth in some way— perhaps by leaving the root, scattering the seeds, or simply thinning them.

When to Pick Herbs

The highest level of vital constituents is achieved just before a new part of the plant manifests. Most of the aerial parts should be harvested in the morning, before the strong heat of the sun causes them to recede and wilt. The leaves should be harvested before the buds and blooms appear, the flowers before the fruit and seeds. Bark and roots may be taken either in the early spring, just as the plant is beginning to show leaf buds, or in the fall. Stripping the bark around its circumference will kill the upper parts of a tree. Discrete patches or whole limbs may be stripped without damaging them.

Drying Herbs

Most herbs should be dried in a well- ventilated, warm, dry environment, by spreading them out in a single layer on a wire mesh or screen. Daily turning will assure even drying and fine quality. Roots should be carefully washed, scraped and chopped into small pieces to assure uniform drying. Bulbs such as onions and garlic may be tied together and strung up to dry.

Storing Herbs

Herbs should be stored in dark glass or earthenware containers. They should be protected from excessive heat, moisture and light, which will cause them to break down and oxidize. In warm, humid environments, the herbs probably should be kept in open wooden drawers so that they can continually dry out. In colder, damp climates, they should be kept in air-tight dry jars. Some herbs, as well as seeds and grains, will eventually attract small bugs. This can be prevented to some degree by adding a few aromatic bay leaves and peppercorns.

Generally, dried leaves lose considerable potency in six months to a year. Non-aromatic roots and barks last longer, from one to two years. Powders generally are good for from one to three months. All these considerations may vary with the individual herb, how it is stored, and other such factors.

---

[1]Aconite is the strongest known metabolic stimulant, of which even a small amount is capable of killing a grown man.

PRINCIPLES OF FOOD THERAPY

In Ayurvedic and Chinese medicine the stomach usually is considered to be the place where all disease originates. What we eat either can support and protect us from disease or gradually pollute our system. If the diet is not properly balanced according to seasonal requirements and the needs of the individual, it is very difficult to maintain health. Further, according to both systems, a diet not aligned with the energetics of the herbs used actually can inhibit their beneficial effects. Conversely, a diet in harmony with the herbal therapy will greatly augment the healing process.

If we begin with the premise that disease expresses an imbalance within the system, diet represents a remedy of fundamental importance. Essentially, insofar as food is concerned, when we follow desires that are in line with our needs, we are promoting optimum health. To the extent this is not so, the contrary will be true.

As "special foods," herbs work by speeding up the innate healing processes of the body; but food itself also is healing. Food therapy provides perhaps the deepest healing. However, someone who is very sick, not only with a weakened body but a weakened will and mind may be unable to follow a strict diet to restore health. Often the imbalance of the individual will express and maintain itself with a poor or imbalanced diet. For such a person, herbal therapy is invaluable.

There is no single diet that is best for everyone, or for all seasons and places. Even the purest diet, if it is not attuned to individual needs, may support rather than counteract a disorder. A therapeutic diet that meets these needs and can be followed for as long as necessary is what is required for true nurturance and healing.

Of course, emotions play a significant part in our health. Our emotions affect our eating patterns and our attitudes literally can pollute the food we eat. The stomach, being the organ of assimilation, relates not only to the assimilation of material food and drink but also to how we assimilate experiences, thoughts and feelings. The Chinese concepts of the theory of yin and yang and the five elements and the Ayurvedic *tridosha* establish an integrated relationship between physical and psychological processes. They also assert the energetic bond between food and herbs.

AYURVEDIC FOOD THERAPY

The vata or air predominant personality is prone to neurological disorders, coldness and dryness. Emotionally, they tend to have an oversensitive, nervous disposition, to be impatient and highly changeable. On the positive side, they are sensitive and responsive.

Foods and herbs that have a cool energy, and dry, rough qualities, with bitter and astringent tastes, aggravate vata. Leafy vegetables also have this effect. On the other hand, substances that are warm, moist and nourishing, with sweet, salty and sour flavors, are beneficial to vata types. Foods that in excess would imbalance a kapha or pitta person are therapeutic for vata disorders.

Following is a building diet for vata-predominant individuals:

93% sweet foods (i.e. nourishing, sweet, complex carbohydrates and
   proteins)
5% sour foods
½ to 1% salty foods
to 1% bitter foods
to 1% spicy and pungent foods
1% astringent foods

Foods beneficial for vata-predominant people include:

Grains: rice, wheat, oats
Beans: kidney beans, tofu and tempeh only
Vegetables: cooked vegetables, onion, garlic, scallions, beets, radishes, cucumbers, peppers, lettuce, carrots, turnips, asparagus
Fruits: sweet fruits, avocados, coconuts, bananas, cherries, melons, peaches, berries, figs, papayas, oranges, mangoes, limes, grapes

Dairy: all dairy products, taken warm
Meat: pork, beef, fish, chicken, turkey, duck, eggs
Nuts: all nuts in small amounts
Seeds: all seeds
Oils: all oils
Sweeteners: all sweeteners in moderation, except white sugar
Drinks: water, tea, warm fruit juice
Spices: ginger, black pepper, cardamon, coriander, cinnamon, cumin, bay leaf

Foods to be limited or avoided for vata conditions are: dried fruits, apples, raw vegetables, cabbage family, nightshade family (including tomato), potatoes and eggplant, sprouts, barley, millet, corn, rye, buckwheat, rabbit, venison, all beans except kidney and aduki beans, tofu and tempeh.

Pitta or fire-predominant individuals have a tendency towards inflammatory diseases, infections, acidity, thirst, intolerance of heat, bleeding and ulcers. They are quick to anger and may be aggressive or overbearing. More positively, they are courageous, vigorous, intelligent and sociable.

Foods and herbs that increase fire are warming, spicy, salty and sour in flavor and are to be restricted in a high pitta condition. Substances that are cooling, sweet, bitter and astringent in flavor are used to treat pitta disorders.

Following is a basic diet for pitta-predominant individuals:

90% sweet foods (see above)
7% astringent foods
2% bitter foods and spices
 to 1% salt
 to 1% spices
½ to 1% sour fruits

Foods beneficial for Pitta-predominant individuals are:

Grains: wheat, oats, rice, barley
Beans: kidney beans and tofu

Vegetables: sweet and bitter vegetables, cabbage, mushrooms, white and sweet potatoes, broccoli, okra, sprouts, zucchini, leafy greens, cucumbers, asparagus
Fruit: sweet fruits, figs, grapes, coconuts, pears, oranges, mangoes, plums, melons
Dairy: milk, ghee, unsalted cheese
Meat: chicken and turkey (white meat), rabbit, venison
Nuts: only coconut
Seeds: only sunflower seeds
Oils: olive, sunflower and soy oils and ghee
Sweeteners: unrefined raw sugar and other sweeteners except molasses and honey
Drinks: cool drinks, water, fruit juice
Spices: only coriander, cardamon, turmeric, small quantities of cinnamon, pepper and fennel seeds

A kapha or water-predominant personality is predisposed to such mucous-type diseases as colds, asthma, coldness, edema, digestive disorders, and arthritic problems. This individual tends to react slowly, and may be dull or less sensitive than other types. The positive traits of kapha are smoothness, steadiness, generosity, forgiveness and patience.

Foods and herbs that increase kapha include mucus-forming foods, dairy, fats and cold foods and substances that are excessively sweet or salty. Thus, herbs and foods suitable for a vata-predominant individual are unsuitable for a kapha-predominant. They are only moderately suited for pitta- or fire-predominant individuals, who may need the cooling aspect of kapha-predominant foods but, because of the oily nature of pitta, may not need the watery qualities of some of them.

Kapha people benefit from foods and herbs that are spicy, bitter and astringent, dry and rough in nature. Hot baths, exercise and fasting also are beneficial for them.

Following is a basic diet for kapha-predominant individuals:

80% sweet foods (this refers to complex carbohydrates and proteins, not strong sweet, sugary things)
15% astringent foods
2½% bitter foods

1 to 2% spicy or pungent things
¾ to 1% sour things
to 1% salt

Foods beneficial for a dry, reducing anti-kapha diet include:

Grains: rye, corn, millet, barley, buckwheat
Beans: mung beans, orange lentils, chick peas, sweet peas, all beans except kidney beans and tofu
Vegetables: all leafy vegetables, flower vegetables, radish, eggplant, potatoes, garlic, asparagus
Fruits: baked apples, guava, persimmon, rosehips
Dairy: baked cheese, ghee and goat's milk
Meat: chicken, turkey, rabbit, venison, eggs (not fried)
Nuts: no nuts
Seeds: only sunflower seeds
Oils: only almond, corn, sunflower oils in small amounts
Sweeteners: none except raw honey
Drinks: water, hot tea, wine (in moderation)
Spices: chili, ginger, black pepper, coriander, bay leaf, fenugreek, cumin, turmeric

Foods to be limited or avoided include: white rice, wheat, oats, bread, flour products, seafood, beef, sweet and juicy vegetables, sweet potatoes, cucumbers, zucchini, tomatoes, sweet fruits, avocados, bananas, melons, coconuts, dates, figs, oranges, grapes and salt.

Since many people are a combination of vata, pitta or kapha, one needs to evaluate each individual and adjust the diet accordingly.

Kicharee: Food of the Gods

Kicharee is regarded in India as the most perfect balanced, healing food. It is said that if *kicharee* is eaten as the sole food for three weeks, it will cure all diseases. Indeed, many wonderful benefits are possible on a two to three exclusive week diet of *kicharee.* The entire blood chemistry, along with organic physiological processes, is brought into balance and harmony. The mind becomes calm and clear and the emotions are regulated. Many Indian yogis and ascetics, in order to further limit their desires and attachment to the world, voluntarily choose to live on a diet of *kicharee* only. It is the ideal food for a fast or to take at the beginning of an herbal program.

This simple dish consists of varying to equal proportions of mung beans and brown rice, mixed with a pinch of sea salt, ghee, coriander, cumin and turmeric powders. During the winter months, dry ginger may be added to help maintain body heat.

To prepare *kicharee,* saute powdered coriander, cumin seeds and turmeric powder in a skillet with approximately a tablespoon of ghee (clarified butter). As the aroma of the spices begins to rise, stir in the precooked mung beans (ideally cooked with a small piece of kombu seaweed for trace minerals). This can be made as dense or thin as desired, depending upon how much water is used to cook the beans. Then add cooked basmati or brown rice, prepared with a pinch of salt. The basic recipe uses approximately one teaspoon each of the spices to one cup of mung beans, but more or less can be added as desired. A pot of *kicharee* may be refrigerated and portions warmed as desired

If one desires to eat only beans and whole grains for a period of time, different types of grains, (such as whole grain noodles, millet and barley) and different types of beans may be substituted. Other spices such as ginger, garlic, and asafoetida may be used.

CHINESE FOOD THERAPY

Chinese food therapy is based upon the principles of yin and yang, the four energies, the five elements and the four directions. With all of these factors to consider, it is somewhat difficult to present an approach to diet and nutrition that can be easily grasped by non-Chinese.

Chinese food therapy addresses six different constitutional types: hot, cold, dry, damp, deficient and excessive. Each of these, like the types in Ayurvedic *tridosha* theory, describes both a constitutional predisposition as well as a disease condition. Thus specific diseases are characterized by one of these six types or a combination of several; or individuals may be born with them as constitutional tendencies. As in Ayurveda, an individual's condition is evaluated by a number of considerations both physical and psychological.

A hot condition will exhibit feelings of heat, redness, preference for cool things, scanty dark urine, hard stools. The tongue will appear red with a yellowish coat and the pulse will be rapid. This type of individual will benefit from generous amounts of fruits and vegetables, cooling, anti-inflammatory herbs, purgatives, cholagogues and alteratives.

A cold condition exhibits feelings of coldness, paleness, preference for warm food and drink, clear and more frequent urination, loose stools. The tongue will be paler, with a thin, white coating. The pulse will be deep and slow. This type of person will benefit from cooked foods, red meat, internally warming herbs, spices, yang, chi and blood tonics.

A dry condition will have greater than normal thirst, dryness of the lips, nose, throat and skin, a dry cough without phlegm, a tendency towards constipation and itchiness of the skin, and will be thin and unable to gain weight. The tongue will be dry and the pulse will feel rough, fine and thready. This type of individual will benefit from soups, cooked foods, sweet fruits, oils, demulcent, yin tonic foods and herbs.

A damp condition will have a tendency towards overweight, heavy feeling of the body, water retention, edema and tiredness. The tongue will appear glossy and greasy, the pulse will feel more slippery and gliding. This type of individual requires a lighter diet, drier foods, fewer rich and heavy foods, no oils or fats, more diuretic foods and herbs. They also benefit from aromatic herbs that aid digestion and promote perspiration.

A deficient condition is underweight, low in energy and spirits and pale in complexion, with a low voice, timidity and has shortness of breath. There is a lack of sexual energy and prolapse of the stomach, intestines, uterus or anus. They will benefit from well-cooked foods, meats, root vegetables and tonic herbs cooked with food. The tongue will appear pale, shriveled or trembling, with a thin white coating. In extreme stages of deficiency there will be signs of *deficient heat* or *false yang* symptoms, the tongue will have no coating and a glazed reddish body and the pulse will be rapid and thready.

An excess type person is physically strong, energetic, high-spirited, loud-voiced, aggressive, excessive in sexual energy and ruddy in complexion. They have a tendency to constipation, hypertension and heart disease. The pulse will feel bounding, full and usually fast. The tongue is full, with a well defined thick coating. These individuals need reducing therapy, more vegetables and fruit, less heavy protein, meat, fats, bread and flour products, and foods with white sugar. They also benefit from removing and reducing therapies, alteratives and purgatives.

Chinese medicine evaluates foods according to their energies, flavors, five element effects and therapeutic properties. Following is a representative sampling of therapeutic properties of foods according to the Chinese system.

Foods that counteract heat are: barley, wheat, millet, buckwheat, mung beans, soybeans, mushrooms, melons, lettuce, mint, watercress, tomatoes, clams, seaweeds, tofu, tangerines, swiss chard, asparagus.

Foods that counteract cold are: glutinous rice, mutton, warm spices, brown sugar, butter, chicken, onion, garlic, peaches, pine nuts, mustard greens, walnuts, shrimp, sweet potatoes, strawberries, sorghum, malt sugar, anchovies, trout, lotus, vinegar, alcohol.

The many foods classified as neutral for both cold and hot types include: rice, eggs, yams, turnips, taro potatoes, squash, shitake mushrooms, plums, pork, beef, pumpkins, raspberries, peas, peanuts, papayas, oysters, tuna fish, grapes, kidney beans, figs, duck, corn, carrots, sesame seeds, cabbage, broccoli, aduki bean, almonds.

Foods that counteract dryness are: millet, agar, amasake, bananas, bamboo shoots, beets, sesame seeds, butter, eggs, milk, cheese, clams, oysters, cucumbers, crab, seaweeds, honey, gluten, barley malt, sugar, salt, kudzu root, apples, mangoes, pineapples, plums, pears, pork, oils, spinach, tofu, tomatoes, melons, citrus fruits.

Foods that counteract dampness are: most spices, turnips, radishes, taro potatoes, barley, string beans, beans, rye, pumpkin, kohlrabi, corn.

Foods that counteract deficiency are: meat, fish, grains, root vegetables, cooked foods, barley malt, unrefined sugar, butter, milk, eggs, sesame seeds, gluten, beans, cooked fruits and vegetables.

Foods that counteract excess are: uncooked foods, fruits, vegetables, bamboo shoots.

Many people have a mixed conformation and therefore require a combination of foods and herbs from different categories.

Abstinence from foods that are cooling is advised while undergoing warming herbal therapy; avoidance of foods that are heating when undergoing cooling herbal therapy. When undergoing lubricating herbal therapy avoid drying foods; when undergoing astringent or drying herbal therapy avoid foods that are moistening. Purging and detoxifying foods should be avoided when undergoing tonification therapy; and tonifying foods avoided when undergoing detoxifying and eliminative herbal therapy.

One of the most important practices in Chinese food therapy is the combination of herbal tonics with appropriate therapeutic foods. Thus, tonic herbs such as ginseng, dong quai and astragalus are boiled into a tea and used as a stock to cook a hearty meat soup or to make *congee,* (rice porridge). This is particularly beneficial for those who are very weak and unable to take more substantial food. Using a slow cooker, approximately one cup of rice is cooked in seven to 10 cups of the tonic herb tea from six to 12 hours.

To clear excess heat, two tablespoons of mung beans are lightly simmered for twenty minutes in a cup of boiling water. The liquid is taken in the morning. Another cup of boiling water is poured over the bean residue at noon and in the evening and each time the fluid is drunk. In the evening the beans also are consumed. This is good for the treatment of hypertension as well.

To counteract dryness and lack of estrogen, two or three salted oysters are eaten daily.

To counteract edema and fluid retention, make a soup of fresh water, carp, catfish or trout with aduki beans. Allow this to cook down, strain off the fluid, and eat the beans and fish.

To treat anemia and hypoglycemia make a soup with ginseng and either bone marrow or ox-tail.

For a blood and female hormone tonic and to alleviate menstrual problems or problems of infertility in women, make a soup with dong quai, ginger and a fresh spring chicken. If a spring chicken is not available, then use any fresh chicken.

To treat impotence in men, prepare lamb stew with daikon radish and Chinese black dates. Drink the broth and eat the lamb.

For morning sickness in women, grind lentils into a powder and take two teaspoons with rice cereal three times daily.

For male prostate problems, eat pumpkin seeds daily.

For the common cold, make a tea of three to six slices of fresh ginger steeped in one cup of boiling water. Add a teaspoon or so of brown sugar. This induces perspiration.

For lowered immune system and low energy, make a soup with ginseng and astragalus with organic beef or wild game. Take once a week.

SUMMARY

George Ohsawa popularized the 10 day macrobiotic diet as a virtual panacea for most diseases. This macrobiotic diet, which is based upon sound Oriental principles of energetic balance, is erroneously thought to consist only of brown rice. This is not so. Ohsawa's number 10 diet included a variety of whole grains and beans, with perhaps an emphasis on brown rice. It was intended to be followed strictly only for ten days, because according to Ohsawa, this is the period of time the blood takes to be renewed.

This idea of a diet using only foods of a neutral energy, such as grains and beans, is one that is universally recognized by traditional herbalists everywhere. Such a diet can balance the blood chemistry and also eliminate any energetic extremes, so that the herbs taken along with it can be more effective.

As we have seen, in Ayurveda the mung beans and rice recipe, *kicharee,* is used for these purposes. In Central America, the West Indies and South America, beans and rice or beans and corn are taken while undergoing herbal therapy. In China rice porridge (*congee*) is combined with apppropriate tonic herbs. This demonstrates the universal application of a diet that emphasizizes foods of a neutral energy and avoids those which are too cold or too hot, too moistening or too drying, too building or too eliminative, as an aid to the herbal strategy.

To patients undergoing herbal treatment, most Chinese herbalists will at least advise the avoidance of all raw foods (because they are too cold), white sugar (because it is too rich and overstimulates the pancreas and liver), strong spices (because they disperse the energy from within to the surface of the body), coffee (because it overtaxes the adrenals), citrus (because it is too moist and cool), shellfish (because they are too cold and moist) and cold dairy foods (because they are too congesting).

Since herbs and foods operate physiologically on the same organic plane, they have the power either to interfere with or enhance each other's action. The herbalist should learn to be a skilled cook, well-practiced complementing the basic energetics of herbs with food therapy.

THE EIGHT METHODS
OF HERBAL THERAPY
How to Use the Planetary Pharmacopoeia

The Planetary Herbal Pharmacopoeia relates traditional diagnoses and the curative action of herbs. That relationship is based upon an energetic connection that classifies diseases and remedies as excess-deficient, hot-cold, external (acute)-internal (chronic).

Thus diseases of an excess nature utilize herbal remedies that are light and eliminative while diseases of a weak or deficient nature require remedies that are tonic. For cold-natured diseases warm or hot-natured medicines are used, while hot-natured inflammatory diseases require cool or cold herbal remedies. Internal diseases require herbal remedies that act more on the internal organs while external diseases need surface-relieving or diaphoretic remedies. All of this is encompassed in the bi-polar principle fundamental to all traditional herbal healing systems.

Classical Chinese herbalism divides the categories of herbal treatment into the Eight Methods of Herbal Therapy:

1. Sweating   5. Harmonizing
2. Emesis   6. Warming
3. Purging   7. Supplementing
4. Removing   8. Reducing

SWEATING THERAPY
(Diaphoresis)

Sweating therapy is used for colds, flu, acute rheumatic complaints, aches and pains, skin diseases. These all are considered external diseases and sweating therapy is used to drive the invading cold, heat, fire, damp, wind, dryness and summer heat out of the body.

Two methods are used: spicy, warm, surface-releasing— called stimulating diaphoretics; and spicy, cool, surface-relieving—called relaxing diaphoretics. A spicy, cool, relaxing diaphoretic is used where the system is hot, the skin dry and the pulse full and quick. If the heart impulse is weak and the skin is cold, then a spicy, warm, stimulating diaphoretic is used. Generally the spicy, warm, stimulating diaphoretic is stronger and better suited for stronger patients. For example, one would not use lemon balm or feverfew if the skin were cold and the pulse slow. In such a condition, fresh ginger or another herb from the warming diaphoretic category would be indicated. On the other hand, if the skin is hot and dry and the pulse full and bounding, use a relaxing diaphoretic such as lemon balm or catnip.

Surface-relieving herbs influence the sudoriferous (sweat) glands. Some also are useful in treating eczema, scarlet fever and other skin diseases. This is because the sebaceous glands are activated through the use of diaphoretic herbs like burdock seeds and sassafras. The oils in both of these herbs are useful in the treatment of dry eczematous skin.

Sweating therapy is used for restoring circulation. Not only herbal teas but saunas and sweat baths are included among the herbalist's strategies for raising body heat and metabolism to burn off toxins and relieve congestion. It has been demonstrated that even certain kinds of cancers have been cured as a result of raising the over-all body temperature. Fever is the body's natural defense against disease and the body can tolerate quite high temperatures as long as the upper cavity (head) is kept cool with the application of cool water packs.

If there is a condition of extreme edema, a hot, dry sauna is preferred. Ayurvedic medicine also recommends sun bathing in the nude or covering the patient from the neck down with heated sand. Usually, a steam or vapor bath is effective for most conditions.

In the case of an acute fever, cold or flu, the patient should take several cups of a sweat-inducing tea, such as elder flower and mint, with two to four tablets of Formula 19 (pg. 129) (Composition powder). They should then rest quietly in bed, warmly covered, until perspiration is induced. Perspiration should be allowed to continue for a short time but not to the point of exhaustion. Then the patient is quickly sponged off with cool water from head to foot and the bedding changed. Warm rice porridge with ginger or a thin meat broth will be strengthening. A simple relaxing diaphoretic tea, such as lemon balm with honey taken in tablespoon doses, is pleasant tasting and will be acceptable to children.

For bronchial and lung infections, a stimulating oil such as camphor or eucalyptus may be rubbed on the chest and back, in addition to the sweating treatment. This will act as a surface counterirritant to help break up the underlying congestion and assist breathing.

For arthritic and rheumatic problems a tea such as those made from angelica root or sassafras may be taken freely before and during the steaming operation. A regular steam bath may be used or a vapor bath can be rigged up by wrapping the patient in several blankets (leaving the head exposed) and seating him over a chair with a pot of boiling water. Formula 19 may be taken every 20 minutes with tea or hot water until the patient is perspiring freely. This is then followed by a brief, cool sponge-bath, after which he or she should recline in a warm comfortable bed. Since the body's energy is being drawn to the surface, only light foods—such as warm juices, soup, grain porridge, or light meat broth—should be taken.

Contraindications for this kind of treatment include extreme weakness, emaciation, surface reddening of the skin, dryness and rapid pulse (yin-deficient heat).

It is interesting to note that just as plants excrete volatile oils to ward off invading pathogenic factors, such as germs and insects, so does the body eliminate its volatile oils (mostly through the pores of the skin), facilitating the process of detoxification.

Stimulating diaphoretics are used to burn away surface toxins in excess conditions. Formula 19, based upon the Composition Powder of the earlier North American herbalists, is a stimulating diaphoretic. The Eclectics considered Composition Powder their most valuable single herbal compound, because of its great effectiveness in stimulating heat, body metabolism and the body's defense systems.

Another important herb used by the Chinese is Ma huang (ephedra), which contains adrenaline-like compounds of epinephrine and norepiniphrine and induces sweating.

Ma Huang Decoction

Ma huang (6-9 gms.)   Apricot seed (6-9 gms.)
Cinnamon branch (6-9 gms.)   Licorice (3-6 gms.)

This preparation is helpful in treating diseases caused by exterior cold and wind, with symptoms of fever, chills, headache, aching, no perspiration and asthma. It is a good treatment for stronger individuals suffering from the common cold and cough. If there is perspiration, headache, nasal congestion or cough with profuse phlegm, eliminate cinnamon from the formula.

For a weaker individual who has profuse perspiration and coldness, the following formula is suggested:

Cinnamon Branch Combination

Cinnamon branch (6-9 gms.)   Jujube dates (3-5 pieces)
Peony root (6-9 gms.)   Fresh ginger (3-4 slices)
Licorice (3-6 gms.)

This formula also is used for the common cold and flu, fever, headache, intolerance of wind, spontaneous perspiration and weakness. It also is helpful for morning sickness, postpartum treatment and various skin disorders such as eczema, frostbite and tinea capitis (a fungal skin disease of the scalp). When stiff neck and shoulders also are present, add pueraria root (kudzu), 6-9 grams.

EMESIS
(Vomiting)

Emesis is used to cleanse the stomach of toxins, mucus and undigested foods. Since mucus originates in the stomach, emetic therapy is the most effective natural method for its elimination. The prevalence of mucus throughout the body can block the channels, giving rise to a condition which in Ayurveda is called *ama,* characterized by a more toxic type of mucus that impedes the flow of nervous energy. *Ama* is considered the primary cause of most degenerative diseases ranging from asthma, arthritis and rheumatism to poor digestion, constipation and general sluggishness. In Ayurvedic medicine, vomiting therapy is considered one of the Five Therapies *(pancha karma)* along with enemas, purgatives, blood-letting and nasal therapy.

In the early American Thompsonian system of herbalism, the use of emetics was considered one of the most effective methods in the treatment of disease. Cleansing the digestive system was considered the first step in arousing the body's recuperative capacities against fevers and acute diseases. Before the properties of lobelia were understood, poisonous substances were used for this purpose. An herb that combines both antispasmodic and stimulant properties, lobelia was considered a near panacea until a controversy arose as to its possible toxicity (which still has not been proven).

Dr. Christopher used acid tincture of lobelia (made with apple cider vinegar) in the treatment of severe asthma. He recommended waiting until the attack reached its zenith, then giving the patient a quart or two of peppermint tea followed by a teaspoonful of lobelia tincture three times at 10 minute intervals to provoke emesis.

In Ayurvedic medicine, emetic therapy is the most direct method for treating kapha conditions. It is used to root out mucus and blockages from the deep channels and tissues of the body. In his book *Ayurveda, the Science of Self-Healing,* Dr. Lad describes the proper method of emetic therapy: "One to three days prior to vaman (emesis), the person should drink one cup of oil two to three times a day until the stool becomes oily, or he feels nauseated. He should also eat a kaphagenic (mucus-predominant) diet to aggravate kapha in the system. Vaman should be given in the morning (kapha time). The person should eat basmati rice and yogurt with much salt early in the morning, which will further aggravate kapha in the stomach. The application of heat to the chest and back will liquify kapha. The person should sit calmly on a knee-high chair, and drink a concoction of licorice and honey, or calamus root tea. This emesis preparation is measured and recorded before being drunk, so that at a later time the amount of vomitis from the decoction can be determined.

After drinking the decoction, the person should feel nauseated. He should then rub the tongue to induce vomiting, continuing until bile comes out in the vomitis. The degree of success in this treatment is measured by: 1) the number of vomitings (8 is maximum, 6 medium, 4 minimum), and 2) the quantity of vomitis (1 quart maximum, 1 ½ pints medium, 1 pint minimum)."

After emesis, resting, fasting, smoking herbs such as mullein, uva ursi and yerba santa and paying heed to all natural urges of elimination should be followed. Contraindications are for small children, those who are feeble and aged, people suffering from hunger, heart disease and lung hemorrhage. Emesis should not be administered to women during menses or pregnancy, nor to people who are emaciated, extremely obese, or in a state of grief.

According to Dr. Lad, emesis is indicated for the following: "cough, cold symptoms of asthma, kapha fever, nausea, loss of appetite, anemia, bleeding through the lower channels, food poisoning, skin diseases, diabetes, lymphatic obstruction, chronic indigestion, edema (swelling), epilepsy, chronic sinus problems, repeated attacks of tonsillitis."

PURGING
(Laxatives)

Purgatives and cathartics are herbal remedies that influence the evacuation of the bowels. Most of them work through stimulating the discharge of bile from the liver and gall ducts. They are called "chologogues" and include the stronger laxative herbs such as rhubarb, cascara sagrada (the tonic-laxative), aloe and buckthorn, the very strong culver's root and mandrake; and several mild herbs, which are classified as *clearing heat,* such as Oregon grape, barberry and dandelion root. Normal evacuation depends upon the normal secretion of bile, the proper mucus secretions in the intestines for lubrication, healthy condition of the bowels and normal peristaltic action stimulated by uninterrupted nerve impulse. This last condition may relate Western physiology to the traditional Ayurvedic designation of the colon as the seat of nervous energy.

Normally one should have at least one bowel movement a day. If this is missed occasionally for two days or so, it is not considered a problem. If this happens more often, or for longer periods, a constipated condition exists. (Conversely, if there are regularly more than two or three evacuations each day, there may be a gradual weakening of the body reserves.) Constipation is a serious disease because it is often the precursor of other degenerative diseases. Still other factors such as liver toxicity and congestion, lack of organic spleen yang chi that would give one the nerve strength to eliminate properly, proper mucous secretion that will lubricate the colon, are also important to proper bowel function.

First, diet should be adjusted to supply a proper balance of whole grains to produce sufficient roughage and green vegetables to gently activate liver function. Fresh fruits are more purely laxative foods, to be used when seasonally available. Only after these dietary needs are supplied should one resort to the use of laxatives.

A cold condition means that there is a lack of energy to push the fecal matter out and this is treated with warming tonics, spices cooked in ghee and the exclusive use of cooked foods. A hot condition is associated with an excess yang state and is directly benefited by the use of herbal purgatives such as rhubarb, cascara, aloe, buckthorn and senna. Sodium sulphate (mirabilitum), a salt sold as epsom salt in pharmacies, is used for the most stubborn cases of congestion. Since nearly all strong laxatives are cold in nature, it would be harmful to over-all body metabolism to prescribe them to individuals suffering from constipation caused by cold and deficient chi.

Symptoms of coldness include spasms, and one of the side effects of purging therapy can be "griping" as a result of the cold energy of the laxative. Herbalists find ingenious methods of adjusting specific purging remedies to suit the needs of the individual. To prevent griping, add a small amount of a warming stimulant herb like ginger to the laxative. (This works well with all the laxative herbs mentioned.) The warming action of the ginger will help protect the energy of the stomach and spleen.

Licorice, which has a cortisone-like action, also has mild laxative properties. Licorice alone works quite effectively for the occasional treatment of constipation in children, especially if manuka raisins also are cooked in the tea. Licorice has a neutral energy and sweet taste, tonifies chi and is often added in small amounts to classical laxative formulas.

Some simple laxative formulas follow:

Rhubarb root (3-6 gms.)
Ginger root (1-2 gms.)
Licorice root (1-2 gms.)

Cascara sagrada may be substituted for the rhubarb if liver stagnation, digestive weakness and general debility are present, since it is more tonic in the Western sense than rhubarb.

If there is liver stagnation, then two to three grams of aloe powder may be added with great benefit. Aloe is specific for the liver and is regularly prescribed in Ayurvedic medicine in a dose of one to two teaspoons of the gel (a milder laxative than the powder) daily for women suffering from premenstrual syndrome, which is most commonly caused by congested liver.

Senna may be used in small amounts, along with other detoxifying and eliminating herbs, to help reduce weight by hastening the transit time of food through the colon.

When severe metabolic coldness is present, a small amount of prepared aconite is added to the rhubarb, ginger and licorice combination; ginseng is added if there is deficient chi. If there is deficient blood, there will be dryness in the colon and six to nine grams of the Chinese herb dong quai is added. Dong quai is not only a blood tonic but its moistening action has laxative effect. Peach seeds, when added to the formula in a dosage of approximately five grams, also serve both to lubricate the intestines and to promote blood circulation.

Finally, various carminative herbs, such as anise, fennel and orange peel, may be added. These help regulate the chi or energy of digestion and elimination.

When dry, hard stools occur, lubricating laxatives are used to increase the mucous secretions in the colon. One of the functions of the colon is to reabsorb back into the system a certain amount of the fluid that was mixed with the digested food and wastes. If the metabolism is too high too much fluid will be reabsorbed and the result will be dry stools and constipation. In such cases, lubricating laxatives like psyllium, flax and cannabis seeds[1] are used to great advantage. A tablespoon of olive or sesame oils taken occasionally before retiring also will provide relief. They help to contract the gall bladder as well as lubricate the intestines.

Enema Therapy

As previously stated, Ayurvedic medicine views the lower bowel as the seat of vata, the air humor that regulates nervous energy. This concept ascribes a broad range of physiological action to an organ which according to contemporary Western physiology has a relatively small and limited scope of activity. In spite of the apparent simplicity of colon function compared to that of other vital organs, Ayurveda recognizes that, as the major organ of elimination, it is vitally important to total physical health.

Enema and purgative therapy differ in that purgatives usually work by discharging bile from the liver and gall bladder, while enemas work directly on the bowel itself. Thus, enema therapy is the primary method of treating air or nervous system derangements in Ayurveda.

Ayurveda considers enema therapy a complete treatment for many diseases, including: constipation, distention, lower back pain, gout, rheumatism, sciatica, arthritis, nervous disorders, chronic fever, colds and flu, sexual disorders, kidney stones, heart pain, neck pains, hyperacidity, nervous headache, emaciation and muscular atrophy.

There are three basic types of enemas:

1. Oil enema, in which a cup of warm sesame or other oil is introduced through the rectum.
2. Decoction enema, in which an herb tea (whichever is indicated orally) is taken rectally.
3. Nutritive enema, which is composed of warm milk, meat broth or bone marrow soup.

Following is a formula for basic Ayurvedic anti-vata enema:

Water (1 ½ qts.)   Castor oil (1 oz.)
Sesame oil (4 ozs.)   Anise seed (2 ozs.)
Honey (4 ozs.)   Rock salt (1 oz.)

Boil the anise seeds and salt from three to five minutes in the water, strain, and stir in the remaining ingredients. When the liquid is lukewarm, pour it into the enema bag. Hang the bag so that it is not more than a foot higher than the syringe. While reclining on a mat on the bathroom floor, insert the syringe slowly into the rectum. Try to retain the solution for at least 30 minutes, or longer if possible.

Enemas are contraindicated for persons with diarrhea or rectal bleeding. Oil enemas should not be given to individuals complaining of cough, shortness of breath, diabetes, severe anemia, chronic indigestion, the aged, or children below the age of seven years. Decoction enemas are contraindicated in cases of acute fever, cold, paralysis, heart pain, severe pain in the abdomen, or wasting diseases.

REMOVING THERAPY
(Alteratives)

Removing therapy refers to anti-inflammatory, heat-clearing methods which use cool substances to resolve conditions of internal heat, such as fever and bacterial and viral infections. These often are treated with blood purifiers or alteratives. The term alterative, or anti-scorbutics, as they sometimes are called, refers to any remedy that gradually alters and corrects impure conditions of the blood.

In Chinese medicine any irritating toxin is called *heat* or fire, depending upon its severity. This would include all of the following: fevers, infections and inflammations, skin eruptions, liver toxicity, jaundice, blood poisoning, boils and carbuncles, gangrene, sore throat, certain kinds of cancers, arthritis, nervousness, burns and the effects of overexposure to the sun.

The Chinese distinguish between full and empty fevers. A full or sthenic fever is caused by external infectious factors and manifests acute inflammatory reactions. These include redness of the face and eyes, high fever, irritability, thirst (with a preference for cool drinks), strong body and breath odor, bitter taste in the mouth, constipation, dark, concentrated urine, dark red tongue and a rapid, strong and full pulse.

An empty or asthenic fever is called *yin weakness with internal fever* or *yin heat or fire*. This condition manifests with strumous or consumptive, wasting diseases and causes hyperfunctional catabolism, dryness and thirst, nervous excitement and metabolically-caused fever. There will be dryness of the mouth, night sweats, a red, fissured tongue and a thin, rapid pulse.

Fevers are classified as being either of the surface or the interior. Surface fevers are accompanied by thirst, fear of wind, perspiration, headache and a rapid, floating pulse. The symptoms of internal fevers are dry mouth, irritability, thirst, dark urine, constipation and abdominal distention.

Antipyretic, anti-inflammatory, antibacterial and antiviral herbs are used to treat internal heat with fever, inflammation, suppuration and dysentery.[2] Chinese herbalism classifies four distinct stages of fevers as follows:

Wei fever

An attack on the defensive immune system. This condition is a surface disease and may progress to a more serious internal heat stage. Its symptoms are sore throat, chills, sweat, thirst, headache, yellow phlegm, floating and rapid pulse and reddish tongue with yellow coating. It is the same as a surface fever or wind-heat condition and is treated by such herbs as echinacea, baptisia, honeysuckle, forsythia and various cooling diaphoretics.

Chi fever

An attack on the internal immune system. Its symptoms are high temperature, intolerance of heat, severe thirst, dark urine and profuse perspiration. This fever is characterized by the presence of physical strength, strong pulse and a red tongue with yellow coating. For this type of fever the mineral gypsum in the White Tiger formula is most often used.

Ying or essence fever

At this stage, the fever has burnt up and damaged the vital fluids. There will have been a degeneration of over-all health, consuming fever, thirst, insomnia, dark red tongue and rapid, thready pulse. In extreme stages there will be loss of consciousness, spasms and dehydration. The herbs used to treat this condition have nutritive, yin tonic properties and include rehmannia, figwort and rhinoceros horn.

Wei, or blood fever

This fever burns up the blood and causes rampant bleeding. This is a further aggravation of the ying stage and includes high fever, insomnia, delirium, coma, hemorrhage, bleeding under the skin, spasms and rapid and thin pulse. It is treated with rhinoceros or water buffalo horn, uncooked rehmannia and other herbs in the clear heat and cool blood categories.

For chi type inflammation, echinacea may be taken every two hours; or a combination of echinacea, garlic, golden seal, honeysuckle and chaparral may be used. Formula 15 (pg. 126) contains herbs that are good for this type of inflammation and is an effective treatment for skin diseases and flu.

A formula better suited for chronic degenerative diseases, including cancers and tumors, is based in South American Pau d'Arco tree bark. See Formula 16 (pg. 127).

Conditions of damp-heat, including hepatitis, jaundice, alcoholism, depression, pre-menstrual syndrom and liver toxicity are treated with cholagogues and herbs for the liver. See Formula 12 (pg. 125).

Venereal and related diseases, such as herpes, are treated with chola-gogic herbs that particularly target the urinary-reproductive organs. See Formula 14 (pg. 126).

Gypsum is specific for lowering rapidly rising and severe high fevers including those associated with meningitis and encephalitis. It also is specific for pneumonia, measles, diabetes and sunstroke. Following is a formula similar to the famous Chinese White Tiger Decoction:

Gypsum and Marshmallow Decoction

Gypsum, powdered (15 gms.) American ginseng (3 gms.)
Rice (10 gms.) Licorice root (2 gms.)
Marshmallow root (5 gms.)

In treating acute diseases, heat-clearing alteratives are most effective if taken along with a light, simple vegetable diet (including thin rice porridge, cereal and warm vegetable soups) so as not to interfere with the healing process. Those with deficient or yin heat may take warm meat broth or boiled warm milk. Those with excess or full heat should have either warm vegetable broth or fruit juices taken at room temperature. The body's recuperative efforts should be supported by conditions conducive to rest.

HARMONIZING

Harmonizing therapy is used when there is a combination of excess and deficiency, internal and external, and hot and cold symptoms. This often occurs with a lingering cold, flu or febrile disease. This therapy incorporates carminative or chi-moving herbs that help balance and regulate energy flow and organ function. It is the method of herbal therapy most commonly used, for example clear-cut symptoms indicating a single approach. Harmonizing therapy combines several approaches for treating complex conditions and apparently contradictory symptoms.

Symptoms indicating harmonizing therapy include: alternating fever and chills, chest distress, subcostal or hypochondriacal pain and distention, nausea, bitter taste in the mouth, abdominal distention and pain, and a taut, wiry pulse indicating stress. It is generally good for treating stress and emotional upset and also is effective for premenstrual depression, tension and pain. It also is effective in treating addictions to substances such as tobacco, alcohol and drugs.

Diseases that have passed the initial, acute phase are said then to penetrate to the liver and gall bladder channels. They are considered half external and half internal. The liver and gall bladder rule the emotions and nervous system.

Hans Selye, in his landmark work *The Stress of Life,* demonstrated how even after a toxin is physically dissipated, the disease cycle persists because of the continuing derangement of the nervous system.

In Chinese herbalism, the reaction the body has to a particular pathogen is called *wind* and in Ayurveda it is described as vata or air humor, which easily combines with either hot (pitta) or cold (kapha) conditions. In these cases, antispasmodics are added to the therapeutic formulas prescribed for the purpose of relieving the nervous reaction and helping to restore homeostasis. Peony root is the most commonly used antispasmodic in Chinese herbalism. North American herbalists add small amounts of lobelia or cramp bark to their formulas to achieve this effect.

Bupleurum falcatum (chai hu) is the principal Chinese herb used for harmonizing therapy. There seems to be no single equivalent herb in the Western herbalist's pharmocopoeia. Bupleurum is a member of the *Umbellifera* (parsley) family, which includes many warming herbs such as the *Angelica* and *Ligusticum* species. Yet it has a cool energy, but with a rising direction, so that it can have an exciting effect as well.

The most important biochemical constituents of bupleurum are its saikosaponins. They give bupleurum its ability not only to alleviate hot and cold external and internal conditions, but to have a deeper action that can affect hormone regulation. Typically, bupleurum is considered an herb for the liver. While it is classified as a cool, surface-relieving diaphoretic, it is most commonly used for chi-regulation. Its indicated use is chiefly for stress and tension, and for pain or tenderness in the area of the liver or transversely from it.

It is important to understand how the action of some herbs is profoundly influenced by their combination with certain others. For instance, the saikosaponins in bupleurum are weakly acidic and are more effective with the addition of a more strongly alkalinizing substance, such as oyster shell. Saponins are best extracted in water. Therefore formulas containing saponins, including most bupleurum formulas as well as many Chinese tonic formulas, are more effectively prepared by long simmering in water decoctions. Saponins are not efficiently extracted in alcohol.

There exists a whole class of bupleurum formulas developed by Chang Chung Ching in the Shang Han Lun (2nd century) and subsequently by other great herbal doctors. "Harmonizing" is not a category in the pharmacopiea because this therapy combines several herbal therapies, according to the treatment indicated for an individual patient. Carminative or *chi-moving* herbs are the main herbs in these formulas.

Minor Bupleurum (see Formula 35, pg. 139) is one of the most commonly used Chinese formulas for acute diseases that tend to become chronic, ranging from the second stages of colds and flu, asthma and digestive problems to hepatitis and hypoglycemia. It also may be taken as a preventative against disease, since it balances organ function (particularly liver with spleen/stomach).

Many modifications of this formula are possible. For deficiency of yin, add powdered tortoise shell and sweet wormwood (*Artemisia apiacea*). For abdominal pains and fullness, supplement with cyperus, corydalis and immature bitter orange. For hysteria, nervousness, spasms and restlessness, add calcium in the form of dragon bone (*Os draconis*) or oyster shell to stabilize the spirit.

The following formula may be used for regulating stagnant chi:

Poria cocos (7 pts.)	Wild yam (3 pts.)
Bupleurum root (4 pts.)	Magnolia bark (3 pts.)
Atractylodes (4 pts.)	Ginger (3 pts.)
Chaste berries (4 pts.)	Licorice root (3 pts.)
Dong quai (4 pts.)	Green bitter orange peel (2 pts.)
Peony root (3 pts.)	*Ligusticum wallichii* (2 pts.)
Cyperus rhizome (3 pts.)	Mint leaves (2 pts.)
Black haw bark (3 pts.)	Gastrodia (1 pt.)

This is used for mood regulation, depression, stagnant liver chi, nervousness, uneasiness, chest pains, digestive upset, abdominal distention, belching, gas, nausea, candida, constipation and many menstrual problems including premenstrual syndrome, irregular menstruation and breast distention. It also is helpful for hypertension and hysteria.

Harmonizing formulas can combine hot and cold, internal and external, and tonic and eliminative herbs in the same formula. They do not cancel each other out because the herbs are used according to the organs and meridians affected. For instance, one might combine a cool herb for the liver such as dandelion root, to help the discharge of bile; with a warm herb, like dong quai to improve blood circulation. In spite of the fact that one is cool and the other warm, in fact, when used together, the desired effect—which is to improve liver function by circulating more blood into the liver—is augmented.

Combining herbs from apparently contradictory categories often gives greater benefits, since most patients have mixed symptoms and respond better to a balanced therapy. Harmonizing therapy, in which one creates formulas that deal comprehensively with the unique symptom complexes of each individual, allows the greatest scope for the art of herbalism.

WARMING THERAPY
(Stimulants)

The purpose of warming therapy is to stimulate circulation, digestion and metabolism. Herbs that warm and stimulate digestion are said to strengthen *spleen yang*. Many of these herbs also promote urination and are said to revive *kidney yang* (essential vitality). Most have a spicy taste, but herbs which warm and raise metabolism may have any of the five flavors.

Warming herbs that act more superficially, such as warming diaphoretics, only disperse energy. The effect of excess of spicy, warm herbs on an individual with insufficient yin essence to counterbalance them will be a dispersion of chi and a core weakening of the individual.

Thus, warm spicy herbs can be used to supplement and strengthen *yang chi* or used to disperse congestion of chi, blood, energy, fluid and food. Indications for warming therapy, which is used to quickly restore over-all vitality, are severe chills, vomiting, abdominal pain, weak pulse and general coldness and weakness.

"Coldness" refers to one's sensitivity to outer climatic cold conditions as well as to general internal hypo-functioning. Thus, individuals with poor health, ineffective digestion, cold extremities, and a weakness of both body and spirit, are said to be cold or *yang* deficient and are to be treated by warming therapy.

Contraindications for warming therapy are signs of internal heat, constipation, bright red or yellow tongue, rapid pulse, spitting of blood and blood in the stools, diarrhea with fever or wasting diseases, with dryness and dehydration.

Among the many common spices used for warming therapy are cayenne, black pepper, cinnamon, cloves, fennel and ginger. Other common foods and spices that are warming are garlic, onions, asafoetida, mustard and horseradish.

Spicy-tasting herbs are anti-mucus in action (anti-kapha in Ayurveda). They frequently are given during the winter season when cold, damp weather often produces an increase in the accumulation of mucus. Since they promote circulation of blood and chi, they also are indicated for people with digestive weakness and rheumatic problems.

Thompsonian herbology, based upon the herbal system of the American nineteenth century herbalist Dr. Samuel Thompson, depended heavily on warming therapy, for which they commonly used cayenne pepper and the vapor (sweat) bath. Raising the over-all body temperature was Thompson's panacea. The Eclectics who followed him, and the late Dr. John R. Christopher, also depended heavily on cayenne to raise physical vitality for fighting off disease.

Indeed, such a strategy is valid for many, but not for those more sensitive individuals who tend towards a deficient state. Such individuals, who are thin or emaciated, and lack sufficient reserves to withstand such stimulation, can be injured by the careless use of strong, pungent, stimulating herbs. However, for individuals whose excess dampness and coldness indicate a lack of *yang chi,* spices are specifically indicated.

The vegetarian diet tends to be yin-predominant and vegetarians suffer from a lack of *yang chi,* with associated symptoms of hypo-functioning coldness and poor digestion. The Hindu people of India, who have adhered to a vegetarian diet for centuries, have learned to master the art of spicing food to maintain strength and digestive power. The curry powder characteristic of Indian cooking was originally a therapeutic blend of spices. It included turmeric, cumin seed, coriander, ginger, asafoetida and chili pepper, along with garlic and onions sauteed in ghee (clarified butter), foods and substances that compensated for the deficiency of yang in their diet.

Ghee is an important component in the East Indian lacto-vegetarian diet, because spices and food cooked in ghee (or in oil) are much more nutritious. The strong yang energy of the spices is counterbalanced by the moist yin quality of oil and ghee.

In the absence of refrigeration, traditional cultures valued spices such as pepper as preservatives for meat—their volatile oils (which serve a similar repellent function in the living plant) demonstrating an antibacterial action. Similarly, spicy-tasting herbs may be used to help the body fight infection and stimulate its immune system. Western, Chinese and Ayurvedic systems of herbology all use pungent and spicy-tasting herbs for these purposes. Following are similar infection-combatting formulas from each tradition.

Western Formulas

Probably the single formula most widely used by the early North American doctors was Composition Powder. This original formula of Dr. Samuel Thompson consisted of a combination of 4 parts bayberry bark, 2 parts white pine bark, 2 parts ginger, ½ part cayenne, ½ part cloves. Formula 19 (pg. 129) is very similar and integrates some of the principles of Oriental herbology and thus includes cinnamon bark and licorice.

A simplified version of Composition Powder combines equal parts of cayenne pepper and ginger root powders. A half to one teaspoon may be taken taken two or three times daily to stimulate vitality, circulation and digestion and to prevent illness.

Chinese Formulas

Chinese herbalism uses cinnamon bark in much the same manner that Western herbalists have come to use cayenne, and for the same indications. Cinnamon, however, is both spicy and sweet and gives a broader, more supportive action. The bark of the tree is used for internal warming, while the stems help to warm and relieve the surface (stimulating diaphoretic). Ginger also is widely used against infection, but is regarded as more effective for digestion. Fresh ginger has a more dispersing energy helpful against colds and fevers; dried ginger warms the center, helping assimilation.

An even stronger warming herb, considered the most yang in Chinese medicine, is aconite root. In its unprepared form, aconite is one of the most deadly plant poisons and as such was used in minute or homeopathic doses by Western Eclectic herbalists. The Chinese, however, have a method of detoxifying it (*Aconitum praeparatum*) which makes it the most yang herb and the strongest metabolic stimulant, with a hot energy. Because of its yang-heating power, it should be used with care, and only for those who are excess yin or yang deficient and complaining of coldness.

An internal warming Chinese formula called **Si Ni Tang** (literally "Warming the Four Limbs Decoction" is prepared as follows:

Prepared aconite (10 to 15 gms.)
Dry ginger (6 to 9 gms.)   Honey-baked licorice (10 to 15 gms.)

This is good for all symptoms of yang depletion, including internal coldness, vomiting, undigested food in the feces, abdominal pain with lack of thirst (indicating excess yin) and general collapse of vitality.

Appropriate variations of this basic yang-stimulating formula may include ginseng and atractylodes for additional chi tonification. For rheumatoid arthritis caused by coldness add cinnamon branch (for warming the surface) and peony root for promoting circulation.

If there is deficiency and dampness of the spleen with symptoms of coldness, edema, bloating after eating and watery mucous discharges, a mild tonic such as codonopsis, along with diuretics like alisma and poria cocos mushroom, may be added.

Formula 42 (pg. 142) is made by grinding prepared aconite, atractylodes, ginger, cinnamon and licorice to a fine powder and mixing them with honey. The resulting paste is taken in quarter to full teaspoon doses. This formula is excellent for those with a yang deficient constitution and accompanying cold extremities. It may be taken daily throughout the cold season.

Ayurvedic Formulas

Ayurvedic medicine uses a basic internal warming, drying and stimulant formula made up of the powders of black pepper (*Piper nigrum*), pippli long pepper (*Piper longum*), and ginger (*Zingiber off.*). It is called *trikatu*, the three spices. There are many variations of this formula, which is designed to raise metabolism, warm the circulation, aid digestion and dry mucus. A milder version, more suitable for children and sensitive individuals, substitutes two parts powdered anise seed for the pippli. The powdered herbs are mixed with honey and taken in doses of one-quarter to one-half teaspoon once or twice a day. Trikatu often is added to other herbal compounds.

Spicy herbs may be used for other purposes than internal warming. Added in small amounts to a formula, they act as a catalyst, intensifying and dispersing the effects of the other herbs. Spicy-tasting herbs may block the liver's tendency to neutralize other herbs and drugs, thus keeping them active in the circulation for a longer period. One reason that spices generally are contraindicated for eruptive skin diseases is that they inhibit the liver's ability to detoxify the blood.

SUPPLEMENTING

Supplementing or tonification therapy is indicated for individuals who are in a deficient, malnourished, weakened state. It also is helpful in preventing symptoms of aging, such as impotence, frigidity, poor memory and failure of sight and hearing.

Generally a tonic is most effective taken with food, since it facilitates the body's ability to absorb nutrients. Tonic herbs such as ginseng, astragalus or dong quai are simmered in soups to which may be added organic meat, grains and root vegetables. Before the discovery of vitamins, traditional peoples would prepare herbs in seasonally adjusted tonic combinations, using them both as preventatives and to augment health.

Most cultures believe that food is the fundamental tonic, and that foods combined with tonic herbs are superior to either used alone. Traditional Chinese families buy a pound each of tonic herbs such as ginseng or codonopsis which tonify the chi; dong quai which tonifies the blood; astragalus root which tonifies the immune system; and lycium berries which tonify the yin. Combinations are made by preparing a stock with one herb or a combination of them, and adding foods according to therapeutic indications. (See section on Food Therapy, pg. 73)

The Chinese herb tonic, Formula 30 (pg. 136), contains 5 kinds of ginsengs and is excellent for most deficiencies. This formula gradually increases energy, improves circulation and strengthens the immune system. It is taken prophylactically, to counteract fatigue and exhaustion, and to aid in recovery from illness. The tea also may be used as stock for soup or cooking rice.

An ancient Ayurvedic formula called *Chyavanprash* (see Formula 27, pg. 133) combines more than 60 finely-powdered herbs in a base of honey, sugar and ghee to make a delicious paste. It is taken in doses of two or three tablespoons in boiled warm milk once or twice a day, for general debility. It is used in much the same manner as ginseng formulas are used by the Chinese but, since the Hindus do not eat meat, they mix their herbal preparations with warm milk to increase their nutritive value.

Formula 6 (pg. 121) is a supplementing tonic formula for women (see Formula 6, pg. 121). It combines a variety of North American and Chinese tonic herbs that strengthen the liver, spleen and blood and the circulatory, nervous and digestive systems. This makes the formula particularly helpful for menstrual and post-partum disorders. It also may be taken occasionally by women for health maintenance, once daily or a few times daily before the menstrual cycle is due.

The yang tonic, Formula 33 (pg. 138), is used to tonify kidney yang. This formula is taken over a prolonged period to tonify kidney yang or that part of the adrenals which governs release of the stimulating hormones of adrenaline, epinephrine and nor-epinephrine. It is effective in treating impotence, frigidity, urinary disorders and lower back and joint pains.

The yin tonic, Formula 32 (pg. 137), nourishes kidney yin, the parasympathetic nervous system. It is helpful for most chronic degenerative diseases and urinary disorders, for diabetes, lower back and joint pains, and sports burnout.

Formula 20 (pg. 129) is particularly useful for the hormonal system. It is used during puberty and menopause as a general hormone tonic for men or women.

Formula 17 (pg. 128) is a tonic for the immune system and supporting the body's internal strength and essence.

In Western herbalism, an alcoholic bitters formula is taken before meals in small doses to stimulate hydrochloric acid and other digestive enzymes and aid digestion and assimilation. It is prepared as follows:

Gentian root (4 pts.)	Citrus peel (orange or tangerine) (2 pts.)
Calamus root (4 pts.)	Ginger root (1 pt.)
Centaury pts.)	Anise seed (1 pt.)
Colombo (2 pts.)	Fennel seed (1 pt.)
Golden seal (2 pts.)	Licorice root (1 pt.)

All of the above herbs are macerated in an alcohol such as vodka or gin for approximately two weeks, using a ratio of four ounces of herbs to a pint of vodka. It is then strained. A teaspoon is taken about 20 minutes before meals to stimulate appetite and increase assimilation.

REDUCING THERAPY

Reducing stagnation therapy is used to treat an accumulation of blocked energy, blood, mucus or food. These accumulations may take the form of lumps, cysts, tumors, congestion, food stagnation, swollen prostate, and urinary and gall stones. Cysts and tumors indicate either blockages of chi, blood or mucus and require reducing therapy.

Kelp softens hardened masses such as enlarged thyroid glands and cancers. Poke root also is used for enlarged glands. Diuretics eliminate fluid stagnation. External poultices reduce cancers and tumors.

The following remedy is used for treating food stagnation and is useful for travel sickness, weak digestion, nausea, vomiting, diarrhea, constipation, morning sickness, bloating and cramps:

Traveler's Joy

Poria cocos mushroom(4 pts.)	Cardamon seed (3 pts.)
Coix seed (4 pts.)	Magnolia bark (3 pts.)
Kudzu (4 pts.)	Rice sprouts (2 pts.)
Actractylodes (3 pts.)	Peppermint leaf (2 pts.)
Wild yam root (3 pts.)	Ume plum (2 pts.)
Cumin seed (3 pts.)	*Gastrodia elata (1 pt.)*
Costus root (3 pts.)	Citrus peel (tangerine or orange) (1 pt.)

In Ayurveda a similar formula is called *hingashtak* for the main herb in the formula asafoetida (hing in Sanskrit). There are several variants to this formula. One is as follows:

Hingashtak

Asafoetida (3 pts.)   Ginger root (2 pts.)
Atractylodes (3 pts.)   Dandelion root (2pts.)
Cumin seed (2 pts.)   Slippery elm (2 pts.)
Caraway seed (2 pts.)   Green citrus peel (2 pts.)
Pippli long pepper (2 pts.)   Rock salt (2 pts.)
Black pepper (2 pts.)

This formula, taken after eating, relieves gas, abdominal swelling, indigestion and food stagnation.

Expectorants, used to loosen and eliminate phlegm from the bronchioles and lungs, may also be helpful in removing stagnation therapy. One decongestant is Formula 1 (pg. 119).

Formula 2 (pg. 120) is very effective in treating bronchiole and lung congestion, asthma, bronchitis, coughs and colds. It serves as a diuretic, alleviating fluid retention, edema, indigestion and abdominal bloating. It also is used to treat bladder and urinary infections.

Urinary and gall stones also are considered to be caused by stagnation. Both may be treated with the same formula, as well as Formula 3 (pg. 120). Taken regularly three times daily, this will help to relieve the pain of urinary and gall stones as well as helping to dissolve and eliminate them safely and painlessly.

Another type of stagnation affects the male prostate gland. The treatment combines clearing heat and removing stagnation. Formula 4 (pg. 120) relieves pain and helps to reduce the swelling of the gland.

Obesity also is treated as a condition of stagnation. Traditional systems of herbalism view overweight as an excess, therefore a condition of toxicity. Such excesses cause the body to make undesirable compensations that often lead to overeating. This in turn puts a heavy burden on the organs of elimination, so that obesity gradually increases as a result of stagnation in such vital organs as the liver, kidneys and colon. When the elimination is poor, the assimilation also will be impaired.

Overweight also involves hormonal dysfunctions such as thyroid and adrenal functions that are too low to maintain metabolism and stimulate digestion and circulation. The aging process brings about a natural diminution of hormonal strength, resulting in a gradual lowering of metabolism which may cause weight gain (or loss depending upon the individual).

The most common cause of obesity is poor digestion with resulting toxic overload of the organs of assimilation and elimination. Overweight people experience hunger because their body is unable to adequately assimilate vital nutrients. Thus they are caught up in a vicious cycle of overeating.

Water retention is a major factor in many overweight conditions. Weakness of the kidneys can cause a gradual build-up and retention of fluids which increases obesity. Drinking a lot of fluids to "flush" the kidneys is a mistaken idea, unless the intention is to dilute and eliminate excess uric acid caused by overeating meat protein. Otherwise, drinking more water than we naturally desire can lead to further exhaustion of the kidneys. In fact, herbalists use sweating therapy, which promotes the elimination of fluid wastes through the pores of the skin, to relieve urinary tract infections.

The best practice is to drink when one is thirsty and, if thirst seems excessive, to find out why, rather than take excess water. While some of them do not take in enough fluids, vegetarians usually do not need so much, because most of their foods have a high fluid content.

Herbs for weight reduction are generally either diuretic or mildly purgative. Large amounts of kelp or other seaweeds are sometimes used because their high iodine content stimulates the thyroid gland, which assists weight loss through increased metabolism.

One type of overweight is due to excess toxic heat, usually caused by eating too much protein and rich foods, such as meat, dairy and sugar. This type responds excellently to a raw food diet with vegetable protein only, in the form of whole grains and beans.

Another kind of overweight is caused by a damp spleen, which means that the body seems to retain a lot of fluid regardless of how much is eaten. This individual may even gain weight on fruit and juices. Such people are most effectively treated with strong diuretic formulas and warming tonic herbs that strengthen spleen chi and general assimilative capacities. The moist, demulcent nature of seaweed is contraindicated for such individuals.

An herb that is helpful for those with obesity caused by deficient spleen yang is *Astragalus membranicus*. This tonic herb, when taken two or three times daily over a period of weeks or months, helps to restore spleen yang, aid assimilation and digestion, and eliminate excess fluid. Approximately four to six slices of astragalus root are boiled in a cup or two of water. Two or three cups are taken daily.

A special formula effective for treating overweight and for detoxification is Formula 26 (pg. 132). This formula mildly stimulates the eliminative organs. It also provides tonic properties to the spleen-pancreas, calms nervous tension, and alleviates hunger.

Reducing therapy also includes a variety of poultices and fomentations used externally to shrink or dissolve growths, tumors and swellings. Inch-thick shredded taro root poultice, applied to breast and changed twice daily, is an excellent treatment to draw out cancers.

---

[1]The seeds of the cannabis plant, unlike its leaves and buds, have no narcotic properties and are considered a food source by rural folk in China.

[2]Surface heat is treated by sweating.

DISEASES AND THEIR TREATMENT

ALLERGIES

Some allergies stem from a weakened immune system, while many others are caused by an injudicious style of living and eating. One of the most effective treatments for allergies associated with mucous conditions is Trikatu, a combination of powdered black pepper, ginger, anise seed and honey. This may be taken daily during the damp, cold seasons; or during allergy seasons to allay or prevent them. Formula 1 (pg. 119) also is very useful for such conditions, since the ma huang in that formula is a very effective adrenal stimulant, helpful in overcoming allergic reactions. Often such diuretic herbs as golden rod are used to treat allergies. In any case, a root tonification treatment using chi, yin or yang tonics as indicated, should be considered. Formula 30 (pg. 140), Formula 32 (pg. 137), and Formula 33 (pg. 138) are also possibilities.

Food allergies are treated with Hingashtak, Draksha or Formula 30 cooked in soup or combined with yin or yang tonics (Formulas 32 and 33 respectively). Formula 12 (pg. 125) helps discharge toxins before beginning tonification therapy, may be indicated.

A good formula for clearing the liver is a tea brewed from Oregon grape, dandelion root and sarsaparilla, with a small amount of ginger and fennel seed. Ginseng may be taken with soups and food and digestive herbs and spices, such as Hingashtak, during or after meals.

ARTHRITIS, RHEUMATISM, SCIATICA AND JOINT PAINS

These conditions are caused by unwholesome foods clogging the channels, poor digestive power, lack of exercise and an excess of rich foods, sweets and meats.

Therapy should begin with a combination of rhubarb, fennel seed, licorice, and ginger to regulate the bowels. Triphala may be taken each morning and night. In addition circulating herbs are needed: angelica root, prickly ash, juniper berries, teasel root or mistletoe with a small amount of licorice. These usually are prepared together as a compound tea formula.

For upper back problems and for releasing neck and shoulder tension pueraria is most specific and effective. It may be taken along or in formula. If there is degeneration of bones and tissues comfrey root should be added; if there is associated nerve injury, add St. Johnswort. If inflammation is present, use echinacea, goldenseal and Oregon grape or barberry. Yucca root is very effective for such conditions as well. Ayurvedic guggul is a specific for nerve and joint pain, including sciatica and arthritis. Shu Jin Chih (see Formula 31, pg 137) is an effective Chinese herb preparation for such problems.

ASTHMA

Asthma is often a difficult disease to treat, but Formula 1 (pg. 119), Ma Huang Combination, Minor Bupleurum and Pueraria Combination are effective remedies. As a root treatment, tonification with either yin or yang tonics, such as yin tonic, Formula 32 (pg. 137) or yang tonic, Formula 33 (pg. 138), can be helpful.

Balancing the stomach and digestion by following sound dietary principles is fundamental to treament. In some cases vomiting, induced by a tincture of lobelia and cinnamon tea, is helpful in interrupting the pathogenesis. Another first-aid measure is to take one or two inhalations of datura leaves.

CANCERS AND TUMORS

Such conditions are difficult to treat but a good remedy is the Planetary Bitters tea taken three or four times daily. It should be accompanied by a generous quantity of kelp—four to six tablets each time the tea is taken. In Chinese medicine, kelp and pokeroot are herbs known to have the ability to dissolve tumors. Pokeroot must be taken dried and aged for six months to neutralize some of its commonly nauseating side effects. A balanced diet, such as is described in this book, based upon whole grains, beans and fresh vegetables, should be followed. Red meats, and usually dairy foods, should be strictly avoided.

Formula 15 (pg. 126) and Formula 16 (pg. 127) may be taken separately or together.

CARDIAC PROBLEMS AND HIGH BLOOD PRESSURE

A universal remedy for the heart is hawthorn berries taken regularly as a tea, a syrup, or in tablet or capsule form. It also is useful for relieving high blood pressure, especially when combined with European mistletoe. Chinese tienchi ginseng is specific for heart problems and circulation and helps clear cholesterol and clogged arteries. An Ayurvedic practice is to drop a piece of gold jewelry into a cup of water before retiring. The water is taken each morning upon arising as treatment for heart problems. A tea of motherwort also may be taken daily to treat and promote normal circulation and ease the heart.

See Formula 10 (pg. 124).

COLDS AND SIMPLE FEVERS

Simple fevers may be treated by fasting or taking only light broths. Only boiled water, which is lighter for digestion, should be used. Ginger, pepper and honey may be added to induce sweating. Lemon balm or sweet basil tea are helpful. Fruit, cold and raw foods, cold dairy and heavy foods should be avoided. When the fever has subsided, give a mild purgative such as Triphala.

Some helpful formulas are: Formula 19 (pg. 129), Trikatu, Pueraria combination and Echinacea.

COUGHS, BRONCHITIS

For coughs, follow the same dietary suggestions as for colds, fevers and flu. Herbs that are warming and expectorant should be given. One combination is made from a grape juice with about 8% alcohol to preserve it. To this is added powdered black pepper, pippli long pepper (if available), cardamon, ginger and cinnamon, giving it a spicy taste. This mixture, called Draksha in Ayurveda, is a basic internal warming remedy good for cold conditions, coughs, weak digestion and related disorders. It keeps a long time. From a teaspoon to a tablespoon may be taken before meals, or several times daily.

A syrup that may be freely taken is made from any or all of these: loquat leaves, wild cherry bark, elecampane root and yerba santa. A simple and easily made syrup blends fresh garlic or onions with honey.

Some formulas to be considered are: Formula 1 (pg. 119), Trikatu and Echinacea.

DIGESTIVE PROBLEMS

Usually the first thing to do is to stop eating, or to eat only very light and liquid-type foods, such as cereals and soups.

Hingashtak is a specific for digestive disorders, including those with symptoms of bloating, gas and acidity. It may be taken before or after meals, or during meals, sprinkled on food. Another simple remedy is a cup of hot ginger tea taken after meals. Finally, it is good to have some Draksha on hand, to take regularly or as needed (see coughs).

HEADACHE

Headaches have many possible causes, making it impossible to find one universal remedy. Willow bark contains salicylic acid, the precursor of aspirin, which may be used without any of the long-term side effects of aspirin. Because of its extreme bitterness, it is better taken powdered in a capsule or in tablet form. Many headaches are caused by stomach disorders and since rosemary contains both aromatic oils good for stomach problems and salicylic acid, it is helpful, used as an occasional tea, for many headaches. Another herb containing salicylic acid is white poplar bark.

Feverfew has recently been discovered to be beneficial for migraine-type headaches. For headaches caused by poor vascular circulation, angelica root is specific.

For relief of many acute headaches, use equal parts of all the above-mentioned herbs for an excellent formula. For more complex types of headaches or more chronic conditions Formula 9 (pg. 123) is recommended.

HEPATITIS AND OTHER LIVER DISEASES

Hepatitis is treated with cholagogic herbs that help promote the regular flow of bile. One of the most effective is dandelion root. Others are Oregon grape, barberry and boldo. Stronger cholagogues are Culver's root *(Leptandra)*, mandrake and greater celandine. Blessed thistle is an excellent and gentle liver and blood detoxifier. In Ayurveda, turmeric is considered helpful as a herb when used with India's species of barberry. The Chinese use many herbs for the liver, chiefly bupleurum and gardenia. Milk thistle *(Sylibum marianum)* is prized for its powerfully regenerative effects upon the liver cells.

A simple but effective tea for the liver is made by combining equal parts of dandelion, blessed thistle, Oregon grape and pipsissewa *(Chimaphilla)* with fennel seed. Three cups are taken daily as a liver tonic and blood purifier.

For the relief of gallstones, a warm tea of fringetree bark with Oregon grape or barberry is very effective. A castor oil pack applied once a day, with the patient lying quietly for 45 minutes, is an additional therapy. Rub a thick coat of castor oil over the gall bladder or liver, cover the area with a thick towel dipped in hot ginger tea, and place a heating pad over the towel.

Formula 3 (pg. 120) is effective in cases of gallstones and urinary tract stones. See also Formula 12 (pg. 125).

IMPOTENCE

Some tonics for impotence are Formula 30 (pg. 136) yang tonic, Formula 30 (pg. 138), Wu Zi Wan and Chyavanprash. Ashwangandha *(Withania somnifera)* is a specific for this condition as well as for most aging symptoms.

INFECTIONS

Fasting or a very light diet is indicated in treating infections. Herbs are applied to the infection site in the form of a poultice, as well as taken internally. Echinacea is probably the single most effective herb for purulent infections, blood poisoning and gangrene. If the infection is severe, it may be taken frequently, initially every half hour, then less often as symptoms improve. Professional guidance is desirable when treating acute infectious conditions.

INFERTILITY

This condition has several possible causes, but usually tonification therapy is indicated, using one or two of the following: Formula 6 (pg. 121), Formula 20 (pg. 129), Formula 30 (pg. 136), Eight Precious Herbs, Chyavanprash, and Szu Wu Tang. The herbs Suma and Damiana also may be helpful.

INFLUENZA

Follow the dietary instructions for colds and fevers. Antibiotic and antiviral herbs are indicated. During the early stages fresh ginger or garlic tea stimulates vitality. A good basic antibiotic tea may be made from a combination of honeysuckle flowers, chrysanthemum flowers, forsythia flowers, echinacea and a small amount of licorice. Echinacea alone may be taken every hour or two.

If influenza continues for more than a week or two, it may have become a mixed hot and cold, excess and deficient, internal and external condition. In such a case, Minor Bupleurum combination should be used.

Some helpful formulas are Formula 15 (pg. 126), Pueraria combination, Echinacea and Minor Bupleurum.

LEUCORRHEA
(Vaginal discharge)

This condition usually is caused by either a mucus-forming diet or general weakness and debility. A toning up of the female reproductive system and a stimulation of blood circulation through the area may be effected by emmenagogue herbs, such as motherwort, dong quai, angelica, pennyroyal and juniper berries. Both Formula 6 (pg. 121) and Formula 12 (pg. 125), taken with a tea of raspberry leaf or squaw vine are very helpful.

A simple vaginal bolus may be made by wrapping a peeled clove of garlic in thin muslin or gauze. Twist the material around the garlic, leaving a tail for removal, dip the bolus in vegetable oil, and insert into the vagina once daily. Also therapeutic is a daily douche of warm water to which has been added a tablespoonful of yogurt or apple cider vinegar as a source of lactic acid. This is a good treatment for trichomonas as well as other common vaginal infections. Since many of these diseases are sexually transmitted, abstinence during the time of treatment is important. The male partner also should take blood purifying herbs, such as Formula 12 (pg. 125), Formula 14 (pg. 126) and Formula 15 (pg. 126). One reportedly effective treatment for trichomonas infection is usnea, usually taken in the form of an alcoholic tincture every two hours for a week or two.

MENSTRUAL IRREGULARITIES

For acute menstrual cramps, steep in a pint of boiling water one handful of chamomile flowers and six slices of raw ginger. The universal remedy for regulating menstruation is dong quai. The North American black haw (*Viburnum prunifolium*) and cramp bark (*Viburnum opulis*) are extremely reliable in alleviating cramps, especially when combined with dong quai or false unicorn (*Helonias*). Another herb frequently used for this purpose is wild yam root (*Dioscorea villosa*).

In Europe, chaste berries (*Agnus castus*) are highly regarded for all menstrual problems, especially those associated with premenstrual syndrome. These may be combined to good effect with cramp bark, false unicorn and dong quai.

A simple tea made of raspberry leaves or squaw vine for delayed periods or excessive menstrual bleeding. For excessive bleeding, one also may use a tincture of fresh shepherd's purse.

It is generally a good practice to take a blood tonic such as dong quai regularly at intervals throughout the month and especially the week before the period is due.

Some helpful formulas include: Formula 6 (pg. 121), Formula 7 (pg. 123), one or both possibly taken with Formula 12.

OVERWEIGHT AND OBESITY

This condition may be caused by any of the following: lack of exer-

cise, day sleeping, overeating of rich, sweet foods, poor digestion, heredi-
tary disorders

Overeating brings about a lack of the vital enzymes necessary for
the digestion of fat. The accumulation of fat then produces a chronic
condition of stagnation and toxicity, that is potentially the underlying
cause of serious diseases.

An overweight condition may result from the digestive fire's being
damaged by a diet of cold, raw foods, or prolonged fasting. This results
in a deficiency of spleen yang (digestive strength) which requires tonification of the spleen, most effectively with a daily dose of astragalus perhaps taken along with a cooling diuretic such as cleavers. Fennel seed
also may be added or taken separately. It will stimulate digestive
enzymes to help digest and prevent fat.

Some helpful formulas are: Formula 11 (pg. 124) and the diuretic,
Formula 2 (pg. 120).

PILES OR HEMORRHOIDS

This condition usually is caused by a poor diet and a sedentary
lifestyle. Suppositories to ease the discomfort may be made by combining in a base of coconut oil to a pie dough consistency various powdered
astringent herbs, such as yarrow, bayberry, oak bark, comfrey root, a
pinch of cayenne pepper and golden seal. This is then rolled into a suppository the width of the middle finger and about an inch and a half
long. Insert each evening before retiring. (Take precautions against leakage on pajamas or bedclothes.)

Liver- and colon-discharging herbs, such as Oregon grape, barberry
and boldo are indicated. Formula 12 (pg. 125), Triphala and guggul are
very useful as root treatments for this condition.

PROSTATE PROBLEMS

During acute phases, heavy, rich foods should be avoided, including
sweets, alcohol, fatty meats and dairy foods. These tend to cause congestion and will aggravate most prostate problems. The basic herbal combination for most prostate problems combines echinacea root and saw

palmetto berries. Tonic diuretic teas such as gravel root or parsley root also may be taken. Formula 4 (pg. 120) combines these herbs with others that are good for this condition.

SKIN DISEASES

There are many causes of skin eruptions but blood toxicity is the most common one. Sassafras tea is excellent for most kinds of skin eruptions, including acne. Planetary Bitters tea helps chronic skin problems. It is composed of equal parts of sassafras, sarsaparilla, dandelion root, burdock root, yellow dock, licorice, red clover, buckthorn, American ginseng, pokeroot, Oregon grape or barberry and echinacea. This is an authentic root beer and can be quite pleasant if the tastier herbs, such as sassafras, sarsaparilla and licorice, are accentuated.

See Formula 15 (pg. 126).

STRESS AND INSOMNIA

Many herbs are effective for these conditions. The nervines and antispasmodics are most commonly used. These include scullcap, valerian, lady's slipper, passion flower, black cohosh and hops. For stronger sedative action, choose herbs from the category of *pacify spirit*. These are heavy mineral substances many of which contain calcium carbonate from powdered oyster shell, or from the ossified bones of prehistoric mammals, "dragon bones". For stress, a simple tincture of hops, valerian, scullcap and, if available, lady's slipper, is effective when taken regularly three times a day. The addition of the mineral calcium to these herbs will make the combination even more effective. See Formula 8 (pg. 123).

A tea of passion flower taken in the evening induces a sound restful sleep. Mix it with boiled warm milk and honey for a deeper more nutritive action.

Be aware of the necessity to detoxify the liver and the colon if there is constipation. If these organs are congested, they profoundly upset the personality and spirit, and the gentle sedative herbs may not then work as effectively.

URINARY INFECTIONS

Bladder infections are treated with teas of watermelon seeds, cornsilk, parsley, uva ursi or cleavers. Unsweetened cranberry juice, which helps alkalinize the urine, making it unfavorable for the proliferation of bacteria, is another well-known treatment for such infections. All sweets, rich foods, alcohol and fruits must be avoided. Diuretic, Formula 2 (pg. 120) is very effective for these conditions and may be taken often throughout the day initially, and with diminishing frequency as symptoms abate. If kidney or bladder stones are present, it may be taken with Formula 3 (pg. 120).

PLANETARY FORMULAS
Their Energetic Conformation, Indications and Counter-indications

UPPER RESPIRATORY
(Lungs, Bronchioles and Sinuses)

Formula 1: warm and clear the lung, tonify spleen

Ma huang (chief herb)
Platycodon (chief herb)
Comfrey root (assisting herb)
Mullein (assisting herb)
Wild cherry bark (assisting herb)
Licorice (assisting herb)

Elecampane (supporting herb)
Ginger (conducting herb)
Cinnamon twigs (conducting herb)
Wild ginger root (conducting herb)

This formula is dispersing, decongesting; good for colds, flu, allergies, asthma and upper respiratory problems. It is excellent to help offset the harmful effects of smoking on the lungs. It has a neutral-to-warm energy.

Dosage: Take two or more tablets, three or more times daily with warm water.

URINARY PROBLEMS

Formula 2: Eliminate internal dampness and relieve heat from the urinary tract

Cleavers (chief herb)   Parsley root (assisting)
Uva ursi (chief herb)   Dandelion root (supporting)
Poria (chief herb)   Ginger root (conducting)
Marshmallow (assisting)

This formula is dispersing, diuretic, harmonizes fluid metabolism; overcomes thirst, swelling, cystitis, and kidney weakness. It has a cool-to-neutral energy.

Dosage: For general fluid balance and elimination take two or more tablets three times daily with warm water. For urinary inflammation take two tablets every two hours with two echinacea tablets.

GALLSTONES AND URINARY STONES

Formula 3: clear gall bladder and urinary heat and eliminate stones

Turmeric root (chief herb)   Licorice (assisting)
Gravel root (chief herb)   Dandelion root (supporting)
Parsley root (chief herb)   Ginger root (conducting)
Marshmallow root (assisting)

This formula has a cool energy and is pain-relieving, dispersing, detoxifying and diuretic for both kidney and bladder stones. Since it helps to regulate blood sugar, it can also treat diabetes.

Dosage: Take two tablets three times daily; for acute conditions take two tablets every two hours and less often as the symptoms subside. Not recommended for pregnant women.

PROSTATE

Formula 4: clear heat, remove dampness and tonify the prostate

Saw palmetto (chief herb)   True Unicorn root (assisting)
Echinacea root (assisting)   Uva ursi (assisting)
Goldenseal (assisting)   Marshmallow root (supporting)
Gravel root (assisting)   Cayenne (conducting)

This formula has a mild-to-neutral energy. It is detoxifying and dispersing, treats prostate problems, promotes the reproductive cycle and strengthens male potency.

Dosage: As a tonic, take two tablets three times daily. For acute conditions take every two hours and less often as symptoms subside.

FOR CHILDREN

Formula 5: calm and stimulate mental and physical development

Chamomile (chief herb)
Catnip (chief herb)
Lemon balm (chief herb)
Semen Zizyphus (chief herb)
Dragon bone (chief herb)
Gotu kola (assisting)
Calcium phos 6x (assisting)
Kali phos 6x (assisting)
Mag phos 6x (assisting)
Hawthorn berries (supporting)
Licorice (supporting)
Stevia (supporting)
Pippli long pepper (conducting)

This formula has a cool energy. It is a soothing, calming, gentle and nourishing nerve tonic. It is recommended for hyper-active children and teething infants. It also assists normal growth and development.

Dosage: Take one or two tablets three times daily or as needed. It may be taken crushed and mixed with honey or maple syrup.

GYNECOLOGY

Formula 6: tonify blood and yin, regulate chi

Dong quai (chief herb)
Lovage (chief herb)
False unicorn (chief herb)
Rehmannia, cooked (chief herb)
Cramp bark (assisting)
Paeonia alba (assisting
    and conducting)
Atractylodes (assisting)
Blue cohosh (assisting)
Moutan (supporting)
Poria (supporting)
Ginger (conducting)

A blood tonic for women, this formula moves blood, regulates the menstrual cycle for deficient blood, and increases estrogen. It has a warm nature and is good for all menstrual disorders: amenorrhea, menorrhagia, and dysmenorrhea. Specifically it is a tonifying pre-ovulation formula, while Formula 7 with chaste tree berries should be used for post-ovulation.

Since the liver is responsible for most gynecological imbalances, Formula 12 may be taken with Formula 6. If there is fluid accumulation, Formula 2 also will be very helpful. Generally, such an herbal program should be followed for a minimum of three months to achieve lasting results.

Dosage: As a tonic, take two tablets three times daily. For acute conditions, take two tablets every two hours with warm water. This formula generally is not recommended for pregnant women.

Formula 7: tonify blood and regulate chi

Chaste tree berries (chief herb)   Cyperus (supporting)
Squaw vine (chief herb)   Poria (supporting)
Dong quai (assisting)   Ginger root (conducting)
Crampbark (assisting)

This formula alleviates menstrual problems and helps to regulate the female hormones. Chaste tree regulates progesterone, helps regulate and smooth liver chi, regulates chi, calms the mind, increases B12, adds calcium, is a diuretic, clears the liver and neutralizes excess hormones. It has a cooling energy and also helps with cramps, premenstrual syndrome, moodiness and anxiety. For difficult, chronic menstrual problems, take this formula after ovulation and until menstruation, and Formula 6 after menstruation until ovulation.

Dosage: As a tonic, take two tablets three times daily as needed. For acute conditions, take more (see above). Usually not recommended for pregnant women.

STRESS AND NERVOUS TENSION

Formula 8: calm wind (nervousness), sedate and settle spirit

Valerian (chief herb)
Dragon bone (chief herb)
Oyster shell (chief herb)
Semen Zizyphus (chief herb)
Scullcap (chief herb)
Wood betony (chief herb)
Black cohosh (assisting)

Chamomile (assisting)
Hops (assisting)
Mistletoe (European) (assisting)
Hawthorn berries (supporting)
Licorice (supporting)
American ginseng (supporting)
Ginger (conducting)

This formula has a mild, neutral and soothing energy and is tonic to the nerves. It relieves insomnia, nervous tension, excessive irritability, anxiety and poor concentration.

Dosage: As a tonic, take two tablets three times daily. For acute conditions, take two tablets every two hours. Not recommended for pregnant women.

Formula 9: relieve head wind and blood stagnation

Feverfew (chief herb)
Semen Viticis (chief herb)
Notopterygium root (chief herb)
Ligusticum (chief herb)
Angelica (chief herb)

Sileris (assisting)
Cyperus (assisting)
Licorice (supporting)
Schizonepeta (conducting)
Tea (conducting)

This formula relieves nervousness, headache, colds and flu. It has a warm energy.

Dosage: Take one or two tablets with boiled warm water every two hours or as needed. Contraindicated for pregnant women.

HEART AND MIND

Formula 10: relieve heart blood circulation, tonify chi and calm spirit

Hawthorn berries (chief herb)
Salvia milthiorrhiza
  (chief and conducting)
Dong quai (assisting)
Tienchi ginseng
  (assisting and conducting)
Motherwort (assisting and conducting)

Polygala (assisting and
  conducting)
Borage (supporting)
Juniper berries (supporting)
Codonopsis (supporting)
Longan berries (supporting)

Acting on the heart and spirit, this formula calms the mind from excessive thoughts, nourishes blood and yin, and assists circulation. It has a warm circulating energy and is useful for arteriosclerosis, restlessness, low energy, palpitations, heart pains and most other heart problems.

Dosage: As a tonic, take two tablets three times daily. For acute conditions, take more as needed. Not recommended for pregnant women.

WEIGHT CONTROL

Formula 11: reduce and remove excess heat and damp, calm spirit and tonify the stomach-spleen

Triphala (chief herb)
Spirulina (chief herb)
Kelp (chief herb)
Cleavers (chief herb)
Astragalus (chief herb)
Cascara (assisting)
Chaparral (assisting)
Echinacea (assisting)
Gambir (assisting)
Rhubarb (assisting)

Watercress (assisting)
Atractylodes (assisting)
Stephania (assisting)
Ma huang (assisting)
Semen Zizyphus (assisting)
Mustard seed (assisting)
Licorice (supporting)
Fennel (conducting)
Ginger (conducting)

This formula gently opens the channels of elimination and assists in a balanced detoxification. It aids assimilation and, therefore, in satisfying hunger. It has a slightly cool, dispersing energy and is good for general detoxification and weight reduction.

Dosage: two to four tablets three times daily. It is excellent taken with a diet of warm soy milk for weight reduction or a tea of cleavers and fennel seed.

LIVER

Formula 12: remove liver stagnation, smooth and regulate chi, tonify liver yin

Bupleurum (chief, assisting
    and conducting
Milk thistle seeds
    (chief and assisting
Dandelion root (chief herb)
Oregon grape root (chief herb)

Angelica (assisting)
Lycii berries (supporting)
Cyperus (conducting)
Fennel seed (conducting)
Ginger (conducting)

A relatively balanced energy, this formula regulates liver metabolism and dredges and detoxifies the liver while supporting liver yin (blood). It is useful for hepatitis, chest pains, colitis due to liver irregularities, constipation, cirrhoses, gynecology, and general blood detoxification. Unlike many other cholagogues, it also helps tonify liver blood, making it especially good for deficient conditions with blood and yin deficiency.

Dosage: two tablets three times daily with warm water.

Formula 13: liver chi regulation, smooth the process of digestion, detoxification, and glycogenesis in the liver

Bupleurum (chief herb)
Cyperus root (chief herb)
Magnolia bark (chief herb)
Chaste tree berries
    (chief and assisting)
White peony root (assisting)
Bitter orange peel (assisting)
Lovage root (assisting)
Cramp bark (assisting)

Wild yam root (assisting)
Poria mushroom (assisting)
Atractylodes (assisting)
Dong quai (assisting)
Gastrodia root (assisting)
Pinellia root (assisting)
Licorice root (supporting)
Ginger root (conducting)

This formula regulates liver chi and relieves abdominal and chest pains caused by an impaired flow of vital energy and blood.

It is useful for relieving depression, stagnation, nervousness, premenstrual syndrome, uneasiness, chest pains, digestive upset, abdominal distention, bloat, belching, gas, indigestion, candida symptoms and constipation.

SKIN AND GENITAL HERPES

Formula 14: remove damp heat from the lower warmer

Echinacea (chief herb)   Poria (assisting)
Yellow dock (chief herb)   Wild yam root (supporting)
Gentian root (chief herb)   Marshmallow root (supporting)
Goldenseal (chief herb)   Myrrh gum (conducting)
Bupleurum (chief and assisting)

This formula has a cool energy and is detoxifying. It disperses damp heat from the lower warmer (the pelvic cavity), making it useful for acute and chronic venereal diseases including herpes, pelvic inflammatory disease, leucorrhea, gonorrhea, syphilis and general skin eruptions. It is good for blood purification and helping to resolve inflammation and pus.

Dosage: two to four tablets three times daily with warm water. While taking this formula, patients should be warned not to use any stimulants, including drugs, alcohol, coffee, sugar and acidic foods such as tomatoes and citrus.

BLOOD PURIFICATION, SKIN AND INFLAMMATORY CONDITIONS

Formula 15: clear heat

Echinacea root (chief herb)   Sarsaparilla root (chief herb)
Golden seal (chief herb)   Yellow dock root (chief herb)
Chaparral (chief herb)   American ginseng (supporting)
Honeysuckle flowers   Ginger root (conducting)
    (chief herb)   Cinnamon twigs (conducting)
Forsythia blossoms (chief herb)

This blood-purifying formula has a cool detoxifying energy. It is useful for inflammatory conditions, skin eruptions, fevers, toxicity of blood and lymph, boils, sores and cancer. It is effective for both bacterial and viral infections.

Dosage: Two to four tablets taken three times daily with warm water. For the treatment of flu, take four tablets with warm water two or three times a day. Follow a simple diet, avoiding heating, dispersing and denatured foods, drugs, stimulants, peppers, sugar (including fruit juices and fruits), alcohol and excess meat.

CHRONIC DEGENERATIVE DISEASES, TUMORS, CANCERS AND CYSTS

Formula 16:clear heat, remove dampness and soften and eliminate tumors

Pau d'arco (chief herb)
Echinacea root (chief herb)
Chaparral (chief herb)
Red Clover blossoms
   (chief herb)

Poria (assisting)
Grifola (assisting)
Kelp (assisting)
American ginseng (assisting)

Cool-natured and dispersing, this formula is a mild diuretic, helping to resolve tumors, cysts and lymphatic congestion. It is specifically useful for chronic degenerative diseases such as cancer, but good also for other chronic conditions. Used with Formula 17, it helps offset some of the negative side effects of chemotherapy and radiation therapy. This formula may be combined with good results with Formula 15.

Dosage: Two to four tablets three times daily with warm water or red clover tea.

IMMUNE SYSTEM

Formula 17: tonify wei (immune system), whi and yin and clear heat

Pau d'arco (chief herb)
Echinacea root (chief herb)
Astragalus (chief herb)
Suma (chief herb)
Siberian ginseng (chief herb)
Reishi mushroom (chief,
    assisting and supporting)

Schizandra berries (assisting)
Ligustrum fruit (assisting)
Chaparral (assisting)
Golden seal (assisting)
Garlic (assisting and
    conducting)

Tonifies both yin and yang as it clears deficient heat, protecting the righteous energy or the immune system. It is to be considered in the prevention and treatment of general weakness, colds, flu, candida albicans yeast overgrowth, cancer, AIDS, and immune-deficiency diseases generally.

Dosage: For prevention take two tablets once or twice daily. For treatment two tablets three times daily with warm water or mild licorice tea.

NATURAL ANTIBIOTIC, BLOOD AND LYMPHATIC CLEANSER

Formula 18: clear toxic heat and promote healing

Pure extraction of: *Echinacea Angustifolia, E. Palida* and *E. Purpurea.*

Cool and detoxifying, this formula counteracts inflammatory conditions of a solid or excess nature. It is useful only as an adjunctive for deficiency heat conditions. Echinacea tonifies the surface immune system, aiding the process of anti-body production. It may be used as an herbal antibiotic, alone or in combination with Formula 15.

Dosage: For acute conditions take two tablets at least every two hours and less frequently as symptoms subside. Continue to use three times daily for a week or two after all symptoms have disappeared. If there is no improvement within the first three days, the inflammation probably is due to a deficient condition. In such cases, also use a small amount of ginseng.

CIRCULATION AND WARMTH

Formula 19: warm and disperse

Ginger root (chief herb)   Bayberry bark (chief and assisting)
Cinnamon twigs (chief herb)   and assisting)
Cayenne (chief herb)   White pine bark (assisting)
Cloves (chief herb)   Marshmallow root (supporting)
                                   Licorice root (supporting)

This formula has a warm, dispersing and drying energy. It is similar to the well-known Composition Powder of early American herbal medical practice. It is a very useful herbal first aid remedy for treating the first stages of colds, flu, congestion, overeating, bloatedness, diarrhea and stagnant circulatory conditions. It may also be used for stimulating hot baths and foot-baths to treat the conditions above. Chiefly an acute remedy for occasional use, this formula is not recommended for chronic inflammatory conditions with deficient heat.

Dosage: Take three to four tablets with warm water or ginger and honey tea at the first sign of cold or flu. Repeat as needed.

GLANDULAR SYSTEM

Formula 20: balance hormones, tonify blood and yin and clear heat

American ginseng (chief herb)   Black cohosh (assisting)
Dong quai (chief herb)   Kelp (assisting)
Chaste tree berries (chief herb)   Golden seal (assisting)
Saw palmetto berries   Wild yam (assisting)
    (chief and assisting)   Licorice (supporting)
Sarsaparilla (assisting)   Ginger (conducting)

This formula has a neutral-to-warm energy, is a general glandular tonic, counteracts aging, preserves youthfulness, is good for pubescent children, helpful in cases of retarded growth and menopause, strengthens hormone function, tonifies both yin and yang, and counteracts impotency and frigidity.

Dosage: As a tonic take two to four tablets two or three times daily.

Formula 21: to aid fasting, neutralize acids and alleviate hunger

Dandelion root (chief herb)   Cleavers (assisting)
Violet leaves (chief herb   Fennel seed (conducting)
Black pepper (chief, assistant   Cardamon seed (conducting)
   and conducting)

Drink this formula during fasting to help alleviate hunger pangs, promote detoxification, neutralize stomach acids and help dissolve fat.

Dosage: Steep one to two teaspoons in a cup of boiled warm water. Honey may be added. Take as often as desired.

FOOD SUPPLEMENT
Formula 22: herbal food

Combine powders of roasted barley, soya protein, yeast, bee pollen, spirulina, astragalus, imperatae herb, wheat germ, psyllium seeds, chia seeds, flax seeds, kelp, rose hips, amla, suma and wheat grass concentrate.

This mixture may be eaten freely. It contains complete and balanced herbal protein, vitamins and minerals as naturally found in wholesome food. It can be used fasting, as an emergency food when traveling and simply as a whole herbal food supplement.

Dosage: Add warm water to two or more tablespoons of the Planetary Herb Food powder to the desired consistency.

BULK NUTRIENT LAXATIVE

Formula 23: lubricate dryness and promote bowel elimination

Equal parts: Psyllium, Flax and Chia seeds

Soak three or four tablespoonsful overnight in a cup of black cherry juice. Drink and eat it in three portions throughout the following day.

AYURVEDIC FORMULAS

Rasayanas

Rasayanas represent a special branch of Ayurvedic medicine which is concerned with the processes of rejuvenation and revitalization. There are a number of extremely valuable rasayanas, of which some of the most important—Triphala, Chyavanprash, Guggula and Shilajit—are described below.

MUCUS, ALLERGIES, DIGESTION

Formula 24: (Trikatu) warm and stimulate the internal and dry wet

Equal parts: Ginger root, Black pepper, Pippli long pepper and Honey

This formula has a hot, spicy energy and is dispersing and drying for damp conditions. It helps overcome mucus, making it useful in treating allergies and colds, helping to reduce fat, aiding digestion and circulation, warming internally. A specific remedy for clear damp discharges that often occur in cold, damp climates, it should be taken in winter by nearly everyone living in such environments and suspended during the warm summer months.

Dosage: One or two tablets three times a day. Patient should be advised to cut down on fluid intake.

Formula 25: (Hingashtak) regulate and tonify digestive chi

Atractylodes (chief herb)
Caraway seed (chief herb)
Cumin seed (chief herb)
Asafoetida (chief herb)
Black pepper (assisting and conducting)

Citrus peel (assisting and conducting)
Dandelion root (supporting)
Slippery elm (supporting)
Rock salt (supporting)
Ginger (conducting)

Having a warm energy, this formula regulates chi, aids digestion, counteracts acidity and digestive weakness, eliminates gas and bloating, and is one of the best formulas to use for hypoglycemia and the symptoms associated with candida albicans yeast overgrowth. It may be powdered and added to food to enhance digestion; or taken either before or after meals with warm water.

Formula 26: (Triphala) eliminate excess, clear heat and protect righteous energy

Equal parts: *Emblica officinalis, Terminalia belerica* and *Terminalia chebula*

Triphala ("tri" three; "phala" fruits), consists of the combination of the fruit of the chebulic, beleric and emblic myrobalan trees, respectively. These are popularly known in India as harad, behada and amla. Triphala is widely regarded as a laxative, but also is considered a rasayana or rejuvenator. Its special value, therefore, is both as a regulator of elimination and a revitalizer of the entire body.

Harada and behada have warm energy, while amla is cool. Triphala, therefore, is quite balanced, making it useful as an internal cleansing and detoxifying formula. It is recommended for everyone, including more sensitive individuals and vegetarians.

Regular, daily use of Triphala will promote normal appetite, good digestion, increase red blood cells and haemoglobin, and aid in the removal of undesirable fat. Triphala can also eliminate what is called *deficient heat* in Chinese medicine. This is a feeling of heat and burning in the chest, legs, palms and soles of the feet, which in Western medicine often indicates a B vitamin deficiency. Taken regularly triphala promotes the absorption and utilization of the B vitamins and will completely relieve the symptoms of deficient heat.

Of primary importance is the use of Triphala as a bowel regulator, for which it is considered to be as safe as food, and non-habit forming even when taken on a daily basis. There is a popular saying in India comparing the importance of Triphala to that of a mother.

Considering triphala's tonic, cleansing and blood purifing actions, it has one more important application, as a strengthener of the eyes. Triphala may be taken daily as an eyewash. It strengthens the vision, counteracts many eye defects, and eliminates redness and soreness.

Dosage: As a blood purifier, reducing and cleansing agent, take two tablets three times daily. As an occasional tonic laxative, take two to six tablets in the evening with a cup of boiled water. For eye problems, crush two tablets and steep in half a cup of boiling water, cool, strain and use as an eyewash.

Formula 27: (Chyavanprash) warm and tonify spleen and stomach chi

This is one of the most potent and delicious tonics known. In Ayurveda it is considered one of the best rasayanas, or preparations used for rejuvenation and longevity. "Chyavan" was the name of the great sage who first created this formula. The legend is that the daughter of a famous emperor was innocently playing blindfolded in the forest when she accidentally stumbled upon the famous saint in the practice of his austerities. Not knowing who it was or what she was doing, she innocently ran her fingers through his hair and garlanded him with flowers. Her father, the emperor, came upon her at that moment and requested the sage to marry his daughter, since it was the custom in India that a woman might touch only one man in all her life. The aged sage asked for some time in which to prepare for the marriage. During this time he created Chyavanprash and lived on it for two months in order to regain his youthful vitality and virility. He then married the young girl, secure in his ability to bestow on his partner conjugal bliss.

Chyavanprash is made only with selected and fresh Indian gooseberries, called amla or amlakis (Emblic myrobalans). These fruits are considered the major health-food herb throughout India. They are the highest known source of easily assimilable vitamin C. Of equal importance, the vitamin C in amla is bound up with certain harmless tannins which maintain the potency of the vitamin content even after the fruit is dried or subjected to heat. Normally, vitamin C is quickly dissipated under such conditions, but not so with amla.

Hundreds of fresh amla fruits go into the making of Chyavanprash. They are first cleaned, washed and tied in a cloth, and boiled in water slowly until reduced to one-sixth the original volume. The decoction is then strained and the seeds are removed and discarded. The remaining fruit is then fried in sesame oil and butter and reduced to a paste. This paste is combined with the strained decoction and further boiled and reduced with jaggury (crude brown sugar with molasses). At this point approximately 34 to 50 herbs, depending upon which variant of Chyavanprash is used, are added in powder form. When the preparation is well cooked, honey is added to complete the process of manufacture.

Chyavanprash is a tonic as celebrated throughout India as ginseng is among the Chinese. The ancient Sanskrit texts prescribe its regular use for weakness and debility of all kinds, including chronic bronchitis, allergies, immune weakness, feverishness, emaciation, chronic cardiac disorders, gout, disorders of the urinary tract, impotence and infertility. It is safely used for young infants, the very old, debilitated or very thin. Because of its great nutritive value, it increases longevity and mental alertness, and promotes a glowing complexion. It clarifies the urine and effects regularity of evacuation. Chyavanprash removes parasites and toxins and cures anorexia, indigestion and dyspepsia when taken over a prolonged period. Regular use of Chyavanprash strengthens sexual strength and vigor in a man. It also is a blood tonic for women.

Many varieties of commercial Chyavanprash are made with excess sugar or white sugar which diminishes its value. Besides amla, the herbs used in Chyavanprash have diuretic, carminative, mildly laxative and tonic properties. They improve circulation, counteract coughs, promote expectoration of phlegm, and tone up the entire system. Some varieties add musk for virility and saffron to stimulate circulation. Added iron, gold, amber, silver or other purified metallic oxides greatly augment its virtues.

Take half to one teaspoonful each morning followed by warm water, herb tea or warm milk to treat low blood sugar, anemia and dyspepsia, build up the tissues and cells of the body, and strengthen the heart, liver and kidneys and the sense organs. Chyavanprash, is truly the king of herbal food preparations.

Formula 28: (Guggula) clear channels, circulate chi and blood

Guggula is made from the resin of *Balsamodendron Mukul;* Sanskrit, guggullu; English, salai tree, gum gugal or Indian bedellium. It is very closely related to myrrh; many books consider the two interchangeable. When fresh, it is moist, viscid and fragrant, with a golden color. It melts in the sun and emulsifies in hot water.

Guggula is considered to be anti-kapha or -mucus and as such reduces fat. Since it also is oily, it alleviates disorders of the nervous system. Since it is mild in nature, it will aggravate pitta or fire after prolonged use. Most importantly, it is considered the most potent remedy against ama: an accumulation of cholesterol, thickened mucus and other materials associated with the aging process. Ama causes various circulatory problems, including arteriosclerosis, arthritis, rheumatism, heart problems, high blood pressure, obesity, enlargement of the prostate and other diseases of old age. Guggula is widely known and celebrated throughout India and, in various forms and combinations, recommended by Ayurvedic doctors for all diseases associated with bone, joint or nerve pain.

Guggula is often combined with Triphala to make Triphala guggula. This is taken morning and evening to counteract obesity, blood disorders, constipation, skin problems, chronic venereal disease, ascites and sores that are difficult to heal. All such diseases are associated with an accumulation of ama which gradually inhibits the natural rejuvenative processes.

Guggula is made according to a traditional method of wrapping the resin in a porous natural fiber cloth and boiling it in a decoction of Triphala to purify the resins so they can easily pass through the system without causing toxicity. The guggul decoction is then further cooked down to a thick paste and spread out on a pan or holder, to dry hard in the sun. This resulting material then can be broken into chunks or powdered for use.

Yogaraj guggula is the most well-known preparation of guggul in India. It is used for many disorders, including sciatica, rheumatism, gout, arthritis, amenorrhea, obesity, painful menses or arrested menstruation, hemorrhoids, worms, fistula and impotence. It is a rejuvenator and, by purifying the blood and promoting normal circulation, allays pain. It increases elimination of wastes through sweat, promotes normal secretion of digestive juices, regulates the bowels, and prevents and eliminates intestinal gases. It has a deep, lasting normalizing effect upon the female menstrual flow: where there is excess it will decrease it and where it is blocked, promote it. Finally, guggula is an excellent circulatory tonic for promoting flexibility, internal strength and stamina, making it very useful for athletes.

Dosage: about 250 to 500 mg. are taken twice daily.

Formula 29: (Shilajit) tonify kidney chi, yin and yang, and overcome wasting

This is the natural exudate of certain rocks and stones found in the Himalayas. It very much resembles and smells like asphalt, which is the English name for it. In its natural state, shilajit is eaten by rats and monkeys. In Ayurveda it is considered the urinary tonic par excellence. It is dark black in color and corresponds to those herbs considered kidney-adrenal tonics in Chinese medicine.

Shilajit is obtained by pulverising the black, greasy-looking stones and boiling them in water. After the boiling, a creamy film develops and this is removed and dried in the sun. To purify shilajit, and thus aid its assimilability, the stones are boiled in a decoction of Triphala.

Shilajit is naturally high in iron and other valuable minerals, making it very helpful for all wasting, degenerative diseases, especially diabetes, chronic urinary tract problems, impotence and infertility. It promotes strong bones and therefore is good for the healing of fractures, osteoarthritis and spondylosis. It is famous for its anti-diabetic properties, reducing blood sugar and countering diabetes in the early stages.

Shilajit usually is prepared as a paste, which is dissolved in a little boiled hot water or hot milk and taken twice daily.

CHINESE FORMULAS

Formula 30: (Tai Chi) to tonify chi, especially of spleen-pancreas and stomach

Panax ginseng (chief herb)   Atractylodes (assisting)
American ginseng (chief herb)   Poria mushroom (assisting)
Siberian ginseng (chief herb)   Fo-ti (supporting)
Codonopsis (chief herb)   Dong quai (supporting)
Tienchi ginseng (chief herb)   Licorice (supporting)
Astragalus (chief herb)

This formula tonifies spleen chi, yang and blood. It has a warm, strengthening energy. It is useful for low energy, fatigue, hypoglycemia, forgetfulness and lowered immune system. It builds stamina gradually over a long period of time.

Dosage: For extreme deficient conditions, simmer four tablets in three cups of water and add some meat, grains or root vegetables to make a soup. This may be taken two or three times daily by those with deficiency and coldness. It can be taken each morning as an herbal energy pill to help maintain energy and youthful vitality.

Formula 31: (Shujin chih) to counteract stiffness and increase flexibility

Dong quai (chief herb)
Ligusticum (chief herb)
Achryanthes (chief herb)
Dipsacus (chief herb)
Chaenomeles (chief herb)
Notoptyrygium (chief, assisting and conducting)

Angelica Tu huo (chief, assisting and conducting)
Gambir (supporting)
Sileris (assisting)
Tienchi ginseng (assisting and conducting)
Lycii berries (supporting)

A tonic for the kidneys and liver, this formula soothes muscles and tendons, increases general body flexibility, improves blood circulation, relieves aches and pains of arthritis, gout and rheumatism, pain of the lower back and legs, numbness and dyskinesia.

Dosage: May be taken either as a tablet or alcoholic-based extract (which is particularly useful for the elderly with circulatory problems). As a tincture, take 30 drops two or three times a day. Use two tablets two or three times a day.

Formula 32: tonifies yin

Rehmannia, cooked (chief herb)
Lycii berries (chief herb)
Chrysanthemum flowers (chief herb)
Polygonum multiflorum (chief herb)
Ligustrum lucidi (chief herb)

Saw Palmetto berries (chief herb)
Cornus berries (assisting)
Moutan peony (assisting)
Poria (assisting)
Alisma (assisting)
Dioscorea (supporting)

A yin tonic with a nourishing, neutral and cool energy, it tonifies kidney yin, strengthens weak kidney urinary function and is useful for the treatment of impotence, ringing in the ears, aching lower back and knees, night sweats, diabetes and involuntary emission. It is also good for night blindness, photophobia, vision weakness, hypertension and regenerating the liver. Supporting the cooling aspect of the adrenal hormones, it may be used for increasing feelings of love and compassion. It is a good tonic for those over the age of forty.

Dosage: Take two tablets two or three times a day with warm water, along with a little miso, tamari sauce or a pinch of salt.

Formula 33: tonifies yang

Ashwagandha (chief herb)
Cornus berries (chief herb)
Psoralea bean (chief herb)
Cuscutae seed (chief herb)
Cistanches (chief herb)
Morindae (chief herb)
Epimedium (chief herb)
Aconitum praeparata
   (chief herb)
Cinnamon bark (chief herb)
Moutan peony (assisting)

Schizandra berries (assisting
   and supporting)
Poria (assisting)
Alisma (assisting)
Rehmannia, cooked
   (supporting)
Dioscorea (supporting)
Saw palmetto berries
   (supporting)
Lycii berries (supporting)
Dong quai (supporting)

This formula, which has a very warm nature, tonifies kidney yang. It strengthens weak adrenal function and is useful in the treatment of general coldness, impotence, chronic nephritis, kidney atrophy, edema, difficult urination, chronic cystitis, diabetes, lower back pains, painful joints and cold, deficient constipation. It increases drive and motivation. This is another useful longevity tonic for those past the age of forty.

Dosage: Take two tablets two or three times a day with warm water and a little miso, tamari sauce or a pinch of salt.

Formula 34: (Pueraria Combination, Ko Ken Tang or Kudzu Root Tea) relieves surface cold, neck and shoulder stiffness

(Ko Ken Tang or Kudzu Root Tea)

Pueraria root (chief herb)	Jujube date (supporting)
Ma huang (assisting)	Licorice (supporting)
Cinnamon twigs (assisting)	Ginger (conducting)
Peony root (assisting)	

This warm-natured formula is helpful for all constitutional types in the treatment of colds, flu, pneumonia, bronchitis, upper shoulder and muscle tightness and soreness, coughs and gastrointestinal diseases.

Dosage: Simmer four cups of tea until it has reduced to two cups in volume. Drink two cups a day.

Formula 35: (Minor Bupleurum Combination or Hsiao Chai Hu Tang) harmonizes half chronic and half acute symptoms, half deficient and half excess

Bupleurum (chief herb)	Jujube date (supporting)
Skullcap root (assisting)	Licorice (supporting)
Pinellia (assisting)	Ginger (conducting)
Ginseng (assisting)	

This is a formula for treating prolonged symptoms of cold, flu, asthma, pneumonia, bronchitis, headaches, nasal congestion, shoulder stiffness, tuberculosis and pleurisy. It is also good for hypoglycemia and hepatitis, and for diseases that are both acute and chronic, weak and strong, internal and external, yin and yang. It is one of the most commonly indicated formulas and may be taken over a long period for promoting general health.

Dosage: Same as Pueraria Combination above.

CHINESE TONIC HERB FOODS

Chinese tonic herb foods provide a different and delicious way to take Chinese herbs. Finely-powdered herbs are specially heated and mixed with honey and ghee, which aid their assimilation into the cells and tissues of the body. Herbs are often taken in this way in China and India because individuals tending towards a yin-damp condition (common among vegetarians) are advised against taking too much fluid, including herb teas.

Formula 36: (Jade Screen or Yipingfeng San) tonifies wei (immune) chi

Astragalus (chief herb)   Sileris (assisting and conducting)
Atractylodes (assisting)

This is a Chinese herb food for tonifying the immune system and treating internal coldness. It energizes and warms all the internal vital organs and strengthens the defensive chi (wei chi). It is good for poor health with frequent colds and flus and perspiration from weakness. This delicious tonic is suitable for young and old and may be taken safely year-round on a regular basis. Most warm-natured tonics are not taken during active, acute, inflammatory conditions, unless specifically prescribed.

Dosage: One half to one teaspoon once or twice daily.

Formula 37: (Strong Blood or Si Wu Tang) tonifies blood

Dong quai (chief herb)   Rehmannia, cooked (chief herb)
Ligusticum wallichii   Peony alba (assisting and
  (chief, assisting and   conducting)
conducting)

This formula tonifies blood, counteracts anemia and regulates menstruation.

Dosage: One teaspoon two or three times daily.

Formula 38: (Four Nobles or Si Junza Tang) tonifies chi

Ginseng (chief herb)   Poria (assisting)
Codonopsis (chief herb)   Licorice (supporting)
Atractylodes (chief, assisting and conducting)

This strengthens the chi, aids digestion, tonifies the spleen chi, strengthens the spleen-pancreas and stomach, and counteracts weakness and fatigue.

CIRCULATION AND WARMTH

Formula 39: warm and disperse

Ginger root (chief herb)   Bayberry bark (chief
Astragalus (chief herb)   Zizyphus seeds (assisting)
Atractylodes (chief and assisting) Polygala root
Jujube dates (chief   Licorice root (supporting)
    and supporting)   Longan berries (supporting)

This tonifies chi, centers the mind, strengthens spleen chi, aids digestion, is calming, alleviates insomnia, palpitations, asthenia, weak heart, poor appetite.

Dosage: One teaspoon two or three times daily.

Formula 40: (Eight Precious Herbs or Bazhen Wan) tonifies blood and chi

Codonopsis (chief herb)   Poria (assisting)
Dong quai (chief herb)   Peony root (assisting
Rehmannia, cooked (chief herb)   and conducting)
Ligusticum (assisting)   Licorice (supporting)
Atractylodes (assisting)

This Chinese herb food is a tonic for blood and energy. This one may be taken as a general tonic or for specific conditions such as anorexia, anemia and weakness.

Dosage: One half to one teaspoon is eaten once or twice daily.

Formula 41: (Wu Zi Wan) tonic for kidney-adrenals

Semen plantago (chief herb)   Cornus berries (chief herb)
Rehmannia, cooked (chief herb)   Poria (assisting)
Semen cuscutae (chief herb)   Alisma (assisting)
Lycii berries (chief herb)   Raspberries (assisting)
Schizandra berries (chief herb)   Dioscorea (supporting)

This is a kidney-adrenal tonic good for both kidney yin and yang. It supports the adrenals, improving health and promoting longevity.

Among the conditions it is used for are urinary weakness, improving the hair and complexion, and counteracting impotence.

Dosage: Take one half to one teaspoon once or twice daily. For those over the age of forty, it is best taken with a tablespoon or so of rice wine once or twice daily.

Formula 42: to counteract excess yin and coldness

Cinnamon bark (chief and
    conducting)
Ginger (chief and conducting)
Licorice (supporting)

Aconitum praeparata (chief and
    conducting)
Atractylodes (assisting and
    supporting)

This raises body metabolism and promotes circulation and digestion as it warms the whole body. Being a hot-natured formula, it is good in the winter and for all yin conditions associated with coldness, clear allergic discharges, clear urine, loose stool, weak digestion, low energy, pallor and chronic bronchitis. It should not be given for excess yang-heat or wasting heat (yin deficient) conditions.

Dosage: Take one-eighth to one-quarter teaspoon one to three times daily.

Formula 43: (Bu Zhong Yin Chi Wan)

Ginseng (chief herb)
Astragalus (chief and assisting)
Atractylodes (chief
    and assisting)
Dong quai (assisting)

Black cohosh (assisting)
Bupleurum (assisting)
Citrus peel (assisting)
Licorice (supporting)

This is the formula for maximum tonification. It treats chronic weakness, tuberculosis, gastroptosis, anorexia, abdominal distention, loss of weight during the summer, neurasthenia, impotence, uterine prolapse, hemorrhoids, rectal prolapse, monoplegia, ephidrosis (abnormal amounts of sweating), hernia, chronic gonorrhea, diarrhea, malaria, suppuration and hemorrhage. The individual in need of this formula will have a weak pulse, with general fatigue, mild fever, night sweats, headache, weak digestion and palpitations at the umbilicus.

Dosage: One half to one teaspoon two or three times daily. As a milder tonic, one may take one-quarter to one half a teaspoon twice a day.

Formula 44: (Ginseng and Antler Combination)

Equal parts: American ginseng and Red deer antler

This is one of the most powerful energy tonics and is especially useful for chi and yang deficiencies in men and women of all ages. It raises body metabolism and treats symptoms of coldness, poor digestion, weakness, aging, arthritic and rheumatic complaints and poor memory. It is also good for weak and sickly children, infants who are not growing, and lack of physical stamina. It is excellent for male and female hormone deficiencies, lack of sexual libido, frigidity and impotence.

American ginseng is the cooler, more yin-tonic ginseng and therefore helps counteract the strong yang qualities of deer antler. It tonifies yin, blood and chi and will balance and complement the effects of the antler

PART TWO

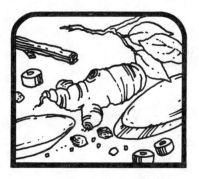

Planetary
Materia
Medica

SURFACE RELIEVING HERBS

Diaphoretics are primarily herbs that treat diseases and release toxins through promoting sweating and peripheral circulation. They repel invasions of pathogens through the surface of the body. Hence in Chinese medicine they are called *surface-relieving* agents.

Specifically these herbs have a dispersing and expelling function, making them useful for: treating superficial colds, flu, coughs and asthma; reducing swelling or edema by means of perspiration and urination; bringing out and quickly terminating measles and skin eruptions; relieving pain caused by energy and blood stagnation.

The Chinese term indicates the area of the body affected. Therefore, the herbs in this category also treat certain skin diseases, acute rheumatic pains and arthritis. These herbs are also said to be *wind relieving* meaning that they relieve the porous and muscular tension that locks the toxins under the skin.

The diaphoretics are divided into two categories, according to whether their energy is warming or cooling. Warming diaphoretics, or warming surface-relieving agents, are used to relieve *wind-chill* conditions characterized by mild fever with chills, lack of sweating, body aches, stiff neck, floating and tense pulse, thin white tongue coating and white phlegm. Cooling diaphoretics, or cooling surface-relieving herbs, are used to relieve *wind-heat* conditions characterized by high fever with chills and possibly sweating, thirst, headache, sore throat, floating and rapid pulse, thin yellow tongue coating and yellow phlegm.

According to Ayurveda, these herbs are largely antimucous and reduce *kapha*. The warming variety also reduces *vata* (wind), while the cooling types are more effective for reducing *pitta* (fire). Ayurveda categorizes the common cold and surface conditions as being largely of a *kapha* (water) nature, though wind *(vata)* is the carrier, but different types are discriminated according to which of the three humors predominates.

Those who are very weak and have signs of excessive physical wasting should avoid excess sweating. (See section on sweating therapy.)

WARMING DIAPHORETICS

(Spicy Warm Surface-Relieving Agents)

This category includes what are called "stimulating" diaphoretics in Western herbalism. They promote sweating by stimulating the surface capillary circulation and are useful for cold diseases. Chinese warm surface-relieving agents also possess stimulating properties, though of a dispersing nature. These herbs treat *wind-chill* conditions mentioned above including not only the common cold but also the initial and acute stages of asthma and arthritis. Herbs in this category are contraindicated in heat conditions, whether excess or deficient.

EPHEDRA   *Ephedra spp.; Ephedraceae*

Energetics: pungent, bitter, warm
Meridians: lung, bladder
Part used: above ground portion
Active constituents: ephedrine alkaloids.
Properties: diaphoretic, stimulant, diuretic, decongestant, antirheumatic, astringent
Uses: In treating colds, flu, lung problems, rheumatic complaints and water retention, this works similarly to ma huang but is less strong. There is a significant difference in stimulating properties between the Oriental ephedra, ma huang, and the American variety, which has little or no ephedrine alkaloids. The more stimulating Chinese ma huang contains plant forms of adrenelin, ephedrine and nor-epinephrine.
Precautions: It is contraindicated for yin deficient conditions or conditions of hypertension.
Dosage: For Chinese ma huang 2-6 grams in decoction; for Western ephedra, four to twelve grams.

ANGELICA   *Angelica archangelica; Umbelliferae*

Energetics: spicy, bitter, warm
Meridians: lung, stomach, intestines
Part used: the root
Active constituents: essential oil with phellandrene, angelica acid, cou-

marin compounds, bitter principle and tannins.

Properties: carminative, stimulant, emmenagogue, diaphoretic

Uses: This is used in treating colds and flu. It induces sweating, warms the body, promotes menses, and also is used for cold digestion. It is similar to the Chinese dong quai *(A. sinensis)* in its blood and chi moving properties, but has less of dong quai's blood building properties.

Dosage: standard infusion or 3-9 grams; tincture, 10-30 drops.

LOVAGE   *Ligusticum levisticum; Umbelliferae*

Energetics: spicy, warm

Meridians: lung, stomach, colon

Part used: root

Active constituents: essential oil with phthalidene, terpineol, carvacrol, isoveleric acid, coumarin, angelic acid, malic and benzoic acid, starch, resin and a sugar.

Properties: carminative, emmenagogue, diuretic, expectorant, stimulant, stomachic

Uses: This is used to treat fluid retention, bloating, gastric catarrh and flatulence; and also may be used to promote perspiration and counteract colds and flu.

Dosage: standard infusion or 3-9 grams; tincture, 10-30 drops.

SCALLIONS   *Allium fistulosum; Liliaceae*

Energetics: acrid, warm

Meridians: lung, stomach

Part used: bulbs

Active constituents: volatile oil consisting mainly of diallyl sulfide.

Properties: diaphoretic, digestant, stimulant

Uses: Use two to five scallions chopped (both the white bulb and greens) and steeped in a cup of boiling water. Add honey and drink freely. Garlic may be similarly used, but because of its strong odor many people prefer to use scallions. This should be taken at the first signs of chills and fevers and to relieve abdominal pain and distention.

Dosage: 2-8 stalks in infusion in a cup or two of water.

MAGNOLIA BLOSSOMS

Magnolia lilifora;
Magnoliaceae

Energetics: acrid, slightly warm
Meridians: lung
Part used: unopened flower buds
Active constituents: essential oil which includes citral, safrole, anethole, estragole, cineol, eugenol.
Properties: diaphoretic, stimulant, decongestant and analgesic
Uses: This treats blocked wind passages, nasal congestion and sinus headache.
Dosage: steep 3-9 grams in a cup and a half of boiling water covered. Combining this with ginger, pueraria, cinnamon and licorice may make it more effective.

HYSSOP

Hyssopus officinalis; Labiatae

Energetics: acrid, warm
Meridians: lung, stomach, colon, bladder
Part used: above ground portion
Active constituents: volatile oil, tannin and a glycoside (diosmine).
Properties: stimulant, carminative, astringent, diaphoretic, expectorant, stomachic
Uses: Hyssop treats sore throat, cold, flu, lung congestion, mucous congestion, gas, dropsy and bruises. Sage may be used in the same way. They are useful as a gargle for sore throat and may be taken as a tea for asthma and chronic bronchitis, which their expectorant properties relieve. Externally, hyssop is very useful for resolving bruises and injuries and promoting the healing of wounds.
Dosage: standard infusion or 3-9 grams; tincture, 10-30 drops.

SAGE

Salvia officinalis; Labiatae

Energetics: spicy, astringent, warm
Meridians: lungs, stomach
Parts used: leaves
Active constituents: essential oil including 30% thujone, 15% cineol, camphor, bitter principle and tannin.

Properties: diaphoretic, carminative, stimulant, antispasmodic, antidiarrheic, promotes estrogen, antigalactagogue.
Uses: Sage is effective against colds, flu and fevers, and as a muscle relaxant for nervous disorders. It also is used to inhibit perspiration. It may be taken as a gargle for sore throats and used as a tea for conditions of gas and indigestion. In my experience, it also is very effective for the treatment of cystitis.
Dosage: standard infusion or 3-9 grams; tincture, 10-30 drops.

OREGANO
and
MARJORAM

Origanum vulgare; Labiatae

Origanum marjorana or Marjoran hortensis; Labiatae

Energetics: Spicy, warm
Meridians: lung, stomach
Part used: aerial portions
Active constituents: essential oil, terpenes (terpinene, terpineol and borneol) and tannins.
Properties: diaphoretic, carminative, expectorant, aromatic and digestive.
Uses: Oregano may be used, like many of the other mint family plants, to promote perspiration and thus treat colds, flu and fevers. It is a familiar condiment, which indicates its effectiveness against digestive disturbances such as indigestion and gas. A tea of oregano, or its near relative marjoram, is excellent to bring on menses and relieve associated discomfort. They also may be used in baths and inhalations to clear the lungs and bronchial passages.
Dosage: standard infusion or 3-9 grams; tincture, 10-30 drops.

SAVORY

Satureja hortensis; Labiatae

Energetics: spicy, slightly bitter, warm
Meridians: lungs, stomach, liver
Parts used: aerial portions
Active constituents: essential oil including 30% carvacrol and 20% cymol.

Properties: diaphoretic, carminative, stimulant, emmenagogue, antispasmodic, astringent.

Uses: The uses of savory are similar to those of oregano and marjoram

BASIL   *Ocimum basilicum; Labiatae*

Energetics: spicy, warm
Meridians: lungs, stomach
Parts used: aerial portions
Active constituents: essential oil, estragol with linalon, lineol and camphor.
Properties: Diaphoretic, antipyretic, antispasmodic, carminative, antispasmodic, stomachic, galactagogue.
Uses: This treats fevers, colds, flu, stomach cramps, vomiting, indigestion, intestinal catarrh, constipation, enteritis, whooping cough, headaches and menstrual pains.
Dosage: standard infusion or 3-9 grams; tincture, 10-30 drops.

YERBA BUENA   *Satureja douglasi; Labiatae*

Energetics: Spicy, warm
Meridians: lungs, stomach, bladder
Parts Used: aerial portion
Active constituents: essential oils and other constituents not identified.
Properties: diaphoretic, aromatic, carminative, diuretic
Uses: It is used against colds, flu, fevers, indigestion and gas. This herb gave San Francisco its original name, which later was changed.
Dosage: standard infusion or 3-9 grams; tincture, 10-30 drops.

COSTMARY   *Chrysanthemum balsamita; Compositae*

Energetics: spicy, warm
Meridians: stomach, lungs
Part Used: leaves
Active constituents: essential oils and other constituents not identified.
Properties: diaphoretic, carminative, aromatic

Uses: This is used to treat colds, flu, fevers, indigestion and gas.
Dosage: standard infusion or 3-9 grams; tincture, 10-30 drops.

OSHA   *Ligusticum porteri; Umbelliferae*

Energetics: Spicy, bitter, warm
Meridians: lungs, stomach
Part used: root
Active constituents: Osha contains several substances some of which
are only partially water soluble. A Chinese variety is used for improving blood circulation, lowering blood pressure, promoting menses, and
slowing postpartal bleeding. It contains volatile and fixed oils, an alkaloid (C27 H37 N3), a lactone glycoside, saponins, phytosterols, and
ferulic acid.
Properties: diaphoretic, stimulant, carminative, expectorant,
emmenagogue
Uses: It is used to treat colds, flu, fevers, cough, cold phlegm diseases,
indigestion, gas, delayed menses and rheumatic complaints. This is one
of the most important herbs of the Rocky Mountains, considered
sacred by the Native Americans and widely esteemed by them for its
broad and effective warm healing power. Many tribes burned it as
incense for purification, to ward off gross pathogenic factors and subtle
negative influences. The energy of this North American herb is immediately apparent from its strong odor, which illustrates superiority of
fresh North American herbs over many of the older and weaker Chinese Ligusticums that are exported for use.
Dosage: standard infusion or 3-9 grams; tincture, 10-30 drops.

GINGER (fresh)   *Zingiberis officinalis; Zingiberaceae*

Energetics: spicy, warm
Meridians: lung, stomach
Part used: rhizomes
Active constituents: essential oil containing terpenes (cineol, philan-
drene, citra and borneol), its acrid, burning taste is due to the phenols
(gingerol, shogaol, zingerone).
Properties: diaphoretic, carminative, stimulant, antiemetic, antispasmodic

Uses: A tea of a few slices of the fresh root is an excellent one-herb remedy to counteract the early stages of a simple cold or flu. It also relieves indigestion, nausea, vomiting and gas. It is one of the most versatile herbs. Taken alone or with chamomile flowers, it is an excellent remedy for regulating the menses. Taken throughout the winter both as a tea and as a condiment with food, it warms up the circulation. Grated ginger can be topically applied externally, as a poultice or hot fomentation to relieve painful aches, sprains and spasms.

Dosage: 2-6 thin slices of the fresh root steeped in a cup of boiling water.

HEDGE NETTLE   *Stachys palustris; Labiatae*

Energetics: spicy, warm
Meridians: lungs, stomach
Part used: leaves
Active constituents: essential oil but otherwise not identified.
Properties: diaphoretic, antispasmodic, expectorant, vulnerary, emmenagogue, mild emetic in large doses (rising energy).
Uses: This is one of the most effective of the sweating herbs, useful in the early stages of colds, flu, and fevers. This is very common and powerful healing herb that deserves more recognition than it gets.
Dosage: ½ ounce steeped in a pint of boiling water or 3-9 grams in infusion.

SASSAFRAS   *Sassafras albidum; Lauraceae*

Energetics: spicy, warm
Meridians: lungs, kidney
Part used: root bark
Active constituents: essential oil with safrol, resin and tannin.
Properties: diaphoretic, diuretic, alterative
Uses: It is effective against skin diseases, acne, arthritic and rheumatic pains, ulcers, colds and flu. Sassafras is an excellent warming diuretic which makes it good for most arthritic conditions.
Dosage: standard infusion or 3-9 grams; tincture, 10-30 drops.

CINNAMON BRANCH

Cinnamon cassia;
Lauraceae

Energetics: pungent, sweet, warm
Meridians: bladder, lung, heart
Part used: the cut twigs and branches
Active constituents: essential oil, eugenol, phellandrene, orthomethyl-coumaric aldehyde, cinnamyl acetate, phenylpropyl alcohol, cinnamic alcohol, and traces of coumarin.
Properties: diaphoretic, aromatic, stimulant, astringent, stomachic
Uses: As a diaphoretic only this Chinese variety is indicated, and specifically the twigs or ramulus. The bark proper is classified as an internal warming stimulant; the more superficial parts of the tree are more suited for treating the more superficial and external diseases. (Its warming properties are similar to that of the North American sassafras, but they should not be used interchangeable.) It is specifically useful for warming the surface, provoking perspiration, treating colds, flu and fevers as well as arthritic and rheumatic complaints. It is also good for any stagnation of chi or blood.
Dosage: standard infusion or 3-9 grams.

COOLING DIAPHORETIC HERBS

(Spicy Cool Surface-Relieving Agents)

This category is similar to the 'relaxing diaphoretics' of Western herbalism. Herbs in this category mildly stimulate the surface capillary circulation, but primarily dilate the pores of the skin to promote perspiration and general relaxation and calmness of surface tension. Cooling diaphoretics are better for dispelling toxins (heat) through sweat, while the warming kinds are better at promoting circulation.

The indications in Chinese medical theory for cooling diaphoretics include symptoms of wind-heat described under the general diaphoretic heading. Wind-heat diseases include colds, flus, rashes, measles, conjunctivitis and other infectious diseases. Many of the herbs in this category help detoxify the liver and treat inflammatory conditions of the eyes. In terms of Western herbalism they often possess alterative and diuretic, as well as diaphoretic properties.

They are contraindicated for individuals with an extremely low metabolism, complaining of coldness when no fever is present; and for individuals whose superficial symptoms of cold, flu or fever have progressed beyond the first stages.

HORSEMINT   *Monarda Punctata; Labiatae*

Energetics: spicy, bitter, cool
Meridians/Organs affected: lungs, liver
Part used: leaves
Active constituents: volatile oil, menthol, menthone, d-iperitone, lemonene, hexenolphenylacetate, ethylamyulacarbinol, neomenthol
Properties: diaphoretic, aromatic, stomachic, calmative, mild alterative
Uses: Horsemint treats colds, flu and fevers.

Mentha arvensis, known in the Midwestern United States as 'poleo', seems to be nearly identical to the variety used by the Chinese.
Dosage: standard infusion or ½-6 gms.

PEPPERMINT   *Mentha piperita; Labiatae*

Energetics: spicy, bitter, slightly cool
Meridians/Organs affected: lungs, liver
Part used: leaves
Active constituents: essential oil, mentol menthone, fasmone, tannic (labiatic acid), bitter principle
Properties: diaphoretic, aromatic, carminative, calmative, mild alterative
Uses: Peppermint is used for colds, flu, fevers, gas and mild digestive disorders.

Spearmint *(Mentha virides)* has almost identical uses to this variety. Spearmint is classified as warm by the Chinese, but these mild mints are effectively neutral and would better fit into this category than the previous one.
Dosage: standard infusion or ½-6 gms.

CATNIP   *Nepeta cataria; Labiatae*

Energetics: Spicy, bitter, cool
Meridians/Organs affected: lungs, liver
Part used: leaves
Active constituents: essential oil comprised of cavracol, nepetol, thymol and nepetalactone.
Properties: diaphoretic, antispasmodic, carminative, emmenagogue, stomachic
Uses: This is effective against colds, flu, fevers, upset stomach, hysteria, insomnia and flatulence. It is very similar to mint, but has more relaxing properties. Although catnip is classified as warm by the Chinese, because of its calming and relaxing properties it is included in this category.
Dosage: standard infusion or ½-6 gms.

LEMON BALM   *Melissa officinalis; Labiatae*

Energetics: sour, spicy cool
Meridians/Organs affected: lungs, liver
Part used: leaves
Active constituents: essential oil with citral, citronellal, geraniol and linalool, bitter principle, acids and tannin (Labiatic acid).
Properties: diaphoretic, calmative, antispasmodic, sedative, carminative, emmenagogue, stomachic
Uses: Lemon balm treats fevers, nervousness, hysteria, insomnia, melancholy, depression, cramps, flatulence, colic and chronic bronchial catarrh. It is one of the best herbs for treating most simple, acute children's diseases; not only because of its excellent properties but also because of its pleasant flavor. Otherwise, its properties are similar to those of catnip. Beginning alchemical students practice making their spagyric tinctures with lemon balm.
Dosage: standard infusion or ½-6 gms.

BURDOCK SEED   *Arctium lappa; Compositae*

Energetics: bitter, sweet, cold
Meridians/Organs affected: lungs, stomach, liver, kidneys

Part used: seed
Active constituents: arctiin, arctigenin, gogosterin, essential oil, fatty oil.
Properties: diaphoretic, diuretic, antipyretic, expectorant, antiphlogistic
Uses: Burdock seed is used in treating throat infections, pneumonia, scarlet fever, measles, smallpox, eczema, psoriasis and syphilis. Western herbalists know it as a treatment for eruptive skin diseases and itching skin from other causes. The Chinese discovered that it was excellent for the treatment of colds and flu.
Dosage: standard infusion or 3-9 gms.

ELDER FLOWERS   *Sambucus nigra; Caprifoliaceae*

Energetics: acrid, bitter, cool energy
Meridians/Organs affected: lungs, liver
Parts Used: flowers
Active constituents: flowers contain an essential oil, with terpenes, glycosides, rutin and quercitrin, mucilage and tannin. The fruits are high in vitamin C. The root has an uninvestigated bitter principle and saponins.
Properties: diaphoretic, alterative, detoxicant, anti-inflammatory
Uses: For colds, flu, fevers and clearing the skin. It is used both internally and externally. Elder flowers, mixed with equal parts of mint and yarrow blossoms, are excellent internal cleansers for detoxification of flu and colds. A tea of the flowers combined with an equal part of sassafras is a good remedy for clearing the skin of such blemishes as acne. Elder flower oil and ointment is made by steeping the flowers in a little olive oil and storing in a warm place for two or three days, then squeezing through a cloth. Heat and dissolve enough bee's wax in the oil to achieve an ointment consistency (test by spooning out a little and cooling to harden) and add some tincture of benzoin to preserve it. This ointment is excellent for burns, cuts, scratches and abrasions. Elder flower oil made with the flower infusion in olive oil is a good remedy for chapped hands and chilblains.

There are many other uses of the sacred elder tree which, besides

being called 'the tree of music', is also called 'the tree of medicine'.
Dosage: standard infusion or ½-6 grams.

FEVERFEW   *Chyrsanthemum parthenium; Compositae*

Energetics: bitter, cool
Meridians/Organs affected: stomach, liver
Parts used: leaves and flowers
Active constituents: essential oil containing camphor, terpene, borneol, various esters and a bitter principle
Properties: antipyretic, carminative, purgative, bitter tonic
Uses: Feverfew treats colds, flu, fevers and digestive problems. It also is effective against headaches, especially migraine, but probably only in those with genuine excess heat conformation.
Precautions: Do not use for migraine resulting from a weak, deficiency condition.
Dosage: standard infusion or 3-9 gms.

CHRYSANTHEMUM FLOWERS   *Chrysanthemum morifolium; Compositae*

Energetics: sweet, slightly bitter, cool
Meridians/Organs affected: lung, liver
Part used: flowers
Active constituents: essential oil, adenine, choline and stachydrine
Properties: antipyretic, carminative, antispasmodic, alterative, tonic
Uses: Generally the yellow-flowered chrysanthemums are preferred. They are used for inflammations, colds, flu and headaches, similarly to feverfew. Chrysanthemum flowers have mild yin-tonic properties and make a healthful beverage that cools and refreshes and has rejuvenative properties.

They also are used both internally and externally as an eyewash for conjunctivitis, dry eyes with tearing, blurred vision, spots in front of the eyes and dizziness. They are indicated for hypertension symptoms. They frequently are combined with honeysuckle blossoms to heighten the antibiotic properties, making this formula, with the addition of a small amount of licorice and cinnamon, very useful for all kinds of influenzas.
Dosage: standard infusion or 3-9 grms.

HORSETAIL
Equisetum species; Equisetaceae

Energetics: sweet, bitter, cool
Meridians/Organs affected: lungs, liver, gall bladder
Part used: above ground portion
Active constituents: silica, starch, volatile oil, resin, equisetic (aconitic) acid
Properties: diaphoretic, diuretic, alterative, hemostatic, anti-inflammatory
Uses: Horsetail Promotes urination, aids general detoxification and promotes healing of bones. It is an astringent for diarrhea and dysentery, enterorrhagia and hemorrhoidal hemorrhage. Externally it is used as a poultice for hemorrhoids and anal fistula. It is also used as an eye wash for eye inflammation and conjunctivitis.
Dosage: standard infusion or 3-9 gms.

DUCKWEED
Spirodela polyrhiza; Lemnaceae

Energetics: acrid, cold
Meridians/Organs affected: lung
Part used: whole plant
Active constituents: not available
Properties: diaphoretic, alterative, diuretic
Uses: It is very useful for all external heat conditions, including fevers, skin diseases and rashes. Also it relieves fluidic swelling and hot superficial edema. It is applied topically and taken internally for bee stings.
Dosage: 3-9 gms.

VERVAIN, BLUE
Verbena hastata; Verbenaceae

Energetics: bitter, cold
Meridians/Organs affected: liver, lungs
Part used: leaves and tops
Active constituents: two glycosides (verbenaline and verbenine), essential oil, tannin, mucilage and a bitter principle
Properties: diaphoretic, diuretic, alterative, emetic, antiperiodic, expectorant, galactogogue, emmenagogue and bitter tonic
Uses: It treats fevers, colds, flu, hysteria, throat and lung congestion,

liver disorders, intestinal worms and irregular menses and cramps. This herb is more detoxifying and exerts its action both on the surface and internally as an alterative.

Dosage: standard infusion or 3 to 9 gms; tincture, 10 to 30 drops.

YARROW   *Achilea millefolium; Compositae*

Energetics: bitter, spicy, neutral
Meridians/Organs affected: lungs, liver
Parts used: leaves and flowers
Active constituents: essential oil, cineol and proaculene; achilleine, which is the bitter component of the herb.
Properties: diaphoretic, carminative, hemostatic, astringent, antispasmodic, stomachic
Uses: It is used to treat colds, flu, fevers and menstrual cramps. For bleeding yarrow is taken internally and topically applied as a poultice. It also treats digestive upset, gas, diarrhea, anorexia, hyperacidity and gastritis. This herb has a long history of association with the occult and mystical. The stalks are used for divining the Chinese *I Ching.*
Dosage: standard infusion or 3-9 gms; tincture, 10-30 drops.

PLEURISY ROOT   *Asclepias tuberosa; Asclepiadaceae*

Energetics: bitter, acrid, cool
Meridians/Organs affected: lungs, colon
Part used: root
Active constituents: asclepiadine, bitter principle, asclepione, cardeno liedes, traces of essential oil, resin, sterol
Properties: diaphoretic, carminative, diuretic, expectorant, cardiac
Uses: Pleurisy root is used to treat colds, flu, fevers, pleurisy and other pulmonary problems.
Dosage: standard infusion of the dried root or 3-9 gms; tincture, 5-40 drops every three hours as needed.

MULBERRY LEAVES   *Morus Alba; Moraceae*

Energetics: sweet, bitter, cold
Meridians/Organs affected: lungs, liver
Part used: leaves
Properties: diaphoretic, alterative
Uses: Mulberry leaves treat colds, flu and fevers. The bark and fruit may be eaten as food.
Dosage: standard infusion or 3-9 gms.

BUPLEURUM   *Bupleurum falcatum; Umbelliferae*

Energetics: pungent, bitter, cool
Meridians/Organs affected: liver, pericardium, triple warmer, gall bladder
Part used: root
Active constituents: furfurol, sterol, bupleurumol
Properties: antipyretic, diaphoretic, carminative, alterative
Uses: It is one of the most important Chinese herbs for treating the liver because it acts on diseases of a mixed conformation, i.e. both internal and chronic, and both external and acute; both hot and cold; both deficient and excess. For more than 2000 years a wide variety of Bupleurum formulas outlined in the early clinical text by the Chinese herbalist Chang Chung Ching have been widely studied and used by both Chinese and Japanese herbalists. Bupleurum seems to be effective against those diseases that tend to begin externally as an acute syndrome and to linger for a prolonged period.

Bupleurum is one of the major *chi regulating* or carminative herbs that help regulate moodiness. It has a strong ascending energy, so that it is also added in small amounts to tonic formulas to raise the yang-vitality, treat organ prolapse and raise sagging spirits.

It is used for hepatitis and all liver disorders and to help resolve and bring out eruptive diseases. In this sense, one of the peculiarities of Bupleurum is its capacity to 'dredge' out old emotions of sadness and anger that may be stored in the organs and tissues of the body.

In Ayurvedic medicine it would be considered to be anti-kapha (water) and anti-pitta (fire) but pro-vata (air). Ayurvedic doctors apparently do not use this herb but, according to David Frawley, achieve a similar action (of releasing the liver) with a combination of turmeric and barberry root.

Dosage: 3-15 gms.

KUDZU ROOT   *Puerariae lobata et thunbergiana; Leguminosae*

Energetics: sweet, acrid, cool
Meridians/Organs affected: spleen, stomach, intestines
Part used: root
Active constituents: a large amount of starch
Properties: diaphoretic, antispasmodic, digestant, demulcent, tonic
Uses: Kudzu root is good for most external, acute conditions and is particularly useful in relieving stiff neck and muscular tension as well as in treating colds, flu, headache and diarrhea. Because of its mild tonic properties and its ability to replenish body fluids, it may be used for the treatment of diabetes and hypoglycemia.

It is sold as a high quality starch thickener for sauces and is highly valued for its health benefits in Japanese Macrobiotic cooking, as well as traditional Japanese cooking. As a simple folk remedy for most acute colds, flu, fevers and digestive problems, it is prepared with ginger root, bancha tea and umeboshi plum (Japanese salt plum)—any one or all of these.

As a starch thickener for sauteed vegetables, mix a small quantity with cold water and perhaps some tamari sauce and stir it into the vegetables. A meal of vegetables prepared in this way is recommended for dieters, since it prevents the hypoglycemic lag that can occur when meals are missed. Dry pan roasted, it is very good for spleen deficient diarrhea and loose bowels.

This herb is presently naturalized in the Southern United States but is regarded as a noxious weed despite its tremendous health and economic potential.

Dosage: 3 to 12 gms.

LAXATIVES

Herbs in these categories increase elimination and regulate colon function. They can all be classified as laxatives, but their strength and the nature of their action varies. Chinese Medicine, like Western herbal medicine, differentiates between degrees of laxative action. Three main categories are recognized. First there are the strong laxatives, also called "attacking herbs", because they strongly attack and dispel toxins and pathogens from the body. These correspond to strong laxatives or "purgatives" in the Western classification, like rhubarb root, which is the main purgative in both traditions. Second are the mild, oily, lubricating or bulk laxatives. These correspond to mild or demulcent laxatives, like flaxseed or psyllium in the Western system. Third is a group of very powerful laxatives and diuretics. These purge not only the feces, the earth element; they also purge water. They are stronger than the first group, often have a certain amount of toxicity, and include some of the herbs most dangerous to use. They correspond to "drastics" in the Western classification, such as mandrake or croton.

In choosing laxatives, therefore, it is important to choose one of appropriate strength. One too strong will deplete energy and through overstimulation cause a long-term weakening of colon function. One too weak will not be ineffective and may further clog and congest the colon. Therefore, care must be taken in prescribing laxatives.

PURGATIVES
(Attacking Herbs)

Attacking therapy is a special branch of Chinese herbalism, similar to certain Western herbal systems which emphasize detoxification rather than tonification as the primary mode of cure. It was generally regarded as part of heat-clearing therapy which was used mainly for febrile diseases and infections. It proved to be of limited effectiveness because often such radical modes of herbal intervention deplete the vital reserves or, as the Chinese say, *injure the righteous chi* necessary to sustain and prolong life. To prevent such a complication, herbs in this category should be used for a limited period of time. Nevertheless, a good herbal strategy is to use attacking and heat-clearing herbs to clean out toxins before utilizing more expensive tonics, such as ginseng. This is especially indicated if there is a yellow coating on the tongue and a full and rapid pulse.

These strong laxative herbs typically exert their action through the presence of anthraquinone glycosides. They included such well known laxative herbs as rhubarb root, cascara bark, senna, buckthorn, aloe and yellow dock. The effectiveness of these herbs is dependent upon the storage of sufficient bile in the liver and gall bladder. Bitter-tasting herbs tend to stimulate bile release, stimulating peristalsis in the intestines. Owing to their cold nature, a small amount of warming carminative herbs like ginger or fennel are added to them to lessen or protect against the griping abdominal pains they tend to cause.

Probably the safest and best herbal remedy for most people with bowel irregularity is the ancient Ayurvedic formula "triphala." This is a mild-acting, internal cleansing combination of three nutritive fruits called "myrobalans", including "amla" fruit, the highest known source of vitamin C. In strength this formula falls between the stronger irritant purgatives of this category and the demulcent laxatives of the category that follows. It is good to use when the former are too strong and the latter are too weak, which often is the case.

While not considered a purgative *per se,* a common effect of triphala is a mild internal cleansing of the blood, liver, digestive tract and colon. Because of its tonic properties, triphala, which emanates from the vegetarian oriented Hindu culture, is particularly adaptable for vegetarians. Its three fruits are beleric, chebulic and emblic myrobalans. Chebulic myrobalan, known as "haritaki" is a wonderfully purifying and strengthening herb regarded as the most potent and sacred herb of the Himalayas. It is depicted as being held in the hand of the Medicine Buddha and is also a sacred herb of Shiva. Haritaki is specifically the most laxative herb in the triphala combination and individuals with more stubborn constipation either may take it alone or in a greater amount than the other two herbs. (See triphala in the planetary formulas section, pg. 132)

A North American herb with effective tonic properties is *Cascara sagrada*. However, the bark of this tree must be aged for at least a year before it can be used without extreme reactions.

Chinese medicine indicates the use of these herbs for excess internal heat, and Ayurvedic medicine similarly uses purgative herbs specifically for pitta or fire imbalances. The colon is said to be the "seat" of the vata or nerve humor, which these herbs stimulate or irritate. Thus herbs in this category can reduce pitta but can aggravate vata. They also tend to reduce kapha (water and earth) by their weight-reducing action.

Contraindications for the stronger herbs in this category are many. They should not be used during lactation, and after the onset of menstruation (purgatives also move the blood and promote menstruation). They are not good for the weak, the very young and very old or the convalescent. They are mainly indicated for severe or acute constipation usually accompanying a febrile disease and exhibiting symptoms of abdominal fullness, distention and pain on palpation, infrequent hard or dry stool, and a strong pulse with a yellow coated tongue.

(See also section on purging therapy, pg. 89)

RHUBARB ROOT   *Rheum palmatum; Polygonaceae*

Energetics: cold, bitter
Meridians/Organs affected: spleen, liver, pericardium
Part used: root
Active constituents: anthraquinones, chrysophanol, physcion, sennidine, rheidine, palmidine, tannins, glucogallin, tetrarin, catechin, gallic

acid, flavone, rutin, starch, pectin, phytosterol

Properties: purgative, astringent (in smaller doses), alterative, anti-biotic, anthelmintic, vulnerary

Uses: It treats constipation, dysentery, hemorrhoids, portal congestion, pin/thread worms, skin eruptions from faulty elimination, blood in the stool and duodenal ulcers. It also is used externally to promote healing, counteract blood clots and promote menstruation.

Precautions: Contraindicated in pregnancy.

Dosage: 1 tsp. of the powdered, dry root infused for a few minutes in ½ cup of water for laxative effect. Generally it is good to combine this with a slice or two of fresh ginger to prevent intestinal griping. As an astringent, anti-inflammatory treatment for diarrhea, use 1 tsp. to ½ cup of water and simmer 20 to 30 minutes. It may be added to any formula when the symptoms of constipation are present. Standard dosage in formulas or 3-9 gms (infused not decocted, as heat destroys much of its laxative properties)

CASCARA BARK   *Cascara sagrada; Rhamnaceae*

Energetics: cold, bitter

Meridians/Organs affected: spleen, stomach, liver, colon

Part Used: bark of tree (aged at least one year)

Active constituents: Emodin glycosides, together with aloin-like glycosides, cascarosides, chrysaloin, chrysophanol, aloe-emodin, bitter principle, tannins, ferment and resin

Properties: laxative, bitter tonic, nervine, emetic.

Uses: This is used for chronic constipation, colitis, hemorrhoids, hepatic torpor and jaundice. It is the tonic laxative par-excellence and daily use will create no laxative dependency.

Dosage: 1 to 2 tsp. of the dried and aged bark infused in a cup of boiling water for 10 minutes, taken at bedtime. Standard dosage in formulas or 3-9 gms.

BUCKTHORN BARK   *Rhamnus cathartica; Rhamnaceae*

Energetics: cold, bitter

Meridians/Organs affected: spleen, stomach, liver, colon

Part used: bark and berries
Active constituents: Various glycosides, rhamnoemodine and shesterine in the fruits; the bark contains rhamnicoside
Properties: laxative, depurative, alterative, diuretic
Uses: Buckthorn bark treats constipation, liver congestion, dropsy, hemorrhoids, colic and obesity. It is milder than its near relative cascara. The two differ so little that either can be substituted for the other. It has a generally calming effect on the gastrointestinal tract and may be used for an extended period of time for chronic constipation. It also is good for treating ulcerative colitis and acute appendicitis. Taken hot, it will induce perspiration and lower fevers. It is used with alterative formulas in small amounts, since its mild laxative effect helps eliminate toxins and treat conditions such as gallstones, itching, lead poisoning, parasites, skin diseases and worms. In ointment form it is very effective in treating warts and various skin problems. The use of this herb is known to antedate the 9th century A.D. The berries prepared with ginger, allspice *(Pimento officinalis)* and honey or sugar were usually made into syrup which was considered one of the finest laxative remedies for children.
Dosage: 1 tsp. of the bark in ½ cup of cool water, let stand for 12 hours; tincture, 5-20 drops; standard dose in formulas.

SENNA   *Cassia acutifolia; Leguminosae*

Energetics: bitter, sweet, cold
Meridians/Organs affected: colon
Parts used: leaf and pods
Active constituents: anthraquinones, flavones, tartaric acid, mucin, salts, essential oil, traces of tannin and resin
Properties: purgative that also inhibits reabsorption in the intestines.
Uses: Senna is used to treat acute constipation only. The leaves are considered to be stronger, while the pods are milder like buckthorn or cascara. Senna, like other strong purgatives, is best combined with carminatives like ginger. It is stronger and more irritating than rhubarb.
Precautions: Overdoses and frequent usage can cause laxative depen-

dency as well as abdominal pains, nausea and vomiting. Contraindi-
cated in pregnancy.
Dosage: 1 tsp. of leaves or pods per cup of boiling water before sleep.
Standard dosage in formulas or 3-9 gms.

BUTTERNUT BARK   *Juglans cinerea; Juglandaceae*
and
WALNUT BARK   *Juglans nigra; Juglandaceae*

Energetics: bitter, cold
Meridians/Organs affected: colon
Parts used: bark, leaves and nut
Active constituents: juglon (also called nucin or juglandic acid
Properties: The bark is laxative, purgative, alterative, astringent and
detergent. The fruit is tonic. The leaves are alterative.
Uses: The several varieties of walnuts all have medicinal properties,
which make them a virtual pharmocopoeia in themselves. Butternut
bark (*J. cinerea*) is commonly used as a mild laxative, but the black walnut (*J. nigra*) also is good for this purpose. Generally, for laxative action
the dried bark is used. It is good for chronic constipation, dysentery and
liver congestion. It also may be used with great effectiveness as a treatment for intestinal worms and parasites. The bark of black walnut also
may be taken in a strong infusion as a purgative. The husk, shell and
peel are sudorific especially if taken green. The unripe nut kills intestinal worms.

The fruit is a mild yang tonic. (See section on yang tonics, pg. 299.)
The leaves are aromatic and may be taken as a tea in the treatment of
chronic eczema and other skin diseases. (The green husks also are
recommended for this purpose.) The dried green husks and leaves are
extremely bitter and are probably more easily taken as a powder in
about two '00' sized capsules three times a day with warm water. Probably because of this intense bitterness, a strong infusion will destroy
various worms and insects in areas of the garden where it is poured.
Dosage: tincture of the bark: 10-30 drops three times a day; powder:
two '00' sized capsules three times a day; tea: steep one ounce of either

the bark or leaves in a cup of water and take two or three times daily.
Standard dose in formulas.

ALOE   *Aloe barbadensis-officinalis; Liliaceae*

Energetics: cold, bitter
Meridians/Organs affected: liver, heart, spleen
Parts used: powder of the leaf, the gel
Active constituents: Two aloins, barbaloin and isobarbaloin which
comprise the crystaline form of aloin which is available in the drug
approximately 10 to 30%. It also contains, amorphous aloin, aloi-
emodin and resin
Properties: purgative, cholagogue, anti-inflammatory, alterative, tonic
anthelmintic, vulnerary
Uses: Aloe powder is a stronger purgative than rhubarb and can be
emetic. The powder is generally used as a laxative whereas the juice is
much milder and functions more as a yin-tonic. The gel is used in
Ayurveda as one of the most important tonics for the female reproductive system, the liver and for regulating pitta (fire). The powder is suitable for stubborn constipation, blood in the stool, liver disorders, pink
eye, headache, tinnitus from liver and gall bladder congestion, irritability from internal congestion. The gel, which is comprised of approximately 50% water may be taken once or twice daily for premenstrual
syndrome, menopause and by women who have had hysterectomies.
According to David Frawley, aloe gel has similar tonic effects to the
Chinese Rehmannia 6 formula (for yin deficiency plus internal heat).
The addition of ginger provides an antidote to its cold nature and
preserves its tonic properties. The fresh gel is particularly effective as a
topical application for the treatment of burns, skin rashes, injuries and
wounds. In Ayurveda, aloe gel is thought to be good for all three
humors.
Precautions: The powder, in any substantial amount, is contraindicated during pregnancy.
Dosage: ½-1 tsp. of the powdered root taken in capsules or steeped in a
cup of boiling water, be warned of its nauseating taste; gel, 2 tsp. mixed
in apple juice or water three times a day.

SODIUM SULPHATE   *Mirabilitum*
(also sold as Epsom salt)

Energetics: acrid, bitter, salty, cold
Meridians/Organs affected: stomach, colon
Properties: laxative, purgative, demulcent
Uses: It is used to treat stubborn constipation; and externally, as a wash for conjunctivitis (pink eye), ulcerated throat and skin lesions.
Precautions: Contraindicated in pregnancy.
Dosage: 10-18 gms.

DEMULCENT OR LUBRICATING LAXATIVES

These herbs are used to counteract dryness and to lubricate the colon, allowing for easier bowel movements. They are suitable for chronic constipation, including constipation in the elderly and bedridden. They also are useful for treating constipation caused by lack of bulk or oil in the diet. They are good for hemorrhoids, which are often aggravated by lack of lubrication. There is a close relationship between herbs in this category and other demulcent and moistening herbs, like blood or yin tonics; and they often are used with them. Any herb with moistening properties will to some extent have laxative action, though the herbs here also tend to stimulate peristalsis to some degree. One of the manifestations of yin deficiency is dryness and this specifically manifests in dryness of the colon, so demulcent herbs usually are used with yin tonics.

In Ayurvedic theory the colon is the site of vata, the air humor. The principal quality of vata is dryness. Hence dryness in the colon is the basis of many vata disorders, including most nervous system disorders and most diseases of old age (the vata stage of life). Therefore these herbs, often taken as enemas, are very important for treating vata disorders. However, their oiliness tends to increase kapha and pitta.

Since these herbs tend to be sweet and oily, they are contraindicated in conditions of water or phlegm stagnation. They sometimes initially need the push of a stronger purgative like rhubarb to get them to function effectively against more long-term constipation. It may take them several days to begin to work efficiently. They are safer to use during pregnancy, but some caution still is advised.

LINSEED (Flaxseed)   *Linum usitatissimum; Linaceae*

Energetics: sweet, neutral
Meridians/Organs affected: spleen, colon
Part Used: the seeds
Active constituents: mucilage, fatty oil including linoleic, linolenic and oleic acids and saturated acids, protein and glycosides
Properties: laxative, demulcent, anti-inflammatory, analgesic and emollient
Uses: Linseed is used for hard, dry stool causing constipation. It is effective also for inflamed ulcerated throat. Ayurveda uses it as a demulcent expectorant in treating bronchial disorders.
Dosage: add one teaspoon to a quart of water and let boil down to ½ quart; in formulas 9-30 gms.

PSYLLIUM   *Plantago psyllium; Plantaginaceae*

Energetics: sweet, neutral
Meridians/Organs affected: spleen, stomach, colon
Parts used: seed and outer husks
Active constituents: mucilage, aucubine, protein, enzymes and fat
Properties: demulcent, laxative. The outer husks are used as a bulk-fiber laxative and are not as irritating as the seeds while the whole seed is a lubricating laxative.
Uses: Taken internally, psyllium treats chronic constipation; externally it relieves skin irritation. They are probably the simplest and most effective bulk laxative.
Dosage: One to two teaspoons of the husks are taken in juice or water once or twice daily as needed, in formulas, 9-30 gms.

CASTOR OIL   *Ricinus communis; Euphorbiaceae*

Energetics: bitter-sweet, neutral, toxic
Meridians/Organs affected: liver, spleen
Part used: expressed oil from the seed. The seed taken internally is a deadly poison).
Active constituents: toxalbumin, chelidonine, chelerythrine, coptisine,

protopine, chelidonic and other acids, saponin, carotenoid pigments, enzymes and traces of an essential oil

Properties: only the oil is non-toxic. It is demulcent, laxative and purgative.

Uses: Taken internally, it treats constipation. Externally, a castor oil fomentation is rubbed over the liver and other areas of the abdomen. A thick towel that has been rung out in ginger tea is then applied over the entire abdomen and a heating pad or hot water bottle is placed over the liver. This will help draw toxins into and through the liver. This treatment is excellent for liver disorders, cysts, growths, warts and other excrescenses. In Ayurveda, castor oil is used in the treatment of epilepsy, paralysis, insanity and many other nervous system disorders. Although the leaves are poisonous, they may be steamed and directly applied externally to relieve pains from bruises, injuries and stiffness.

Dosage: 1-2 tablespoons before sleep.

MARIJUANA SEEDS   *Cannabis sativa; Cannabinaceae*

Energetics: sweet, neutral

Meridians/Organs affected: spleen, stomach, colon

Part used: seeds

Active constituents: 19% protein, 31% lipids, choline, trigonelline, zylose, inositol, phytin, enzymes (lipase, maltase, emulsin, linamarase, amylase, urease, nuclease, erepsin, tryptase, calalase)

Properties: demulcent, nutritive, laxative

Uses: The seeds do not have any of the intoxicating properties of the leaves and flowers. In fact, they are used as a healthful peasant food in China. As a laxative, marijuana seeds are very good in cases of constipation associated with wasting diseases (yin deficiency), for older people, intestinal, febrile illnesses, post-partum women and those with anemia.

Dosage: 1 ounce of the pounded seed meal is simmered in one quart of water until the liquid reduces down to a pint. Take this in three doses throughout the day. In formulas, 9-30 gms.

SESAME OIL   *Sesamum indicum; Pedaliaceae*

Energetics: sweet, neutral
Meridians/Organs affected: spleen, liver, lungs
Part used: oil from seeds
Active constituents: (see black sesame seeds under yin tonics, pg. 319)
Properties: demulcent, emollient, nutritive, yin tonic, laxative
Uses: Sesame oil if used for dryness of the bowel, for which a table-spoon of the oil taken in the evening is quite effective. Like olive oil, it is commonly used as a medium for therapeutic oils in which other herbs are prepared according to indications.

OLIVE OIL   *Olea europea; Oleaceae*

Energetics: sweet, neutral
Meridians/Organs affected: spleen, liver
Part used: oil of fruit, leaves
Active constituents: fatty oil, with linoleic, oleic, palmitic, stearic and arachidic acids; also small amounts of free fatty acids, phytosterin, enzymes, bitter principle, pigment and a trace of lecithin
Properties: demulcent, emollient, nutritive, laxative; the leaves are antispasmodic, vasodilating and astringent, and they lower blood pressure.
Uses: Olive oil is used like sesame oil. One or two tablespoonsful taken in the evening are an efficient demulcent laxative. Both oils also are excellent to apply externally to counteract abrasions and dryness.

CATHARTIC LAXATIVES

This category has very strong irritating, laxative properties and is recommended only for occasional use. Cathartics sometimes are called "drastics" or "hydragogues" because they also eliminate excess abdominal fluid. Many have toxic properties. Their main traditonal usage was for acute dropsy or ascites. In terms of Ayurveda, these herbs greatly aggravate vata (air) and irritate the nervous system. They are contraindicated during pregnancy, menstruation and lactation, and in any condition of debility.

POKE ROOT
Phytolacca spp.; Phytolaccaceae

Energetics: bitter, cold, toxic
Meridians/Organs affected: lung, spleen, kidneys
Part used: root
Active constituents: saponin, formic acid, tannin, fatty oil, resin, sugar and phytolaccin
Properties: cathartic, alterative, antitumor, anodyne
Uses: Poke root treats constipation and glandular and lymphatic congestion. In the latter conditions it may be taken in regular small internal doses of the tincture of the fresh root. Take only 2 to 5 drops two or three times daily. If it causes nausea, stop and begin again with even smaller doses. Poke is one of the best blood and lymphatic purifying herbs. It is excellent for the treatment of cancer, tumors, arthritis and degenerative diseases, but should be used with respect and preferably in combination with other herbs in a formula to offset its powerful detoxifying effects. Externally it is applied as a poultice for sores and boils and to relieve difficult urination.
Precautions: Because of its toxicity, do not take more than 1 gm. per day.
Dosage: infusion, 1 tablespoon to a pint of water, take one mouthful several times a day

JALAP
(Morning Glory Seeds)
Ipomoea jalapa (syn. Pharbitis hederacea); Convolvulaceae

Energetics: bitter, cold, toxic
Meridians/Organs affected: lung, kidney, colon, small intestine
Part used: seeds
Active constituents: pharbitin, rhamnose, angelic acid, pelargonic and cyanin
Properties: cathartic, laxative, carminative; narcotic and emetic in large doses, vermifuge
Uses: Jalap is used to treat acute constipation, congestion of phlegm in the chest with constipation, food congestion. This herb is not as toxic or as strong as others in this category. It sometimes is used for unblocking stuck chi and moving food stagnation, particularly when associated

with heat in the intestines. It may also be used for intestinal parasites.
Dosage: 1 tsp. to a cup. Only one cup should be taken daily, a mouthful at a time several times throughout the day. In formulas, 3-6 gms.

MANDRAKE ROOT   *Podophyllum peltatum; Berberidaceae*

Energetics: bitter, cold, toxic
Meridians/Organs affected: liver, colon
Part used: the dried rhizome
Active constituents: a neutral crystalline substance, podo-phyllo-toxins, podophylloresin, and amorphous resin, picro-podophyllin, quercetin, starch, sugar, fat and yellow coloring matter
Properties: cathartic, counterirritant, antibilious, hydragogue
Uses: This herb taken internally is a powerful stimulant to the liver and intestines. It is a very strong glandular stimulant and useful for treating chronic liver diseases, promoting bile flow and digestion, and in the elimination of obstructions and skin problems. It has been studied as a possible natural plant treatment of cancer, since clinical tests seem to indicate its capacity to destroy cancer cells in test animals. It appears to be an effective treatment for female sterility. It is commonly used for severe constipation and as a topical application to stimulate the removal of venereal and other kinds of warts.
Precautions: This is a powerful herb and can cause intestinal irritation and other aggravations if it is not used carefully. Care also should be taken when it is applied externally. It should never be used during pregnancy.
Dosage: 10-30 grains of the powdered root or 1-10 drops of the alcoholic tincture, once or twice daily. In formulas, 1-3 gms.

CROTON OIL   *Croton tiglium; Euphorbiaceae*

Energetics: spicy, hot, toxic
Meridians/Organs affected: stomach, colon
Part used: the oil
Active constituents: a powerful and strongly irritating resin, glyceride of tiglic acid, triclinic plates, rods, spicy odor, vesicant, protoplasmic

crotin poison, phenol phorbol which has been identified from the resin
Properties: cathartic
Uses: It treats acute constipation.
Precautions: This is one of the most toxic and violently irritating oils
and therefore is not recommended. It is employed as a strongly violent
purgative in cases of lead poisoning.
Dosage: 10 drops of the oil

GAMBOGE   *Garcinia hanburyi; Guttiferae*

Energetics: spicy, hot, toxic
Meridians/Organs affected: stomach, colon
Part used: the hardened resin
Active constituents: resin, gum, garonolic acids, vegetable matter. The
gum is similar to gum acacia.
Properties: cathartic, drastic hydragogue
Uses: This powerful cathartic is used for reducing dropsical conditions
and for lowering blood pressure when there is danger of cerebral con-
gestion. Combined in small amounts with other purgatives, it increases
their effectiveness.
Precautions: It is never given alone. Other herbs, such as licorice and
ginger, are always added to counteract its tendency to cause nausea,
severe vomiting, and intestinal griping. Use cautiously.
Dosage: 2-6 grains of the powder in an alkaline solution.

ELDER BARK   *Sambucus canadensis; Caprifoliaceae*

Energetics: bitter, toxic
Meridians/Organs affected: stomach, colon
Part used: the aged bark for cathartic action
Active constituents: an unknown bitter principle, saponins,
hydrocyanic acid and sambuline
Properties: cathartic, laxative, diuretic
Uses: Elder bark treats acute constipation and fluid retention
Precautions: Only bark that has been aged for a year or more should
be used or cyanide poisoning may result. The Western species are
more toxic.

Dosage: aged inner bark, 2 ounces in 1 quart of water, simmered down to a pint, take 2 to 4 fluid ounces at a time.

BROOM, SCOTCH   *Cytisus scoparius; Papilionaceae*

Energetics: bitter, cold, toxic
Meridians/Organs affected: colon, kidney
Part used: flower tops
Active constituents: an alkaloid (Sparteine), secondary alkaloids consisting of cytisine and others, tannin, bitter principle and traces of an essential oil
Properties: cathartic, diuretic
Uses: This is used for acute constipation, fluid retention and edema causing heart problems. It often is combined with diuretic herbs, such as uva ursi or dandelion, to enhance its effectiveness.
Precautions: Large doses can cause vomiting, purging, weakening heart, lowered nerve strength and low blood pressure. Advanced stages of toxicity can cause complete respiratory collapse.
Dosage: 1 tsp. of the flowers steeped in a cup or 1-10 drops of the tincture.

HEAT-CLEARING HERBS

Heat has many meanings in Chinese medicine. First it refers to fevers, infections and inflammations. It also refers to hypermetabolic conditions that are caused either by excess or by deficiency. It is easy to see how *excess heat* relates to such symptoms as constipation, high fever, deep ruddy complexion, fast and strong pulse, severe pains and a red tongue with yellow coating. It is the condition of most acute fevers and infections.

The concept of *deficient heat* is harder to understand. It can produce symptoms similar to those of excess heat, but associated with an over-all pattern of weakness. It is characteristic of many chronic low grade fevers and wasting diseases like tuberculosis or consumption, and also is common in chronic urinary tract infections. The symptoms include low grade afternoon fever with sensation of heat in the palms of the hand and soles of the feet, night sweats, insomnia, anxiety, thirst, rapid thready pulse and red tongue with little or no coating.

Heat disorders are primarily to febrile diseases, but all fevers are not treated in the same way. Fever with chills and body ache, as in the common cold, is regarded as a *surface fever* and treated with diaphoretics, with sweating induced to lower the fever. The herbs in the heat-clearing categories treat *internal heat,* a condition in which the pathogen has invaded the interior, producing a constant high fever without chills. The method of treatment in this case, much like the use of antibiotic drugs, is to cata-lyze the fever with cooling herbs. These herbs function as "natural antibiotics" and many possess demonstrable in vitro antiviral or antibac-terial action. Yet they are not as depleting as antibiotic drugs. They may be safely used for longer periods, and are not as deranging to the immune system, although they are not always as effective in acute con-ditions. It should be noted that antibiotic herbs such as echinacea and goldenseal can cause the same side effects as antibiotic drugs, if they are used incorrectly or to excess.

All traditional cultures have had their favorite, usually bitter, yellow antibiotic or antifever herbs. For the Native Americans it was golden seal; in Europe, barberry; in India, chiretta; and in China, coptis. Such herbs were used to treat high fevers, epidemics and contagious diseases and, like antibiotic drugs, saved many lives. Quinine, for example, which was used to treat malaria, came from the cinchona tree, an herb of this type.

As new diseases like AIDS arise in the modern world, largely through an excess use of antibiotic drugs that cause a rapid mutation in disease-causing viruses and bacteria, natural antibiotics are again becoming important. These are the herbs that will be used to treat acute conditions when antibiotics fail. In terms of Western herbalism, these herbs possess alterative, antipyretic, anti-inflammatory, antiperiodic and bitter tonic properties. They cleanse the blood and the liver.

Ayurvedic medicine classifies them as strongly anti-pitta (fire). They are the main herbs for acute high pitta conditions. High pitta causes heat in the blood, which is considered the internal cause of infectious diseases. Heat-clearing herbs also decrease kapha (mucus) and many of them are cleansing to the lymphatics (high kapha often manifests as lymphatic congestion and bronchial disorders). However, they all increase vata (air) and must be used with care for vata or nervous, hypermetabolic types.

The Chinese divide this category into at least five subsections indicating the different lines of heat-clearing action.

Contraindications for these herbs include surface fevers or internal deficiency. They usually are used only symptomatically, and administration should be discontinued after the fever is resolved.

As most herbs of this class are bitter or otherwise unpleasant in taste they often are more easily taken in capsule or tablet form, rather than in tea form. There also are a number of good patent medicines for clearing heat.

(See also section on removing therapy for more information on the functions of these categories of herbs, pg. 93)

CLEAR HEAT AND PURGE FIRE

These herbs are largely antipyretic, which means, literally, "anti-fire". In

Chinese medicine they are considered to be the best herbs for acute high fever, particularly when associated with severe thirst, sweating and a strong flooding pulse. This condition occurs in many febrile diseases including encephalitis, meningitis and pneumonia.

The Chinese use gypsum, a mineral, as the chief herb for lowering dangerously high fevers. Since this and other mineral herbs are commonly used, it seems appropriate to include them in our pharmacopoeia.

Without this substance, this category would not be well defined. Otherwise it might be confused with the other heat-clearing categories. Many of the herbs that clear heat and dispel damp are used for high fever and fire, as are many of the herbs that detoxify the blood. The difference is that the herbs in this category are generally better for high fever where there is burning up of body fluids, as many of them have moistening properties. Generally speaking, they have the coldest nature of any used in Chinese medicine. To avoid damaging the spleen, they should not be used in excess. Otherwise, indications and contraindications are the same as for the heat-clearing category in general.

GYPSUM   *Calcium sulfate*

Energetics: spicy, sweet, cold
Meridians/Organs affected: stomach, lung
Properties: antipyretic, antiphlogistic, vulnerary
Uses: Gypsum clears and lowers heat. It is used for excess conditions with high fevers and without chills, for meningitis, thirst, profuse sweating, red tongue with yellow coating and full pulse. It is effective for cough and wheezing with heat signs; for toothache and swollen and painful gums; and for headache characterized by what is called *stomach fire*. Externally, it is applied to eczema, burns, ulcerated sores. Gypsum is non-toxic and only one part in four hundred is absorbed internally. In Chinese medicine only the decoction is taken. The gypsum is allowed to settle to the bottom (though it does not hurt if some gets in the water). In small doses it is safe and effective for children or infants.
Dosage: 9-30 gms. (or as much as needed). Boil the powdered stone for 30 minutes before adding other herbs.

CALCITUM

Energetics:spicy, salty, cold
Meridians/Organs affected: stomach, kidney
Properties: antipyretic, antiphlogistic, vulnerary
Uses: Calcitum treats high fever, irritability, thirst, yellow-coated tongue. It also may be applied externally as a powder for burns.
Dosage: 9-30 gms. Boil the powdered stone for 30 minutes before adding other herbs.

SELF-HEAL   *Prunella Vulgaris; Labiatae*

Energetics: bitter, spicy, cold
Meridians/Organs affected: liver, gall bladder
Part used: aerial portions
Active constituents: essential oil, bitter principle, oleanolic acid, rutin, caffeic acid, ursolic acid, hyperoside, vitamins C, B1, K and tannin
Properties: antipyretic, alterative, cholagogue, astringent, diuretic, styptic
Uses: Self-heal is used for fevers, hepatitis, jaundice, high blood pressure, fluid retention and edema. One of the best and most common herbs for liver heat, in China it also is used in the treatment of cancer because of its antitumor properties. In Western herbalism it is commonly used externally to stop bleeding and improve the healing of sores and wounds and is valuable for this purpose in the wild, where it is commonly found.
Dosage: 9-15 gms. in infusion

BITTERSWEET   *Solanum dulcamara; sonalaceae*

Energetics: bitter, sweet, cold, toxic
Meridians/Organs affected: liver, lungs, stomach
Part used: leaves
Active constituents: It contains the alkaloid, solanine, an amorphous glucoside dulcamarine which imparts its bittersweet taste; also gum, starch, sugar and resin.
Properties: antipyretic, alterative, antispasmodic, narcotic

Uses: It is mainly useful as an alterative for eruptic skin diseases and ulcers. It has a very cool energy and is useful for most inflammatory conditions, including ulcerative colitis and inflammatory rheumatic diseases. It also is used for severe high fevers with extreme excitability and acts as a cooling sedative for hysteria and anxiety as well as chronic jaundice.

Precautions: Berries can be toxic but unlike its near relative deadly nightshade (*Atropa belladonna*) it has only feeble narcotic properties and does not dilate the pupils of the eyes.

Dosage: 1 oz. dried and infused in ½ pint, taken in ½ cup doses 2 or 3 times a day. In formulas, 3-6 gms.

HEARTSEASE (PANSY)   *Viola tricolor; violaceae*

Energetics: bitter, sweet, cool
Meridians/Organs affected: lungs, stomach, liver, heart
Part used: the aerial portions
Active constituents: saponins, salicylates, a flavonic glycoside called violaquercetin and other biochemical agents
Properties: antipyretic, alterative, antispasmodic, anodyne, demulcent, aperient, vulnerary, expectorant
Uses: It is commonly used in an infusion as a treatment for skin eruptions in children, fevers, hypertension, anxiety and nervousness, dry throat, cough, and diarrhea and urinary inflammations.
Dosage: standard infusion or 3-9 gms.

SWEET VIOLET   *Viola odorata;Violaceae*

Energetics: sweet, bitter, cool
Meridians/Organs affected: lungs, stomach, liver, heart
Part used: flowers and rhizome
Active constituents: saponins an alkaloid called odoratine. The flower also contains an aromatic compound called irone, and a blue pigment.
Properties: antipyretic, alterative, expectorant
Uses: Very similar to its near relative, heartsease, except that this herb is particularly used to soften hard lumps and counteract cancer. It can be

made into a syrup mixed with honey and used for chronic coughs and asthma. The flowers lower blood pressure and in large doses are emetic.
Dosage: standard infusion or 3-9 gms.

GARDENIA   *Gardenis florida; Rubiaceae*

Energetics: bitter, cold
Meridians/Organs affected: heart, liver, stomach, triple warmer
Part used: the fruit
Active constituents: gardenin, crocin, chlorogenin, tannin, mannitol
Properties: alterative, antipyretic, hemostatic, stomachic
Uses: Hepatitis, jaundice, hypertension, depression, restlessness, ulcers, urinary tract infections, anti-inflammatory and promotes healing in soft tissue injuries. This herb is sometimes called the "happiness herb" because it relieves liver congestion and along with it, blocked emotions. A good general herb for febrile disease, it treats heat in any of the three warmers. The fragrance of the flower is very calming to the heart.
Dosage: 6-12 gms.

LOTUS PLUMULE   *Nelumbinis nuciferae; Nymphaceae*

Energetics: bitter, sweet, neutral
Meridians/Organs affected: heart, spleen, kidney
Part used: the plumule
Active constituents: Raffinose, oxoushinsunin, N-norarmepavine, calcium, iron
Properties: antipyretic, alterative, nervine
Uses: It calms excessive mental activity, relieves insomnia, irritability and anxiety, and cools fevers. The plumule is the sprout that comes out of the seed, sometimes called the "heart" of the lotus.
Dosage: ½-6 gms.

DWARF BAMBOO   *Lophatheri gracilis; Graminaceae*

Energetics: sweet, bland, cool
Meridians/Organs affected: heart, stomach, bladder

Part used: stem and leaves
Active constituents: cyulindrin, arundoin, taraxerol, friedelin
Properties: alterative, antipyretic, diuretic
Uses: It treats urinary infections with scanty urine, mouth and gum sores, and inflammations and irritability
Dosage: 6-9 gms.

REED GRASS   *Phragmites communis and spp.; Graminaceae*

Energetics: sweet, cold
Meridians/Organs affected: lung, stomach
Part used: root
Active constituents: 51% glycosides, 5% protein, 0.1% asparagin, vitamins B1, B2 and C
Properties: antipyretic, alterative, stomachic, antiemetic
Uses: Reed grass is used for inflammation of the stomach and lungs with acute symptoms of yellow phlegm, cough, expectoration, gastritis, belching and vomiting. It also is effective in treatment of urinary tract inflammations with dark and scanty urine. It is used for eruptive rashes, helping them to come out fully and terminate more efficiently. All of these symptoms tend to be accompanied by irritability and thirst.
Dosage: 15-30 gms.

CELOSIA (Cockscomb)   *Celosiae argentea and C. cristata; Amaranthaceae*

Energetics: sweet, cool
Meridians/Organs affected: liver
Part used: seeds
Active constituents: potassium nitrate and nicotinic acid
Properties: antipyretic, alterative, astringent, opthalmic, vulnerary
Uses: It is used specifically in decoctions for retinal hemorrhage and conjunctivitis. It is also very effective in lowering blood pressure.
Dosage: 3-15 gms. in decoction; often combined with herbs such as chrysanthemum flowers

DEMULCENT FEBRIFUGES
(Herbs to Clear Heat and Cool and Nurture the Blood)

This category treats more advanced stages of febrile disease, wherein the fever has already burnt up the vital fluid (yin) and the blood and caused an acute internal deficiency. Hence these herbs combine demulcent and blood-nourishing properties along with heat-clearing action. Many of them have tonic properties and are related to yin and blood tonics. They treat the most severe febrile diseases (which may necessitate intravenous feeding), by preventing dehydration. As the fever burns up the blood it causes rampant bleeding, most typically subcutaneous hemorrhage. Symptoms include high fever, thirst, delirium, rapid thready pulse and dark red or purple tongue with no coating.

These herbs also treat less serious disorders of *deficient heat.* They are useful for chronic low-grade febrile or infectious conditions. Often a demulcent febrifuge is added to the more typical strong heat-clearing herbs to help protect the body fluids.

According to Ayurveda, these herbs are better for treating fevers in vata (air) constitutions, who benefit from their moistening action. They reduce pitta (fire) but tend to increase kapha (water).

Contraindications include cold conditions or conditions of phlegm and damp stagnation.

REHMANNIA (raw)   *Rehmannia glutinosa; Scrophulariaceae*

Energetics: sweet, bitter, cool
Meridians/Organs affected: heart, kidney, liver
Active constituents: glycosides, saponins, arginine, b-sitosterol, manintol stigmasterol, campesterol rehmannin, catapol, glucose, tannin, resins, coloring matter and a substance similar to myrtillin
Part used: dried root
Properties: demulcent, alterative, hemostatic, yin tonic
Uses: It is commonly used in Chinese herbology and also is found as a perennial in many parts of North America. It is important in this category. Rehmannia is used for diabetes, tuberculosis and wasting diseases, continuous low-grade fever, hemorrhage during high fever, with heat entering the blood level, thirst, mouth and tongue sores, irritability,

insomnia, yin deficient sore throat.
Dosage: 9-30 gms. (also see rehmannia under blood tonics, pg.313)

FIGWORT   *Scrophularia nodosa; Scrophulariaceae*
(Carpenter's Square)

Energetics: bitter, sweet, cool
Meridians/Organs affected: lung, stomach, kidney
Active constituents: stereoptene, propionic and acetic acid
Part used: root
Properties: demulcent, alterative, yin tonic, anodyne
Uses: The root is used for nearly all the conditions treated by rehman-
nia, as well as for the following: deobstruent to the glandular system,
hepatic diseases, skin eruptions, dropsy, struma (an inflammatory con-
dition with associated depravity of fluids and solids), externally for
ringworm, bruises, piles, swelling, itch, cutaneous conditions of a vascular character. It may be used alternately with rehmannia.
Dosage: 9-30 gms.

WATER BUFFALO HORN   *Bubalus bubalis*

Energetics: bitter, salty, cold
Meridians/Organs affected: heart, liver, stomach
Active constituents: keratin, eukeratin, various proteins, peptides, free
amino acids, arginine, guanidine and cholesterol (It is similar to rhinoceros horn)
Properties: alterative, antipyretic, cardiotonic, hemostatic
Uses: It is used to treat very high fevers with delirium, tremors, bleeding, vomiting of blood, convulsions. Rhinoceros horn was the herb of
choice for such conditions; but considering its scarcity and expense, this
is the best substitute.
Precautions: Not to be used for patients with deficient energy conditions but only with excess.
Dosage: 3-9 gms.

MARSHMALLOW ROOT (see yin tonics, pg.319)

One of the best herbs for this category and also an effective tonic.

STILLINGIA   *Stillingia sylvatica; Euphorbiaceae*

Energetics: acrid, bitter, cool
Meridians/Organs affected: lungs, kidney, liver
Part used: the root
Active constituents: stillingine, which is an alkaloid, gum, starch, both a fixed and a volatile oil and coloring matter
Properties: alterative, astringent
Uses: Stillingia treats skin diseases, strumous disorders (yin deficient heat signs), syphilis, chronic laryngeal and bronchial inflammations, leucorrhea, chronic coughs, rheumatism, and chronic liver affections. This herb must be used fresh and can be extracted in alcohol to make a tincture, using two ounces of the bruised root to a pint of diluted alcohol.
Dosage: tincture, 10-30 drops; a decoction may be made of the fresh bruised root, using one ounce of the root and one and one quarter pints of water boiled down to a pint. One or two fluid ounces is taken several times daily.

TREE PEONY   *Paeonia suffruticosa; Ranunculaceae*

Energetics: acrid, bitter, cool
Meridians/Organs affected: heart, liver, kidney
Part used: the root
Active constituents: ketone paeonol, glycosides and benzoic acid
Properties: alterative, antipyretic, antispasmodic, emmenagogue
Uses: It stops excessive bleeding caused by inflammatory conditions, including nosebleed, vomiting of blood and bleeding under the skin. It also is specific for removing false yang or heat caused by strumous or deficient conditions. It promotes blood circulation and helps to dissolve tumors, lumps and masses, as well as bruises. It will promote menses, relieve headache, eye pains and painful menses, and bring down swelling and help drain pus from abscesses. Tree peony is a common ornamental grown here and native to China.
Dosage: 6-12 gms.

GROMWELL

Lithospermum arnebia and L. rudrale; Boraginaceae

Energetics: bitter, sweet, cool
Meridians/Organs affected: pericardium, liver, heart
Part used: whole plant
Active constituents: two crystalline coloring matters, shikonin and acetyl-shikonin
Properties: demulcent, alterative, antipyretic, depurative
Uses: It is particularly effective, used both internally and externally for excess type skin rashes, bringing out and eliminating rash. It also lubricates the intestines and promotes bowel movement. Externally it is a very effective wash for poison oak and ivy dermatitis, and a douche for purulent leucorrhea, genital itching and herpes. An important anticancer herb in China, particularly for skin cancer, it often is added to oils for moistening or nourishing the skin. The Shoshone Indian women used this plant to induce temporary sterility for contraception.
Dosage: 3-9 gms.

LYCIUM ROOT

Lycium chinensis and spp.; Solanaceae

Energetics: sweet, cold
Meridians/Organs affected: lung, liver, kidney
Part used: the root
Active constituents: betaine, cinnamic acid, sitosterol, linoleic acid, linolenic acid psyllic acid
Properties: alterative, antipyretic, demulcent
Uses: It is used for deficiency heat with night sweats, fever, chronic low grade fevers, lung heat with cough and wheezing, nosebleed, vomiting blood, blood in the stool and urine. It also is used both internally and externally for skin rashes, including various forms of dermatitis (poison oak and ivy), for which it combines very effectively with gromwell (see above). It also may be used as a douche for leucorrhea, genital itching, herpes rashes. (See also lycium under blood tonics, pg.311)
Dosage: 9-15 gms.

CLEAR HEAT AND COUNTER TOXINS

This is perhaps the most important sub-category of heat-clearing herbs, since they tend to have a broad antibiotic action. Some are directly antibacterial and antiviral, while others work indirectly through activating specific organs and processes of detoxification. A few have mild tonic properties. They include the main line alterative or blood-cleansing herbs of Western herbalism, like echincacea. However, those Western alteratives, like garlic or sassafras, which work by improving circulation rather than by cooling the blood, will not be found here. The herbs in this category lend themselves to combination, since each will tend to principally affect only one of the many conditions for which detoxification is needed.

These herbs are more specifically antitoxin than the other categories of heat-clearing herbs and work more directly on cleansing the blood and the lymphatics. Some even have diaphoretic properties for wind-heat surface conditions. They are particularly useful in treating infectious and contagious diseases.

From the Ayurvedic standpoint, they reduce pitta (fire) and kapha (water) but will increase vata (air).

Contraindications are similar to those for heat-clearing herbs in general. Many of these herbs are used only symptomatically relative to particular toxins.

ECHINACEA   *Echinacea spp.; Compositae*

Energetics: bitter, pungent, cool
Meridians/Organs affected: lungs, stomach, liver
Parts used: root and aerial portions
Active constituents: According to herbalist Steven Foster there are approximately nine species of echinacea, all of which are native to North America. The variety preferred by the Eclectic physicians of the early part of this century is *E. angustifolia* but other varieties, including *E. pallida,* and the most common and domesticated *E. purpurea,* are of relatively similar therapeutic effectiveness. Additional varieties include *E. simulata* and *E.paradoxa.*

The biochemistry, according to Steven Foster, is as follows: "an essential oil containing the oncolytic hydrocarbon (z) -1, 8- Penta-decadiene; polysaccharide 1 (a heteroxylan) containing arabinose, xylose, glactose, glucose and 4-0- methylgluronic acid; polysaccharide 2 (an arabinorhamnogalactic) containing rhamnose, arabinose, galac-tose, and glucuronic acid; echinacen (an isoabutylkylamide comprising 0.01% of the dried root of *E. angustifolia* and 0.001% of the dried root of *E. pallida);* echinolone (appolyacetylene compound from *E. angustifolia);* echinacoside (a glycoside found in *E. angustifolia,* at concentrations of 1% of root preparations); echinacin B; an unsaturated aliphatic sesquiterpene, betain; inulin; inuloid; fructose; sucrose; higher fatty acids; 6.9% protein in air dried roots of *E. angustifolia,* 5.3% in *E. purpurea;* tannin; vitamin C; enzymes; an unidentified glucoside; resin; acids and thirteen polyacetylene compounds."

Properties: alterative, carminative, stimulant, vulnerary

Uses: Echinacea stimulates the body's immune system against all infec-tious and inflammatory conditions, counteracts pus, and stimulates digestion. It specifically strengthens the immune system against patho-genic infection by stimulating phagocytosis, T-cell formation, and by inhibiting the hyalurinadase enzyme secreted by bacteria to effect the breakdown of cell walls and the formation of pus. Echinacea is one of the most powerful and effective remedies against all kinds of bacterial and viral infections. It should be taken frequently, every hour or two during acute stages of inflammation, tapering off as symptoms improve. There are no generally recognized side effects of echinacea overdose, but the author has noted a peculiar scratchy, tickling sensa-tion in the throat from excessive use.

Dosage: standard infusion or 3-9 gms.; tincture, 10-30 drops

RED CLOVER   *Trifolium pratense; Leguminosae*

Energetics: sweet, salty, cool
Meridians/Organs affected: liver, heart, lungs
Part used: flowers
Active constituents: These have not been very well studied, but it is apparently high in many important nutrients, including vitamins and minerals. It contains blood-thinning coumarins, which make it very

effective for many chronic degenerative diseases. These are quite mild, however, and generally are more regulatory than specific in blood-thinning qualities. Laboratory tests seem to indicate that it has some estrogenic activity and is antibiotic against several bacteria including those of tuberculosis, which are more characteristic in strumous or wasting diseases.

Properties: alterative, antispasmodic, expectorant, antitumor

Uses: It is used to treat cancer, to clear the skin, to counteract fevers, to treat inflamed lungs, whooping cough and inflammatory conditions associated with arthritis and gout. For cancer it is combined with chaparral for greater effectiveness.

Dosage: 6-15 gms. in infusion

BLUE FLAG   *Iris versicolor; Iridaceae*

Energetics: acrid, bitter, cold

Meridians/Organs affected: liver, gall bladder, colon, stomach

Part used: rhizome

Active constituents: starch, gum, tannin, bolatile oil, 25% acrid, resinous matter, isophthalic acid, traces of salicylic acid, an alkaloid and oleoresin to which it owes most of its therapeutic properties

Properties: alterative, cholagogue, diuretic, laxative; emetic, and cathartic in large doses

Uses: Blue flag is used to treat liver diseases, jaundice, hepatitis, skin diseases. The fresh root is very acrid and will produce nausea, vomiting, purging and intestinal pains. The dried root is less acrid but still has emetic, diuretic and cathartic properties. Only small doses are used for clearing the liver, usually in combination with other alterative herbs.

Dosage: 1 tsp. dried root powder steeped in 1 cup of cold water for 8 hours. Strain and take ½ cup a day, 2-4 tbls. at a time, warm. Tincture, 1-3 drops; in formulas, 1-3 gms.

CHAPARRAL   *Larrea divaricata; Zygophyllaceae*

Energetics: slightly salty, acrid, bitter, cool
Meridians/Organs affected: kidneys, lung, liver
Part used: leaves
Active constituents: Chaparral is famous for its primary constituent
NDGA (nordihydroquaiaretic acid) which has pronounced antioxidant
and anticancer effects. It relieves pain, has vasodepressant properties
and has been found to increase ascorbic acid levels in the adrenals.
Properties: alterative, antitumor, laxative
Uses: Chaparral is used to treat cancer, skin diseases, arthritis and rheu-
matic complaints. A mouthwash used on a daily basis will prevent den-
tal caries.
Dosage: ½ ounce infused in a pint of boiling water or 3-6 gms.; tincture, 10-30 drops

BURDOCK ROOT   *Arctium lappa; Compositae*

Energetics: bitter, slightly sweet, cool
Meridians/Organs affected: lungs, stomach, kidney, liver
Part used: root
Active constituents: essential oil, nearly 45% inulin
Properties: alterative, diuretic, diaphoretic, nutritive
Uses: Burdock root treats skin diseases, boils, carbuncles, fevers, inflam-
mations and fluid retention. It may be used as a food and is especially
good for preventing excesses in yang or fire types.
Dosage: standard decoction or 3-9 gms.; tincture, 10-30 drops

DANDELION ROOT   *Taraxacum officinale;*
                                              Compositae

Energetics: bitter, sweet, cool
Meridians/Organs affected: spleen, stomach, kidney, liver
Part used: root
Active constituents: lactupicrine, a bitter principle, tannin, inulin and a
latex-like substance
Properties: alterative, cholagogue, diuretic, stomachic, aperient, tonic

Uses: It is used for all heated liver conditions, breast tumors, abscesses, boils, fluid retention, stomach disorders, constipation. Dandelion root is one of the best remedies for the treatment of hepatitis and a possible preventative for breast cancer.

Dosage: standard decoction or 3-9 gms.; tincture, 10-30 drops

YELLOW DOCK   *Rumex crispus; Polygonaceae*

Energetics: bitter, cool
Meridians/Organs affected: liver, colon
Part used: root
Active constituents: rumicin and from the root, chrysarobin
Properties: alterative, cholagogue, astringent, aperient, blood tonic
Uses: It is used to treat skin diseases, liver disorders and iron deficiency. According to herbalist Michael Moore, it liberates iron that is stored in the liver. It is used for anemia during pregnancy and anemia generally. It has a tonic-laxative effect good for treating rheumatism and bile congestion. As an astringent, it treats hemorrhoids and bleeding from the lungs. It functions similarly to rhubarb as a purgative, but has a milder action. It is specific for a variety of chronic and acute skin diseases including psoriasis, urticaria and eczema (all of a hot and inflammatory nature). To take it is as a syrup, boil ½ pound of the crushed root in two pints of water until the liquid reduces to one half, then add half a pint of blackstrap molasses, which enhances its blood tonic action. Take one tablespoon or teaspoon two or three times a day. It combines well with sarsaparilla as a tea for chronic skin problems.

Dosage: standard decoction or 3-9 gms.; tincture, 10-30 drops

SARSAPARILLA   *Smilax officinalis; Liliaceae*

Energetics: sweet, mildly spicy, neutral
Meridians/Organs affected: liver, stomach, kidneys
Part used: root
Active constituents: saponins, parillin, sarsaponin, glycosides, sitosterol stigmasterin, traces of essential oil, resin, sugar and fat
Properties: alterative, diuretic, diaphoretic, tonic

Uses: It is used to treat skin disorders, liver problems, rheumatism and hormone excesses. The species of this herb vary in different areas; and many herbs with somewhat similar properties also have become known as sarsaparilla. A related species called China root *(S. china)* is commonly used in Chinese medicine as an alterative and diuretic for syphilis, gout, skin disorders and rheumatism. Generally the best quality sarsaparilla is the Jamaican. Honduran and Mexican are also very good. The roots with the deeper orange-red color are considered to be of superior quality. Sarsaparilla is excellent for chronic hepatic disorders, for venereal diseases like gonorrhea and syphilis, and for female leuchorrea, herpes and other skin disorders caused by blood impurities. It combines well with other alteratives and especially with yellow dock, sassafras, burdock, dandelion and red clover. It also is of some help for epilepsy and other nervous system disorders.

Because of its saponin content and pleasant flavor, it is used alone or with sassafras to make root beer. A simple recipe is to brew a combination of sarsaparilla and sassafras in boiling water for 20 minutes, about four ounces to a gallon. Strain and add a pound of honey or sugar to sweeten, and live baking or brewing yeast. Keep covered in a warm place (about 68 degrees Fahrenheit) for an hour or two until small bubbles start to rise, showing that fermentation has begun. Decant into bottles and tightly cap. Wait 24 hours before drinking.

Dosage: 6-15 gms. in decoction; tincture, 10-30 drops

PULSATILLA   *Anemona pulsatilla; Ranunculaceae*

Energetics: cold, bitter
Meridians/Organs affected: stomach, colon
Part used: root
Active constituents: saponins, protoanemonin wich polymerizes to give anemonin
Properties: alterative, antispasmodic, nervine, diaphoretic
Uses: This is another interesting example of the same or similar herbs being used quite differently in different traditions. Such cross-cultural comparisons give a greater understanding of the therapeutic effects of herbs and their uses. In Traditional Chinese medicine, pulsatilla is used

as an anti-inflammatory and is considered specific for amoebic and bacterial dysentery. Externally, it is used as a douche for trichomonas.

Western herbalists and homeopaths, on the other hand, use minute doses of pulsatilla as an important remedy for premenstrual syndrome. Curiously, mainly fair and blue-eyed women are responsive to this remedy. It is generally used as an emmenagogue and to increase blood and energy circulation for both men and women. It strengthens sexual sensitivity while lessening the tendency towards morbid preoccupation. It is a good remedy to consider for disorders of the reproductive organs and the prostate, associated with nervous and emotional problems. Characteristically, the symptoms treated are nervousness, restlessness and an active imagination or fear of impending danger or disease. For menstrual irregularity or delayed menstruation, it is used to treat simple suppression due to atony or shock. It is also good for some cases of heart disease, again with strong mental symptoms.

Pulsatilla is used for various inflammatory conditions, but especially if accompanied by nervousness, despondency, sadness, unnatural fear, weepiness and depression. It is used also for headache, insomnia, neuralgia in the anemic, thick tongue coating with a greasy taste, stomach disorders from over-indulgence in fats and pastries, various alternating and shifting signs such as diarrhea/constipation, amenorrhea and dysmenorrhea, pain from exposure to wind, toothache and styes.
Precautions: It is not recommended for individuals with a cold or deficient type diarrhea.
Dosage: Pulsatilla is prepared only from the fresh herb. Macerate two pounds in four pints of strong alcohol. Two to three drops of the tincture are taken three or four times a day in a spoonful of water. Owing to the delicate nature of its constituents, the tincture must be used within a year after preparation. In formulas, 6-15 gms.

ISATIS   *Isatis tinctoria; Cruciferae*

Energetics: bitter, salty, very cold
Meridians/Organs affected: stomach, colon, liver, heart
Parts used: root, leaves

Active constituents: Indoxyl-glucoside, sitosterol, isatin, arginine, glutamine, proline, tyrosine
Properties: alterative, antibiotic, cholagogue, anodyne
Uses: This is a broad spectrum antibiotic agent effective against many kinds of infections and inflammations. It is not much used in Western herbology but is widely appreciated by the Chinese who use the roots and leaves for acute laryngitis, lymphoadnitis, encephalitis, mumps, sudden high fevers, swellings that are inflamed, hepatitis, diphtheria, dry throat, scabies, thirst from heat and heat rash. It is similarly used in Ayurveda (called *nila*).
Dosage: 9-30 gms.

BAPTISIA   *Baptisia tinctoria; Leguminosae*

Energetics: bitter, extremely cold, toxic
Meridians/Organs affected: liver
Parts used: leaves, root
Active constituents: baptitoxine (baptisine); two glucosides; baptin, a cathartic; a yellowish resin
Properties: alterative, antibiotic, antiseptic, emmenagogue, emetic
Uses: It is used to treat for inflammatory conditions associated with septicemia, severe disintegration of tissues due to capillary congestion, putrid ulcerations and malignant ulcers, mouth sores, sore nipples, erysipelis, scrofula, malignant sore throat, diptheria, scarlatina, tonsillitis, typhoid dysentery, typhoid pneumonia, cerebro-spinal meningitis, fetid leucorrhea and ulceration of the cervix. Foul discharges with a dark purplish discoloration are definite indications for baptisia. Ointments using baptisia are excellent for inflamed tumors, cancers, boils and ulcers.
Dosage: half an ounce of the root boiled for 10 minutes in a pint of water. Take one tablespoon every three or four hours. If nausea or sick feelings result, lessen the dose. For children, give half or less according to size and age. In standard infusion 3-9 gms.

HONEYSUCKLE   *Lonicera japonica; Caprifoliaceae*

Energetics: sweet, bitter, cold
Meridians/Organs affected: lung, stomach
Part used: flowers
Active constituents: Luteolin, inositol, tannin
Properties: alterative, antibiotic, diuretic, refrigerant, diaphoretic
Uses: Honeysuckle is used for infections and inflammations and has broad spectrum antimicrobial activity against salmonella typhi, pseudomonas aeruginosa, staphylococcus aureus and streptococcus pneumoniae. It is very effective against fevers, colds and flus and is regarded as a reliable antibiotic herb, for which use it is often combined with forsythia fruit. It is similar to the echinacea of Chinese medicine. Recent studies in China have found it to be effective in the treatment of certain cancers, especially of the breast. It is useful for sore throat and conjunctivitis, as well as inflammations of the intestines, urinary tract and reproductive organs. This is the same plant as the commonly known ornamental flower.
Dosage: 9-15 gms.

FORSYTHIA   *Forsythia suspensa; Oleaceae*

Energetics: bitter, slightly acrid, cool
Meridians/Organs affected: lung, heart, gall bladder
Part used: seed
Active constituents: oleanolic acid, matairesinoside, saponin, flavonoid glycoside
Properties: alterative, antibiotic, antiemetic
Uses: Forsythia is used to treat the common cold, fevers, flu, high fevers with thirst, urinary tract infections, skin diseases, abscesses and allergenic purpura. It usually is combined with other antibiotic herbs like honeysuckle for a basic remedy for acute infectious diseases. Like honeysuckle, it has broad spectrum antiviral and antibacterial properties. It too is commonly cultivated as an ornamental plant in this country.
Dosage: 6-15 gms.

PURSLANE   *Portulaceae oleracea; Portulacaceae*

Energetics: sour, cold
Meridians/Organs affected: colon, liver, spleen
Part used: leaves
Active constituents: noradrenaline, calcium salts, dopamine, DOPA, malic acid, citric acid, glutamic acid, asparagic acid, nicotinic acid, alanine, glucose, fructose, sucrose
Properties: alterative, refrigerant, bactericide
Uses: Purslane is used to treat boils, sores, pain of bee stings, snakebite, postpartum bleeding, bacillary dysentery, diarrhea, hemorrhoids and enterorrhagia. This herb, a common garden weed, is steamed and eaten as a vegetable in many parts of the world. It is a good cooling food for the summer.
Precautions: It is contraindicated during pregnancy and for individuals with cold and weak digestion.
Dosage: 15-30 gms.

BEAR LICHEN   *Usnea barbata; Usneaceae*

Energetics: sweet, cold
Meridians/Organs affected: lungs, liver, colon
Part used: entire plant
Active constituents: usnic acid
Properties: alterative, antibacterial, antifungal
Uses: It is effective against most streptococcus and staphylococcus infections, and for trichomonas in women (for which it needs to be taken in tincture form every two hours for a week). It is also good applied full strength to infected cuts, fungus infections, impetigo, gastrointestinal tract and urinary tract and streptococcus infections. This is an important new natural antibiotic.
Dosage: tincture, 10-30 drops

ST. JOHNSWORT   *Hypericum perforatum; Hypericaceae*

Energetics: bitter, cool
Meridians/Organs affected: liver, kidney, spleen, stomach

Part used: aerial portions
Active constituents: essential oil, hypericine (a glycoside that is a red pigment), a polyphenolic favonoid derivative (hyperaside)
Properties: alterative, antispasmodic, anti-inflammatory, astringent, vulnerary
Uses: Taken internally, it is a pain relieving sedative used in the treatment of neuralgia, anxiety and nervous tension. Externally, it is a specific treatment for diseases directly affecting the spine. It is applied as a liniment or poultice for sciatica, neuralgia and rheumatic pains; and as a lotion to relieve the pain and inflammation of bruises, varicose veins and mild burns. St. Johnswort oil is made by soaking the herb in olive oil and allowing it to stand in a warm place for a few days.
Dosage: One to two teaspoons per cup of boiling water, taken two to three times daily. Standard decoction or 3-9 gms.

GOTU KOLA

Centella asiatica and
Hydrocotyle asiatica; Umbelliferae

Energetics: bitter, sweet, cool
Meridians/Organs affected: heart, liver
Part used: root
Properties: alterative, antipyretic, diuretic, antispasmodic, nervine, tonic
Uses: Gotu kola is an alterative for sore throat, measles, tonsillitis, hepatitis, venereal diseases and urinary tract infections. In Ayurveda it is considered the prime nervine tonic and is used to treat insomnia, stress, nervousness and disturbed emotions, and many nervous system disorders. It promotes mental calm and clarity and assists in the practice of yoga and meditation. It possesses tonic properties and could be considered a yin tonic like eclipta. It is used with eclipta for strengthening the nerves and promoting the growth of hair.
Dosage: 6-15 gms.

CLEAR HEAT AND DISPELL DAMPNESS
(Bitter Tonics)

This category specifically treats conditions associated with *damp-heat,* which is primarily congested bile. It is drained by using herbs with cholagogic properties like Oregon grape or golden seal. Damp-heat also may refer to the presence of purulent yellow-colored discharges and hence to infectious conditions. Many of these herbs are used for general heat-clearing and fire-purging action, like those in the other categories. Indeed, the most typical and strongest of the heat-clearing herbs used in various herbal traditions tend to be found here, as heat and infection usually go together.

This is the category of typical cold bitter herbs, many of which are yellow in color and contain related bitter principles like berberine. They are the main line and strongest of the antibacterial herbs. From a Western persective, they also possess alterative, febrifuge, antipyretic, antiperiodic and anti-inflammatory properties.

Damp-heat conditions treated by these herbs include diarrhea, dysentery, urinary tract infections, jaundice and hepatitis, boils, septicemia, eczema and herpes. The herbs here combine well with other alteratives, especially those that clear heat and clean toxins. Many are good for fevers, particularly malaria. They also treat ulcers and other inflammatory conditions of the gastrointestinal tract.

Many of the herbs in this category are classified by Western herbology as tonics, but this is a concept of tonics that is different from that of traditional Chinese medicine. A small amount of so-called tonic "bitters" taken before meals will stimulate digestive secretions, while taking them after meals tends to hinder them. Bitter herbs cleanse the digestive tract and stimulate digestion, so that the food is better assimilated and more strengthening in its effect. On the other hand, the Chinese tonics, like ginseng, contain important deep activating hormonal precursors and usually have a sweet or pleasant taste. Tonic bitters, however, are very effective and the Chinese agree that they have the capacity of *clearing the yang,* i.e. drying and clearing.

According to Ayurveda, the herbs in this category are the strongest herbs for lowering high pitta (bile). They also help reduce kapha (phlegm), and many are effective in weight reduction. They help regu-

late liver and pancreas function and aid in the digestion of sugar and fat.
They increase vata (air) and therefore are contraindicated for conditions
of nervousness and debility.

Herbs in this category are contraindicated for individuals who suffer
from cold, fluid deficiency, emaciation and weak digestion.

WAHOO   *Euonymus atropurpureus, E.*
(Burning bush)   *europoeus; Celastraceae*

Energetics: bitter, cold
Meridians/Organs affected: lung, liver, gall bladder, stomach
Parts used: bark and roots
Active constituents: bitter principle, euonic acid, crystalline glucoside,
asparagins, fat, culvitol, 14% ash and resins
Properties: alterative, cholagogue, diuretic, expectorant, laxative,
cardiac
Uses: It is basically a stomach bitter that removes liver congestion and
thus relieves pains and congestion in the chest. A decoction of the bark
will stimulate bile flow and have a mild laxative action; and also is useful for treating venereal diseases, uterine discharge, skin ailments and to
induce vomiting. It also is a remedy for dandruff and scalp problems.
Dosage: ½ tsp. two or three times daily; tincture, 5-10 drops; 3-9 gms.
in formulas

WILLOW   *Salix nigra, S. alba; Salicaceae*

Energetics: bitter, cold
Meridians/Organs affected: liver, kidneys, heart
Part used: bark
Active constituents: the glycosides salicine (salicoside) and salicortine
and tannin. The European white willow is very similar in properties to
the North American variety but contains more tannins.
Properties: alterative, anodyne, febrifuge, astringent, antiperiodic and
vermifuge
Uses: It is used to treat headache caused by dampness and heat in the
gastrointestinal tract, rheumatic aches and pains, recurring fevers,
gonorrhea, ovarian pains, dyspepsia, dysentery, chronic diarrhea,

worms and edema. It also may be taken as a bitter tonic in small doses before meals, to hasten convalescence from acute disease.

Dosage: 1-3 tsp. of bark in 1 cup of water, soak for 2-5 hours, 1 cup daily, a mouthful at a time; standard decoction in formulas, 3-9 gms.

CINCHONA BARK   *Cinchona succirubra; Rubiaceae*

Energetics: bitter, cold
Meridians/Organs affected: stomach, heart, liver
Part used: bark
Active constituents: catechins combined with 20 alkaloids which include quinine, quinidine, cinchonine and cinchonidine
Properties: bitter tonic, antiperiodic, astringent, antiseptic
Uses: It is used for malaria, fevers, typhoid, diarrhea, dysentery; and, similarly to willow, as a tonic bitter. It relieves inflammation and is therefore effective as a treatment for rheumatic pains. Cinchona bark may be taken as a powder, tincture or wine.
Dosage: tincture, 10-60 drops 3-6 gms. in formulas

POPLAR   *Populus spp.; Salicaceae*

Energetics: bitter,cold
Meridians/Organs affected: liver, lungs, stomach
Parts used: bark and leaves
Active constituents: There are many varieties of poplars. The buds of the balsam poplar (*P. balsamifera*) yield a high quality resin called Balm of Gilead, which is used for lung problems. Other varieties are the quaking aspen (*P. tremuloides*), the black poplar (*P. nigra*) and *P. fremontii*, which has a slightly bitter mucilage bark similar to slippery elm bark.
Properties: alterative, antipyretic, anti-inflammatory, diuretic, bitter tonic
Uses: Poplar is used to treat fevers and inflammation, and also as a bitter digestive stimulant. A tincture of the bark and buds of *P. balsamifera* is used to treat lung, stomach and kidney disorders, as well as gout and rheumatic problems. The fresh flowers of this species are steeped in cold water and strained off and taken as a blood purifier.
Dosage: tincture, 10-60 drops; standard decoction or 3-9 gms.

GENTIAN   *Gentiana lutea; Gentianaceae*

Energetics: bitter, cold
Meridians/Organs affected: liver, gall bladder
Part used: root
Active constituents: There are many local species of gentians, including various North American and European varieties. They all are bitter-tasting to some degree and have similar uses. Of *G. lutea* or yellow gentian there are three bitter glycosides. This plant is used as the standard for other bitter plants and in dilution of one part to 12,000 the bitter taste is still apparent.
Properties: alterative, antipyretic, bitter tonic
Uses: Its most common use is as a digestive bitter with alcohol, taken in small doses before meals. The Chinese use one of their species for pelvic inflammatory diseases and venereal diseases. It also is useful in treating hepatitis, jaundice and most liver disorders.
Dosage: tincture, 10-30 drops approximately 20 minutes before meals as a bitter tonic; standard decoction in formulas or 3-9 gms.

GOLDEN SEAL   *Hydrastis canadensis; Ranunculaceae*

Energetics: bitter, cold
Meridians/Organs affected: heart, liver, stomach, colon
Part used: root
Active constituents: hydrastine, berberine, resin, traces of essential oil, chologenic acid, fatty oil, albumin and sugar
Properties: alterative, anti-inflammatory, antiperiodic, astringent, diuretic, laxative, bitter tonic
Uses: It dries and cleanses the mucous membranes, inhibiting excessive flow, counteracts inflammation, regulates menses, aids digestion, treats liver diseases, cleanses the blood and counters infection. It also is a stimulant to the uterine muscles, contracts the blood vessels and inhibits excessive bleeding. Golden seal is effective against flu, fevers and infections of all kinds; and in treating hemorrhoids, vaginal yeast infection and as an eyewash for inflamed eyes. It also alleviates gastroenteritis, indigestion, gas and heartburn; and is effective in treating amoebic dysentery (giardia) when used over a 10 day period. It proba-

bly is the strongest and most typical of the Western herbs in this category and may be used as a general antibacterial or a general anti-inflammatory, externally as well as internally.

Precautions: Long-term or excessive use can weaken the flora of the colon.

Dosage: infusion, one teaspoon in a cup of boiling water; tincture, 10-30 drops; 3-6 gms. in formula

BARBERRY   *Berberis vulgaris; Berberidaceae*

Energetics: cold, bitter
Meridians/Organs affected: liver, stomach, colon
Part used: root

Many species of this plant are found throughout the world. They all are used for similar therapeutic purposes by the different traditions.

Active constituents: berberine alkaloid, chelidonic acid, resin, tannin, wax

Properties: alterative, hepatic, laxative

Uses: This is one of the mildest and best liver tonics known, good for jaundice, hepatitis and diabetes. Since it is milder than some of the other herbs in this category, it is safer to use and can help clear deficient heat. A combination of barberry and turmeric is used in Ayurvedic medicine to regulate liver energy in a way that is very similar to the use of bupleurum in Chinese herbalism. Barberry is useful as a bitter tonic to stimulate digestion, as a mild laxative, and in the treatment of inflammatory arthritic and rheumatic complaints.

Dosage: tincture, 10-30 drops; standard decoction or 3-9 gms.

OREGON GRAPE   *Mahonia repens; Berberidaceae*

Energetics: cold, bitter
Meridians/Organs affected: liver, stomach, colon
Part used: root
Active constituents: alkaloid berberine
Properties: same as preceeding
Uses: This is the Pacific Northwest variety of barberry and was used by the indigenous mountain folk of California as the preferred treatment

for all chronic degenerative diseases, especially cancer and arthritis. Combined with dandelion root in a tea, it is an excellent treatment for hepatitis and jaundice. It also is good for chronic skin problems caused by blood toxicity.

There are several related varieties of this plant, which appear to have similar properties. This herb is known in the Spanish-American tradition as Yerba de la Sangre, "herb of the blood", indicating their widespread use of it as a blood purifier. It was used by them in this way in the treatment of syphilis and as a mild diuretic laxative. They also used it very similarly to yellow dock in the treatment of anemia. This is not because of the significant presence of iron in the plant but rather its ability to release iron stored in the liver. Women would drink it first thing each morning to stimulate menses.

Dosage: tincture, 10-30 drops; 3-9 gms. in formulas

BOLDO   *Peumus boldus; Monimiaceae*

Energetics: bitter, cool
Meridians/Organs affected: liver, spleen, kidneys
Part used: leaves
Active constituents: essential oil with ascaridol alkaloids and flavanoides
Properties: alterative, cholagogue, diuretic, antiseptic
Uses: Boldo is used to treat hepatitis, poor digestion and urinary infections. It stimulates uric acid elimination, and gastric and bile secretion.
Dosage: tincture, 10-40 drops; 3-9 gms. in formulas

FRINGETREE   *Chionanthus virginicus; Oleaceae*

Energetics: bitter, cool
Meridians/Organs affected: gall bladder, liver, spleen
Parts used: root bark and bark
Active constituents: glycoside phyllirine, saponin
Properties: alterative, cholagogue, laxative
Uses: It stimulates bile secretion and is used to treat hepatitis, jaundice and gall stones
Dosage: tincture, 10-30 drops; standard decoction or 3-9 gms.

BITTERROOT   *Lewisia rediviva; Portulacaceae*

Energetics: bitter, sweet, cool
Meridians/Organs affected: liver, spleen
Part used: root
Active constituents: It contains a bitter principle and starch which is used as a nutritive substance like arrowroot and was commonly eaten by the natives of Montana.
Properties: alterative, cholagogue
Uses: It once was a primary food source of the Western Native Americans who evolved rituals for gathering it and mythologies to explain its origin. One story of the Flathead Indians tells of an old woman who had no meat or fish to feed her sons. Fearing that they would starve to death, she wept each morning on the banks of the river. The sun sent a guardian spirit in the form of a red-feathered bird, which consoled her by saying that from each of her tears that fell on the earth there would rise a beautiful flower to feed her people. Legend says that the plant's silvery appearance comes from the old woman's hair and the redness of the flower is from the crimson feathers of the sun bird's wings. The plant, although a staple food, will always be bitter in flavor because of the old woman's sorrow.

The roots are crushed and leached in water to remove most of their bitterness (some always remains). It is then cooked into a starchy, jelly-like gruel. The Indians boiled the roots and used it for angina pains, pleurisy, impure blood, skin problems and to increase mother's milk.
Dosage: tincture, 10-40 drops; in formulas, 6-15 gms. in decoction

CULVER'S ROOT (Black root)   *Leptandra virginica;*
                                          Scrophulariaceae

Energetics: bitter, cold
Meridians/Organs affected: liver, colon
Part used: root
Active constituents: The alkaloid, leptandrin, a bitter principle, a resin and other unidentified substances
Properties: alterative, cholagogue, laxative

Uses: It cleanses the liver, stomach and intestines. The fresh root is too drastic a purgative. Dried, it becomes more of a cholagogic laxative that does not debilitate the intestines but gently stimulates and regulates normal activity. In small doses of 2 drops or so of the tincture, it counteracts hepatic torpor and restores liver function. The cathartic action is beneficial in the early stages of acute fever and dysentery. It is very good for chronic dysentery and enteritis with dizziness, cold extremities, headache, abdominal and liver pains with depression. General conformation, according to King, is "drowsiness, coldness of the extremities, hot, dry skin, sluggish circulation, abdominal plethora, aching pains in the hepatic region, and in the left shoulder, and dull frontal headache, sallow or yellow skin, with a pale, white coated, broad, thick tongue, and a bitter, disagreeable taste." All these are symptoms of hepatic malfunction.

It also may be used for hepatitis, malaria, dropsy and ascites.

Dosage: fluid extract, 2 drops to one teaspoon; powder, ¼ to one teaspoon; in formulas, 3-6 gms.

FUMITORY   *Fumaria officinalis; Papaveraceae*

Energetics: bitter, cool
Meridians/Organs affected: liver, gall bladder
Part used: aerial portions
Active constituents: Fumarine and other alkaloids, fumaric acid, bitter principles, resin, mucilage
Properties: alterative, cholagogue, bitter tonic
Uses: It treats liver congestion, constipation, stomach disorders, eczema, dermatitis and exanthema
Dosage: infusion, one teaspoon in a cup of boiling water; standard dosage in formulas, 3-9 gms.

CENTAURY   *Erythraea centaurium; Gentianaceae*

Energetics: bitter, cool
Meridians/Organs affected: liver, stomach
Part used: aerial portions

Active constituents: bitter principles, including gentiopicrine and erythrocentaurin, valeric acid, wax, etc.

Properties: alterative, febrifuge, stomachic, bitter tonic

Uses: It serves as a blood purifier, working on the kidneys and liver. It also is used for digestive weakness as a bitter tonic taken before meals. People who have sluggish digestion with a tendency towards heartburn, gas and abdominal fullness may take it before meals with great benefit for a period of time. It is used as a treatment for muscular rheumatism. It kills worms as do most bitters.

External, the juice applied to the eyes will clear the vision, and applied to wounds will help promote healing. The decoction applied to the skin regularly will clear the skin of freckles and spots. In ancient times it was a primary cure for intermittent fevers and malaria, as well as a remedy for snake poison and other animal bites. A decoction externally applied also will destroy lice and other parasites in the hair.

Dosage: one teaspoon steeped in a cup of boiling water; tincture, one teaspoon taken before meals; standard decoction, 3-9 gms.

CASCARA AMARGA

Picramnia antidesma and spp.; Simurubaceae

Energetics: bitter, cool
Meridians/Organs affected: liver, stomach
Part used: bark of the root
Active constituents: bitter principle and a bitter sweet amorphous alkaloid;
Properties: cholagogue, alterative, purgative, diaphoretic, bitter tonic
Uses: It is used for diarrhea, dysentery, indigestion, toning the intestines and relieving intestinal spasms. In large doses it is emetic and will cause vomiting and nausea.
Dosage: tincture 10-30 drops; standard infusion or 3-9 gms.

GREATER CELANDINE   *Chelidonium majus; Papaveraceae*

Energetics: bitter, cool
Meridians/Organs affected: liver, colon

Part used: whole herb
Properties: alterative, diuretic, purgative, antispasmodic, diaphoretic, anodyne, narcotic
Uses: It is used for liver problems, hepatitis, jaundice, eczema, cancer and skin problems. Only the dried herb should be taken internally. The fluid extract is made with the fresh herb. The toxic, orange-colored, acrid juice is directly applied to stimulate the removal of warts, ring-worm and corns, but it should not be allowed to come into contact with other parts of the skin. The fresh juice mixed with milk is used to help remove cataracts and the white spots that form on the cornea. An ointment of the roots and leaves boiled in oil or lard is an excellent treatment for hemorrhoids.
Dosage: a teaspoon of the dried leaves steeped in a cup of water is taken two or three times daily; tincture, 8-10 drops; standard dosage in formulas or 3-9 gms.

CLEAR SUMMER HEAT

This category is the least used of the heat-clearing herbs because it is strictly associated with climatic conditions, particularly those indigenous to China and areas where there is humid heat. Summer heat also refers to various conditions associated with the season, including dysentery, diarrhea, sunburn, sunstroke and common colds and summer flu. These herbs most resemble refrigerants in Western herbalism, those herbs possessing a strongly cooling and often refreshing nature. They usually also have diuretic, diaphoretic or alterative properties. In terms of Ayurveda, as with other antiheat herbs, they are good for pitta and kapha but may increase vata.

HIBISCUS   *Hibiscus rosa-sinensis; Malvaceae*

Energetics: sour, sweet, cool
Meridians/Organs affected: liver, stomach
Part used: flowers
Active constituents: not available
Properties: refrigerant, anti-inflammatory, astringent
Uses: It is used for fevers and minor stomach and intestinal complaints. It also makes a refreshing summer beverage.
Dosage: standard infusion or 3-9 gms.

BORAGE   *Borago officinalis; Boraginaceae*

Energetics: bitter, sweet, cool
Meridians/Organs affected: lungs, heart
Part used: leaves
Active constituents: mucilage, tannin, traces of essential oil
Properties: refrigerant, diaphoretic, febrifuge, aperient, galactagogue
(promotes the flow of breast milk), pectoral
Uses: It lowers fevers, promotes coolness, and is a decongestant for
the lungs
Dosage: standard infusion or 3-9 gms.

HOUND'S TONGUE   *Cynoglossum officinale; Boraginaceae*

Energetics: cool, bitter, astringent
Meridians/Organs affected: lungs, intestines
Part used: leaves
Active constituents: alkaloids, allantoin, heliosupin, tannins, essential
oil and mucins
Properties: anti-inflammatory, astringent, demulcent
Uses: It is used for bronchial and lung problems, coughs, colds,
phlegm, diarrhea and dysentery. Hound's tongue soothes the digestive
organs and relieves hemorrhoids. Used externally it promotes the healing of wounds, burns and bites. It is used like its relative comfrey for
these purposes. Culpepper claimed that he cured rabies from the bite of
a mad dog with this herb. Legend has it that if the leaves are laid under
their feet, it prevents dogs from barking. Hence its name.
Dosage: standard infusion or 3-9 gms.

MUNG BEAN   *Phaseolus munginis; Leguminosae*

Energetics: sweet, cold
Meridians/Organs affected: heart, stomach
Part used: the green bean
Active constituents: protein, starch, calcium, iron, phosphorus, caro-
tene, thiamine, nicotinic acid, riboflavin, phosphatidic acid,

phophatidylserine, phosphatidylglycerol, phophatidylinositol, phos-
phatidylinositol, phosphahti dylethanolamine, phosphaitdyl
Properties: nutritive, alterative, anti-inflammatory, diuretic
Uses: It neutralizes acids, lowers and regulates blood pressure, heals
ulcers, relieves heat of the stomach and hot-natured dysentery. A special fast using only this food is excellent for clearing all diseases-causing
pathogens and toxins. (See kicharee in section on food therapy, pg. 77)
Dosage: 9-30 gms. in decoction

SOUTHERNWOOD   *Artemisia abrotanum; Compositae*
  and
WORMWOOD, COMMON   *A. Absinthium;*
                                          Compositae

Energetics: bitter, cold
Meridians/Organs affected: liver, gall bladder
Part used: leaves
Active constituents: absinthol which is common to all wormwoods,
in addition to other essential oils including pinene, cineol borneol phenol cuminic aldehyde, artemisia ketone
Properties: alterative, cholagogue, emmenagogue, astringent,
vermifuge
Uses: It is used to counteract fevers, regulate the liver and menses and
treat anemia and arthritis. It also is abortive. It is taken as a bitter tonic
and given to eliminate intestinal worms and parasites. A wash of the
tea will relieve itching from rashes.
Precautions: Contraindicated during pregnancy.
Dosage: one teaspoon of the dried herb infused in a cup of boiling
water or 3-9 gms.

WATERMELON   *Cucurbita sativus,*
                           Citrullus vulgaris; Cucurbitaceae

Energetics: sweet, cool
Meridians/Organs affected: heart, stomach

Parts used: rind of the fruit, fresh juice
Active constituents: citrulline, betaine, arginine, lycopene, phytofluene, vitamin C, bromine, fructose, dextrose, sucrose, malic acid, phosphoric acid. Citrulline is thought to be part of the process of forming urea from ammonia and carbon dioxide in the liver. It stands between ornithine and arginine which are two other amino acids that produce urea.
Properties: diuretic, refrigerant
Uses: It treats discomfort from heat, irritability, fevers and fluid retention
Dosage: one cup of the fresh juice or 15-30 gms. of the rind

CUCUMBER   *Cucumis sativus; Cucurbitaceae*

Energetics: sweet, cool
Meridians/Organs affected: heart, stomach
Parts used: fruit and seeds
Properties: refrigerant, alterative, diuretic
Uses: It counteracts summer heat, clears the skin and promotes fluid elimination
Dosage: 15-30 gms. or one cup of the juice of the fruit

LOTUS LEAF   *Nelumbinis nuciferae; Nymphaceae*

Energetics: bitter, slightly sweet, neutral
Meridians/Organs affected: heart, liver, spleen
Part used: leaf
Active constituents: starch, vitamin C, asparagin, nelumbine
Properties: alterative, astringent, refrigerant
Uses: It is used to treat fever, irritability, excessive sweating, scanty urine, dysentery and diarrhea. It also stops bleeding and is an antidote for mushroom and alcoholic poisoning.
Dosage: 15-30 gms.

IMPATIENS
(Jewelweed)

Impatiens palida, I. aurea,
I. biflora; Geraniaceae

Energetics: sweet, bland, cool, toxic
Meridians/Organs affected: liver, stomach
Part used: plant
Active constituents: tannin
Properties: it is cathartic, emetic and diuretic and is considered danger-
ous to use internally
Uses: It is applied externally and directly for skin rashes, poison oak
and ivy dermatitis.
Dosage: 1-3 gms. or the juice can be applied as often as needed

DIURETICS
(Herbs to Regulate Water-Metabolism)

Diuretics are herbs used to eliminate excess fluid, aid the process of detoxification through the kidneys and treat urinary affections. These include difficult, painful or burning urination, urinary tract infections or stones, and urinary dribbling or turbid urination. They also are used for various disease conditions associated with aging, lymphatic congestion, clear mucous discharges, skin diseases, venereal diseases and arthritic and rheumatic complaints. Increasing diuresis, moreover, aids in the purification of the blood and the relieving of infections, including jaundice and hepatitis. These herbs help drain damp-heat downwards and thereby can be useful in treating febrile diseases. Since excess fluid in the abdominal cavity can weaken the power of digestion, some are helpful for gastrointestinal disorders, including diarrhea.

The general rule in Chinese medicine is that if there is edema or water retention in the upper half of the body (above the navel) it should be dispersed upwards through evaporation, using diaphoretic herbs. If it is in the lower part of the body (below the navel) it should be dispersed downwards thorugh diuresis, using the herbs in this category.

The traditional Chinese concept of permeating wetness indicates not only the ability of herbs to eliminate fluid waste but also to properly hydrate bodily cells by effecting an electrolytic balance of sodium and potassium ions. Hence the herbs in this Chinese category are more specialized and would not include all herbs classed as diuretics in Western herbalism, though the most typical would be included here. Some herbs here are mild water-metabolism regulators, like poria, and safe for general use. Others are more powerful and good for acute conditions like stones. The stone-dissolving herbs are called lithotriptic. The strongest diuretics are classed as cathartic diuretics (see the laxative section).

When water retention is caused by kidney deficiency, additional kidney tonics may be required. When water retention is caused by internal cold, warming the yang or stimulant herbs may be necessary. It is not always effective to use water-reducing herbs to treat water retention. The whole condition must be examined and treated comprehensively.

According to Ayurveda, diuretics tend to reduce kapha (water). Most tend to reduce pitta (fire) by their capacity to drain damp-heat. However, they usually increase vata (air) and so must be used with care on individuals suffering from nervous or wasting disorders (vata diseases).

Ayurveda holds that flushing out the kidneys with diuretic herbs is an important therapy not only for treating disease but for maintaining health. It purifies the water element and prevents the buildup of toxins. It is used in Ayurveda for treating lower back pain, sciatica and kidney disorders.

Diuretic therapy is a form of attacking therapy, like purgation, but less strong. As such, it must be used with care when there is deficiency or debility. Diuretics are contraindicated for individuals with symptoms of fluid deficiency, wasting and dryness (particularly yin deficiency). As they can irritate the mucous membranes of the urinary tract they usually should be combined with demulcents like marshmallow, licorice or gelatin. This is required particularly when there is blood in the urine.

The role of Polypore Mushrooms in Normalizing Fluid Metabolism

To accomplish the dual function of eliminating excess fluid while increasing absorption into the deep tissues of the body, traditional Chinese medicine uses certain polypore mushrooms, including poria *(fu ling)* and grifola *(zhu ling)*. These are classified as having a bland and sweet taste and a relatively neutral energy. Many representatives of this family of mushrooms are abundant in our natural forests. Some, called shelf or punk mushrooms, have seldom been used by Western herbalists. A small one called *Coriolus versicolor,* however, currently is being used in Western countries, as well as in Japan and China, for its anticarcinogenic properties. These colorful mushrooms, known as "turkey tails" in the West, grow on the sides of decaying tree trunks. They may be dried and powdered and taken in dose of up to 20 gms. 3 times a day.

A related species, *Ganoderma lucidum (ling zhi)*, also has been shown to have antitumor properties. According to Chinese practitioners, their main actions are to regulate blood circulation and to relieve nervousness, insomnia and dizziness. They have been shown to be useful adjunctive treatments for AIDS and cancer. The use of these mushrooms for cancer is evidence of a traditional Chinese medical theory that holds that it often is a disease of "water-stagnation."

PORIA (Tuckahoe) (also called Hoelen and Fu ling)

Lycoperdon solidum (Gronovius), Polyporus tuberaster; Polyporaceae

Energetics: sweet, neutral
Organs/Meridians affected: heart, lung, spleen, stomach, kidney
Part used: the scletotium of the fungus. It usually is found adhering to the roots of pine trees.
Active constituents: tetracyclic triterpenic acid (eburicolic acid, pachymic acid), polysaccharide (pachyman), ergosterol, choline, fat, glucose, lipase, protease
Properties: diuretic, sedative, tonic
Uses: It eliminates excess fluid retention, aids tonification of chi by dispelling dampness, helps digestion, and calms the mind and emotions. It is good whenever a mild diuretic is needed and may be used safely by children, the elderly and the deficient. It is serviceable also in more excess conditions.

This is one of the many valuable North American therapeutic herbs that have fallen out of general use here. It was described more than 100 years ago in *King's Dispensatory* as follows: "Tuckahoe - A peculiar formation found upon fir- tree roots, believed to be an alteration of the same, produced by a fungus. It is found in the Southern portion of the United States, where it is known as Tuckahoe, or Indian Bread. It is also found throughout the Eastern U.S. and Canada and apparently in Europe where it is sold as food. In China, where it also grows, it is called fu-ling. It has a long or irregularly globose body, often weighing many pounds. It has a rugose, ashy-black surface, and a whitish, firm, but apparently spongy interior. It has a starchy appearance, internally and breaks into irregular fragments. The name 'tuckahoe' refers to the custom of searching for the mushroom by poking into the ground at the base of coniferous trees with the handle of a hoe. In China and Asia this mushroom is highly prized for its antitumor and antihepatitis effects and often cultivated. The large underground tuber, called a sclerotium is used medicinally. It contains pectose, glucose, gum, cellulose, nitrogen and salts."

Dosage: 6-18 gms. in decoction.

DANDELION LEAF   *Taraxacum officinale; Compositae*

Energetics: bitter, cold
Organs/Meridians affected: bladder, liver
Part used: leaf
Active constituents: taraxin, ceryl alcohol lactucerol, taraxacerin, inosite, choline, vitamins A and B, nicotinic acid, arnidiol and faradiol
Properties: diuretic, alterative
Uses: Dandelion leaf has been clinically tested and shown to be as effective a diuretic as any drug. It may be eaten steamed, or used as a healthful pot herb. It has a very high potassium and vitamins A and C content. Dandelion leaf is effective for bladder and kidney infections and hepatitis.
Dosage: standard infusion or 3-9 gms.

PARSLEY   *Petrosellinum sativum; Umbeliferae*

Energetics: sweet, bland, warm
Meridians/Organs affected: lung, stomach, bladder, liver
Parts used: seeds, leaf and root
Active constituents: the root contains essential oil, apiin, bergaptein, isoimperatorin, mucilage, sugar. The seeds are stronger in essential oil with apiol, myristicene, pinene and other terpenes, flavone glycoside apiin, furanocumarin bergapten, fatty oil and petroselinic acid; the leaves are similar but weaker in the above constituents.

Properties: diuretic, carminative, anthelmintic, stimulant, emmena-gogue (especially the seeds), expectorant
Uses: It is used for edema, fluid retention, frequent urination, bed-wetting, rheumatic complaints, menstrual disorders, indigestion, gas and intestinal worms.
Dosage: standard dosage or 3-9 gms.

CORIANDER   *Coriandrum sativum; Umbelliferae*

Energetics: spicy, neutral (seeds), cool (leaves)
Meridians/Organs affected: bladder, stomach
Parts used: leaves, seeds
Active constituents: essential oil which consists of a linalol called cori-androl (60 to 70%), geraniol, borneol and terpenes
Properties: carminative, aromatic, diuretic, diaphoretic
Uses: It is a specific for strengthening the urinary tract. Both the seeds and the leaves may be used in infusion for urinary tract infections. It also is good for stomach upset, indigestion and gas. Coriander is one of the basic ingredients in Indian curry, along with turmeric and cumin seed. The leaves, called cilantro, often are added to hot spicy dishes to offset the strong pungent flavors of Indian dishes.
Dosage: standard infusion or 3-9 gms.

BUCHU   *Barosma betulina; Rutaceae*

Energetics: pungent, warm
Meridians/Organs affected: bladder, stomach, lung
Part used: leaves
Active constituents: essential oil with barosma camphor
Properties: diuretic, aromatic, carminative, diaphoretic, stimulant
Uses: Buchu treats fluid retention, gravel, catarrh of the bladder, indigestion and bloat. It is found in the Southwest region of Cape Colony in South Africa, where its use was first learned of from the Hottentots. Buchu brandy is their stimulant tonic and stomach remedy, made by infusing it in brandy.
Dosage: A standard aqueous infusion is made from the leaves, and a half cup is taken three or four times daily; tincture, ½ to 1 teaspoon is taken three or four times daily; standard infusion in formulas, 3-9 gms.

PLANTAIN   *Plantago spp.; Plantaginaceae*

Energetics: bland, bitter, cold
Meridians/Organs affected: bladder, small intestine, gall bladder
Parts used: seeds, leaf
Active constituents: mucilage and a heteroside, aucuboside that hydro-lises into aucubine and sugar
Properties: diuretic, alterative, astringent, refrigerant, vulnerary
Uses: It treats urinary infections, hepatitis, and other inflammatory dis-eases. The leaves are used externally to stop bleeding and as an anti-inflammatory. Taken internally they are antitoxin.
Dosage: 5-10 gms. in infusion.

GRAVEL ROOT   *Eupatorium purpureum,*
                                            also Epigea repens; Compositae

Energetics: bitter, pungent, neutral
Meridians/Organs affected: kidney, bladder, stomach, liver
Part used: root
Active constituents: euparin, which is yellow, neutral and crystalline (C 12, H 11, O 3); eupurpurin is an oleoresin that is precipated from an alcoholic tincture of the herb
Properties: diuretic, lithotropic, nervine, carminative
Uses: It is used to treat fluid retention, frequent and night-time urina-tion and poor digestion. It also strengthens the nerves, dissolves and eliminates stones and treats hematuria (blood in the urine)
Dosage: Using an infusion or decoction, taking 1 cup every two hours for excess uric acid. Use one ounce to a pint of water or ½ to 1 teaspoon of the tincture three times daily. For chronic weakness, less may be used over a prolonged period. Standard decoction in formulas, 3-9 gms.

CLEAVERS (Bedstraw)   *Galium aparine; Rubiaceae*

Energetics: bitter, cool
Meridians/Organs affected: bladder, gall bladder
Part used: aerial portions
Active constituents: a glycoside, asperuloside

Properties: diuretic, alterative, aperient
Uses: It eliminates excess fluid, counteracts inflammations, and urinary infections, hepatitis and venereal disease. In the East Indies, the sucus (juice) of the herb taken in teaspoonful doses is considered a very effective treatment for gonorrhea. It is a blood purifier as well as an effective diuretic. Thus it is excellent for inflammations, both taken internally and applied topically in the form of a poultice. It has a good reputation as an external application for cancerous growths and tumors. A decoction sponged on the face with a soft cloth is useful for sunburn and freckles. A tea is considered excellent for the treatment of psoriasis and various skin diseases. The ancient Greeks matted it together to make a natural, rough sieve, supposedly for straining milk.
Dosage: standard infusion or 3-9 gms.

HYDRANGEA *Hydrangea arborescens; Saxifragaceae*

Energetics: pungent, cool
Meridians/Organs affected: kidney, bladder, colon **Part used:** root
Active constituents: two resins, gum, starch, sugar, albumen, soda, lime potassa, magnesia, sulphuric and phosphoric acids, a protosalt of iron and a glucoside, hydrangin. There seems to be no tannin present.
Properties: diuretic, lithotropic
Uses: It treats fluid retention and stone formation in the kidneys and bladder (for which it was extolled by the Cherokee Indians). It also is excellent for chronic penile discharge (non-specific urethritis) in men and mucousal urinary irritation in the aged.
Precautions: Overdose can cause vertigo and stuffiness in the chest (chi congestion).
Dosage: 30 grains of the root and 30-100 drops of the tincture; standard decoction in formulas or 3-9 gms.

PELLITORY OF THE WALL *Parrietoria officinalis; Urticaceae*

Energetics: acrid, cool
Meridians/Organs affected: bladder, kidney, colon

Part used: whole plant
Active constituents: contains nitre in abundance.
Properties: diuretic, laxative, refrigerant, demulcent
Uses: It treats fluid retention, stones and gravel, dropsy and other urinary complaints. It combines well with parsley or wild carrot seed or root. It counteracts mucus and is useful for chronic coughs.
Dosage: tincture 10-30 drops; standard infusion, 3-9 gms.

WATER PLANTAIN   *Alisma plantago; Alismaceae*

Energetics: sweet, bland, cold
Meridians/Organs affected: spleen, stomach, kidney, bladder
Part used: root
Active constituents: volatile oil, 23% starch, a very acrid resin
Properties: diuretic, antipyretic
Uses: It is used for fluid retention, urinary disorders, gravel and calculus, dysentery and epilepsy. Water plantain is commonly used in Chinese medicine and widely available in different areas of the United States where it ought to be harvested and made commercially available. It is useful in treating the weak and elderly for whom other diuretics may be too strong, and is particularly good for chronic urinary tract infections or yin deficient heat.
Dosage: 6-15 gms. in decoction.

COUCHGRASS   *Agropyron repens; Graminae*

Energetics: sweet, cool
Meridians/Organs affected: bladder, lung, heart, small intestine
Parts used: underground rhizome and stolons
Active constituents: a mucilaginous substance, triticine which is a fructosan, an antibiotic substance that is derived from agropyrene, vanilloside (glucovanilline) and mineral salts
Properties: diuretic, demulcent
Uses: Couchgrass is used for urinary infections, including cystitis, nephritis and urethritis. It also is useful for urinary calculi, gall stones and jaundice, as well as gout and rheumatic complaints. It is said to

clear damp heat in the lower warmer, according to Traditional Chinese Medicine.

This herb is considered to have equivalent properties and actions to *Juncus effusus* used in Chinese medicine.

Dosage: Given in the form of a standard infusion and taken three times daily.

WILD CARROT   *Daucus carota; Umbelliferae*

Energetics: sweet, pungent, warm
Meridians/Organs affected: spleen, kidney, stomach
Part used: root and seed
Active constituents: volatile oil and other unidentified constituents
Properties: diuretic, anthelmintic, carminative, emmenagogue, astringent
Uses: It treats fluid retention, chronic urinary tract problems, gout, jaundice, intestinal parasites, gas and indigestion. The seeds are more warming and stimulant and are useful for gas, hiccoughs, dysentery, chronic coughs and urinary calculus complaints. They also are useful for jaundice and gall bladder stones, as well as menstrual disorders.
Precautions: Contraindicated in pregnancy.
Dosage: standard dose in infusion, 3-9 gms.

KNOTWEED   *Polygonum aviculare; Polygonaceae*

Energetics: bitter, slightly cold
Meridians/Organs affected: bladder, small intestine
Part used: whole plant
Active constituents: silica, mucilage, tannins and various flavonic derivatives, quercitol and kaempferol
Properties: diuretic, lithotriptic, astringent, hemostatic, vulnerary
Uses: It is used for all urinary infections, pyelitis, stone formations in the urinary tract, jaundice, weeping eczema, mucus and bloody discharge from the urinary and reproductive organs of men and women, enteritis, diarrhea and dysentery. It also is used to treat bronchitis with bleeding.
Dosage: 9-15 gms. in decoction.

WATERMELON SEEDS
Citrullus vulgaris;
Cucurbitaceae

Energetics: bland, neutral
Meridians/Organs affected: bladder, stomach, heart, small intestine
Part used: seeds
Active constituents: Not specifically identified but the fruit contains amino acid, citrulline, aminoacetic acid, lycopene, carotene, vitamin C, bromine, fructose, dextrose, sucrose, malic acid and phosphoric acid.
Properties: diuretic, refrigerant, sialagogue
Uses: It is used to treat fluid retention, urinary inflammations, summer heat, dysentery, fever, dry heaves, thirst.
Dosage: 6-15 gms. in decoction.

UVA URSI
Arctostaphylos uva urse; Ericaceae

Energetics: bitter, astringent, cold
Meridians/Organs affected: heart, bladder, small intestine, liver
Part used: leaves
Active constituents: arbutin, methyl-arbutin, ericolin, ursone, gallic acid, ellagic acid myricetin, and a yellow principle resembling quercetin. Tannin is present up to 6 to 7 percent.
Properties: diuretic, astringent, antiseptic
Uses: It is used as a urinary antiseptic for bladder infections, and to treat blood in the urine, kidney infection and womb problems (very good as a post-partum remedy to prevent infections).
Dosage: 3-6 gms. Do not boil.

PIPSISSEWA
Chimaphilla umbellata; Ericaceae

Energetics: bitter, astringent, cool
Meridians/Organs affected: heart, bladder, small intestine, spleen
Part used: aerial portions.
Active constituents: ursolic acid, the glycosides arbutin, ericolin and chimophilin, excreted in the urine as disinfectant substances similar to uva ursi
Properties: diuretic, alterative, astringent

Uses: It has the same properties as uva ursi but far fewer tannins, making it superior in treating urinary problems, arthritis and most other conditions in which either of these herbs might be used. It aids liver and kidney detoxification and helps the heart by eliminating excess fluid.

Dosage: standard infusion or 3-9 gms.

WATERCRESS   *Nasturtium officinalis; Cruciferae*

Energetics: spicy, bitter, warm
Meridians/Organs affected: kidneys, bladder, stomach, lungs
Parts used: flowers, leaves
Active constituents: vitamins A, B2, C; minerals iodine, iron, phosphorus, manganese, copper, zinc, calcium, sulphur
Properties: diuretic, expectorant, laxative, stimulant, stomachic, nutritive.
Uses: It is used to treat fluid retention, mucus in the lungs and indigestion. It also stimulates metabolism, promotes bile metabolism and helps dispel gas.
Dosage: standard infusion, 3-9 gms.

AZUKI BEAN (Aduki bean) *Phaseolus calcaratus; Leguminosae*

Energetics: sweet, sour, neutral
Meridians/Organs affected: spleen, heart, small intestine
Part used: bean
Active constituents: protein, fat, carbohydrates, nicotinic acid, vitamin B 1, B 2, calcium iron, potassium
Properties: diuretic, alterative, nutritive
Uses: It is used to treat urinary problems, urinary infections, edema, suppurative skin infections and eczema.
Dosage: 9-30 gms. in decoction.

CORN SILK   *Zea mays; Graminae*

Energetics: sweet, bland, neutral
Meridians/Organs affected: bladder, small intestine, liver
Part used: stylus
Active constituents: cryptoxanthin, resin, saponins, alkaloids, ascorbic acid, vitamin K, sitotsterol, stigmasterol, malic acid, palmitic acid, tartaric acid, oxalic acid, pantothenic acid
Properties: diuretic, lithotriptic, cholagogue
Uses: It treats edema, urinary dysfunction, urinary tract stones, jaundice and hypertension. Even though it is effective for kidney stones, it is one of the milder and safer diuretics. This is an example of a Western herb currently being incorporated into the Chinese herbal system.
Dosage: 6-20 gms.

ANTIRHEUMATICS
(Herbs for Dispelling Wind and Damp)

Antirheumatics are used to counteract arthritic and rheumatic joint pains. Some are cool and anti-inflammatory, others possess a spicy warm stimulating property. These properties describe what is therapeutically required to treat arthritic and rheumatic complaints, respectively: one being a condition of poor circulation while the other is one of congestion and inflammation.

Draft or *wind* in Chinese medicine refers to diseases that are manifested primarily by the nervous system and characterized by spasmodic pains and derangement of movement. *Damp* is the congestion of fluids, primarily lymphatic fluid, that can increase and become aggravated by excessively damp foods and climate. According to Chinese medicine when wind-damp blocks the channels of energy circulation it causes pain which condition Western medicine calls arthritis. Though wind-damp usually is associated with cold, which causes contraction, it can become heat through stagnation. When wind is the major factor in blockage of the channels, the pain is migratory and fluctuating. When damp is the chief factor, the pain is associated with swelling and water retention. When heat is the chief factor, the pain is fixed and severe. When heat is the main factor, there is inflammation and feverishness. Different types of arthritis are distinguished according to these symptoms.

The herbs in this category possess combinations of diaphoretic, diuretic, anti-inflammatory, antispasmodic and stimulant actions. Many are related to warming diaphoretic herbs. Some strengthen the tendons, ligaments and bones and have a tonic action.

In the Ayurvedic system, most of these herbs would be said to reduce kapha (dampness) and regulate vata (wind). They also are anti-ama, ama being a more toxic type of mucus described by one practitioner as attaching itself to the nerves. Ayurveda calls arthritis *ama-vata,* a toxic wind condition.

As arthritis may create or be based upon an underlying deficiency, tonification also may be required in treating it. The herbs in this category more specifically target the pain of arthritis. Herbs from other categories may be necessary for additional action, such as improving circulation (blood-moving herbs). As a general rule, holistic treatment is best.

These herbs are contraindicated for deficient and wasting diseases, owing to their reducing and drying nature.

GUIACUM   *Guiacum officinalis; Zygophyllaceae*

Energetics: bitter, cool
Meridians/Organs affected: lungs, colon, bladder
Parts used: resin, bark and wood
Active constituents: volatile oil, resin, but otherwise not identified
Properties: antispasmodic, diaphoretic, diuretic, stimulant
Uses: It is used to treat rheumatism, arthritis, gout, catarrh, syphilis and skin diseases
Dosage: 30-60 grains of wood shavings; resin, 5-15 grains; standard decoction in formulas for bark and wood

POLYPODY FERN   *Polypodium vulgare; Polypodiaceae*

Energetics: bitter, sweet, warm
Meridians/Organs affected: liver, kidney
Part used: rhizome
Active constituents: a resinous bitter principle; essential oils; a sweet, sugary mucilage
Properties: diuretic, antirheumatic, anthelmintic, carminative, vulnerary
Uses: It treats arthritic pains in the limbs and lower lumbar region. It is applied externally as a poultice or liniment for trauma and injury, growths and excrescenses.
Dosage: 5-10 gms. in decoction

WINTERGREEN   *Gaultheria procumbens; Ericaceae*

Energetics: spicy, warm
Meridians/Organs affected: liver, lungs
Part used: leaves
Active constituents: glycoside, gaultherin (which is comprised of about 99% methyl salicylate) an enzyme gaultherase, aldehyde 1 alcohol, 1 ester, tannin, wax and mucilage
Properties: antirheumatic, antispasmodic, anodyne, diuretic, antiseptic, expectorant, rubefacient
Uses: It is both applied externally and taken internally to relieve pain and allay rheumatic complaints. The leaves contain methol salicylate which has anti-inflammatory properties similar to aspirin, making it useful for a wide variety of painful syndromes from headaches to arthritis. It also is used for urinary problems, as a gargle for sore throat and as a decongestant for the lungs. It is one of the most commonly used ingredients, worldwide, in analgesic oils and balms.
Dosage: standard infusion or 3-9 gms.

BLACK COHOSH   *Cimicifuga racemosa;*
Ranunculaceae

Energetics: sweet, pungent, slightly bitter, cool
Meridians/Organs affected: liver, spleen, stomach, large intestine
Part used: root
Active constituents: various glycosides such as actaeine, cimicifugin, bitter principles racemosin, estrogenic substances, triterpenes, isoferulic acid, tannin
Properties: antispasmodic, expectorant, emmenagogue, diaphoretic, alterative
Uses: It is useful for rheumatic and arthritic complaints accompanied by feelings of heaviness. It also is used to ripen and bring out skin rashes such as measles. In Chinese medicine it is used to raise the chi and counteract prolapsed conditions of the stomach, intestines, bladder and uterus. It improves blood circulation and is used in treating delayed and painful menses. Combined with other parturient herbs such as

squaw vine and raspberry, it is used during the last two weeks of pregnancy to facilitate childbirth. Black cohosh is classified in traditional Chinese medicine as a cooling diaphoretic but it is used more by Western herbalists for its antispasmodic properties.

Dosage: 2 tsp. of dried root in a pint of water, take 2 or 3 tbsp. 6X daily, cool; tincture, 10-60 drops; standard decoction in formulas, 3-9 gms.

DEVIL'S CLAW
(Grapple plant)

Harpagophytum procumbens; Pedeliaceae

Energetics: bitter, cool
Meridians/Organs affected: liver, stomach
Part used: root (preferably secondary root)
Active constituents: blycoside, hapagosie, hapagide, procumbine, sugar, stachyose
Properties: anti-inflammatory, antirheumatic
Uses: Devil's claw treats arthritis, rheumatism, diabetes, stomach disorders
Dosage: powder, tsp. is taken three times daily; tincture, 10-30 drops four times a day; standard dosage in formulas, 3-9 gms.

WHITE BRYONY

Bryonia alba and B. dioica; Cucurbitae

Energetics: bitter, warm, toxic
Meridians/Organs affected: spleen, liver
Part used: mostly the root
Active constituents: resin (bryoresin), a bitter glucoside (bryonine); the stems and leaves contain an alkaloid (bryonicine); the toxic berries a carotenoid pigment (lycopin)
Properties: antirheumatic, analgesic
Uses: It treats connective tissue pain anywhere in the body and rheumatic pains in the chest caused by fluid accumulation and chronic cough. It is good for pleurisy, bronchitis, pneumonia, blood-streaked expectoration and glandular enlargements with chronic inflammations. It is the remedy for inflammation of the serous tissues and is also useful for peritonitis and synovial inflammations. It will help to control the

cough and pain associated with influenza. It is particularly useful for conditions that are caused by cold.

It is most safely and widely used in homeopathic medicine where its specific indications are symptoms aggravated by motion. This is in contrast to *Rhus toxicodendron* (poison ivy), whose symptoms are ameliorated by movement. This tends to indicate its use for phlegmatic individuals with a tendency towards lethargy.

Precautions: White bryony is quite toxic and irritating and will cause blisters when in contact with the skin; although a plaster of the crushed roots serves as a soothing rubefacient and may be used in place of a mustard plaster. It can cause uncontrollable diarrhea, gastrointestinal inflammation, vomiting, vertigo, reduction of temperature, and even eventual collapse and death.

Dosage: While it is safest to use homeopathically, the Eclectics successfully used it internally for all the above conditions by mixing 5-20 drops of Bryonia tincture to four ounces of water. Of this a teaspoon is taken three or four times daily. Of the tincture, no more than a fraction to one drop is taken at a time.

POISON OAK, POISON IVY
Rhus toxicodendron; Anacardiaceae

Energetics: acrid, bitter, hot
Meridians/Organs affected: liver
Part used: leaves
Active constituents: toxicondendrol and a yellow resin, toxicondendrin
Properties: toxic, rubefacient, antirheumatic
Uses: The fresh leaves may be made into a fluid extract, which is particularly helpful for stiffness associated with arthritis and rheumatism; its classical indications for use being conditions that improve with movement. It also is specifically indicated for conditions associated with edema. Edema can occur when the supply of blood to an area is inadequate, causing an excess of histamines and serous fluids to accumulate.

Precautions: It should not be overused internally as it can cause gastric irritation, drowsiness, stupor and delirium.

Direct contact with practically any part of the plant can cause a severe rash, Although some people have a natural immunity to it. There are many remedies for poison oak dermatitis, including grindelia used as an external wash, impatiens juice applied externally, a wash of yellow dock root tea, a tea of willow bark taken internally, and an external wash of mugwort. One of the most effective remedies for poison oak rash is tincture of echinacea both taken internally and applied externally.

Dosage: The tincture may be taken in doses of 5-30 drops according to Grieve, the smaller doses being more sedative. The best preparation is from the fresh green plant using 1 to 4 strength. The dose of 25% tincture is given in 1-5 drops three times a day.

YUCCA   *Yucca spp.; Liliaceae*

Energetics: sweet, bland, cool
Meridians/Organs affected: liver, stomach
Part used: root
Active constituents: saponins
Properties: anti-inflammatory, antirheumatic, laxative, alterative
Uses: Yucca is used for arthritis, rheumatism, gout, urethritis and prostatitis. Herbalist Michael Moore is the principal authority for information in the use of this and other plants of the North American desert and Western mountain regions. The most important variety of yucca is a desert plant sometimes known as Spanish bayonet. Its root has a high content of natural saponins. When it is chopped up in water it makes a natural lather and is an effective soap substitute. It may be added to shampoo or used by itself for washing hair. One half to a cup of the chopped fresh or dried root is boiled in one and a half cups of water until suds form.

Perhaps it is these same saponins that account for the effective anti-inflammatory action of yucca in the treatment of arthritis and rheumatism. In some clinics in the Sonoran desert region of Arizona, yucca is the remedy routinely prescribed against arthritis, with impressive results. The root is split lengthwise before drying (it should be used only after it has been dried). At one time it was considered an important source of phytosterols and used in the manufacturing of steroidal hormones. According to Michael Moore, one-fourth ounce of the dried root boiled in a pint of water for fifteen minutes may be taken in three or four doses throughout the day. It has the ability of relieving pain for several days.

A good general arthritis formula is as follows:

Yucca root (6pts.)   Prickly ash bark (2 pts.)
Devil's claw (4 pts.)   Ginger root (2 pts.)
Black cohosh root (3 pts.)   Licorice root (2 pts.)

Make into a standard decoction and take one cup two or three times daily.

Precautions: Occasionally there are some purgative side effects that may be accompanied by intestinal cramping. This can be prevented by adding as an antidote some ginger and prickly ash bark, which also will aid its antiarthritic properties. Long term use is said to slow absorption of fat-soluble vitamins, but these findings require further study.
Dosage: The quantity of yucca root taken by itself is about one-half ounce per day.

COCKLEBUR   *Xanthium strumarium; Compositae*

Energetics: sweet, bitter, warm
Meridians/Organs affected: lung
Part used: fruit
Active constituents: Xanthostrumarin, resin, fatty oil, alkaloids, organic acid, vitamin C, ceryl alcohol
Properties: antispasmodic, diuretic, analgesic, alterative, antibacterial, antifungal
Uses: Cocklebur is used to treat arthritis and rheumatism, to open the nasal passages and sinuses, for allergic rhinitis with headache, chronic lumbago, leprosy and pruritis (severe itching) of the skin. This herb is very obnoxious to contact in its natural state, as the seed pods tend to

adhere to animal fur and human clothing. It is, however, a very valuable therapeutic agent widely used by the Chinese for rheumatic aches and pains as well as sinus blockage.
Dosage: 5-10 gms. in decoction

CLEMATIS   *Clematis spp.; Ranunculaceae*

Energetics: spicy, salty, warm
Meridians/Organs affected: bladder
Part used: root and stem
Active constituents: anemorin, anemonol, protoanemonin, oleanolic acid
Properties: antirheumatic, analgesic, antispasmodic, stimulant
Uses: It circulates blood and chi, treats arthritis, rheumatism and stiffness, dilates blood vessels, and relieves headaches. This is very important herb for arthritis in traditional Chinese medicine.
Dosage: 3-12 gms. in decoction (usually with complementary herbs, such as angelica, which also activate circulation of the vessels and channels)

CHINESE QUINCE   *Chaenomelis lagenariae or*
                                      Cydonia oblonga; Rosaceae

Energetics: sour, slightly warm
Meridians/Organs affected: liver, spleen
Part used: fruit
Active consituents: mucins, amygdalin, hydrocyanic acid, enzyme emulsion, vitamin C, malic, tartaric and citric acids, fatty oil, tannin, protein
Properties: antirheumatic, anti-inflammatory, laxative, analgesic, astringent, tonic
Uses: Quince is used for ligament pains, congestion of the blood and nerve channels, weakness in the lower back and extremities, severe cramping pains, abdominal pains, spasms of the calves and swelling of the legs
Dosage: 3-12 gms. in decoction

KAVA KAVA
Piper methysticum; Peperaceae

Energetics: pungent, bitter, warm
Meridians/Organs affected: liver, kidneys
Part used: root
Active constituents: resin including lactones, kawahin, yangonin, methysticin, glycosides, starch
Properties: analgesic, antispasmodic, antiseptic, sedative, diuretic, tonic
Uses: It relieves pain in rheumatic complaints, and alleviates insomnia and nervousness. It is used as an intoxicating beverage in certain South Sea islands. It can induce lethargy, drowsiness and dreams. Kava kava is one of the best pain-relieving herbs.
Dosage: 4 tbsp. simmered 10 minutes in 1 pint of water; standard dosage in formulas, 3-9 gms.

BIRCH
Betula alba or *B. lenta; Betulaceae*

Energetics: spicy, warm
Meridians/Organs affected: stomach, spleen
Part used: bark and leaf buds
Active constituents: saponins, traces of essential oil, tannin, bitter principle, glycosides
Properties: antirheumatic, stimulant, astringent, diuretic, anthelmintic
Uses: Birch treats rheumatism, boils, urinary problems and intestinal worms
Dosage: One teaspoon of the inner bark or leaf buds is steeped in a cup of boiling water; one to two cups is taken daily. Of the tincture, -½ teaspoon is taken three times a day. Standard dosage in infusion, 3-9 gms.

MEADOWSWEET
Filipendula ulmaria; Rosaceae

Energetics: bitter, astringent, cool
Meridians/Organs affected: liver, bladder, colon
Part used: aerial portions
Active constituents: salicylic aldehyde and spireine both in the form of a glycoside; methyl salicylate, gaultherine and spiraeoside, a flavonoid glycoside, sugar and tannin

Properties: antirheumatic, analgesic, diaphoretic, diuretic, astringent, antispasmodic
Uses: It is used for gout, rheumatism, arthritis, fever and urinary tract infections
Dosage: ½-1 tsp. of fluid extract; in infusion 3-6 gms.

JEFFERSONIA   *Jeffersonia diphylla; Berbidaceae*

Energetics: bitter, acrid, warm
Meridians/Organs affected: liver, kidney
Part used: rhizome
Active constituents: bitter substance, an acrid and nauseating constituent, pectin, fatty resin, tannic acid, gum, starch, sugar and mineral matters
Properties: antirheumatic, alterative, diuretic, antispasmodic, diaphoretic
Uses: It is used to treat chronic rheumatism, nervousness, excitability, tension, spasms and cramps, It also is effective for inflammatory symptoms, sore throat, ulcers, ophthalmia and indolent ulcers. It may be used during pregnancy for any of the above conditions. It is specifically indicated for head pains with dizziness and feelings of tension.
Dosage: 10 drops to 1 tsp. of the tincture; in decoction, 3-9 gms.

PINE   *Pinus tabulaeformis* and *P. sylvestris; Pinaceae*

Energetics: bitter, warm
Meridians/Organs affected: liver, kidney
Part used: knots in the wood
Active constituents: lingin, a-pinene, camphene. The oil of P. sylvestris contains terebenthine and the young resinous branches contain oil consisting of esters, phellandrene and pinene. It also produces various glycosides (pinicrine, piceine and coniferoside).
Properties: analgesic, antispasmodic, stimulant
Uses: The knot of the wood is used in decoction with dong quai *(Angelica sinensis)* and angelica for rheumatoid arthritis. It also is used in com-

bination with such other herbs as clematis, acanthopanax, quince and mulberry branches. Other pines possess similar properties, particularly in the resin, but also to some extent in the leaves. The oil of pine makes one of the most effective external treatments for local relief of rheumatism, sciatica, chronic bronchitis, coughs, pneumonia (applied over the chest) and nephritis.

Dosage: 9-15 gms. in decoction

MULBERRY BRANCH   *Morus alba; Moraceae*

Energetics: bitter, sweet, slightly cold
Meridians/Organs affected: liver
Part used: small branches
Active constituents: mulberrin, fructose, glucose, arabinose, xylose, stachyose, sucrose
Properties: antirheumatic, antispasmodic, diuretic, alterative
Uses: It is used for rheumatic and arthritic pains, especially through the extremities of the body. A native Chinese plant, it is a common ornamental tree in this country.
Dosage: 15-30 gms. in decoction

STAR JASMINE   *Trachelospermum jasminoides;*
Apocynaceae

Energetics: bitter, cool
Meridians/Organs affected: liver, kidney
Parts used: stem and leaves
Active constituents: resinous substance, fatty material, tannins, glycosides. The stem is mildly toxic.
Properties: antirheumatic, analgesic, emmenagogue
Uses: Star jasmine treats rheumatic and arthritic pains and inflammation and spasm. It also is used as an alterative for poisonous sores, ulcers and painful abscesses. It may be combined with other alterative, anti-inflammatory agents, such as echinacea and honeysuckle, to treat pain and spasms in the extremities. It may be combined with other antispasmodics and nervines to relieve pain and spasms. In combina-

tion with dandelion and echinacea, it is used to treat boils and abscesses. It is a common ornamental in warmer regions of this country.

Dosage: 6-15 gms. in decoction

RHEUMATISM GINSENG   *Acanthopanax gracilistylus and spp.; Araliaceae*

Energetics: acrid, sweet, warm
Meridians/Organs affected: liver, kidney
Part used: bark of the root
Active consituents: essential oils including 4-methyl salicyladehyde, palmitic and linoleic acid, tannin, vitamins A and B 1
Properties: antirheumatic, analgesic, diuretic, antispasmodic, tonic
Uses: A close relative of Siberian ginseng, it is very beneficial for rheumatic and arthritic complaints. It is usually available at Chinese pharmacies and also is an excellent treatment for other complaints of the elderly. In China it is often soaked in rice wine and sold as Wu Jia Pi wine. The alcohol enhances its circulating properties and a small amount is taken daily, especially through the cold seasons. It is also variously combined with clematis, angelica, teasel and blue gentian for pains and muscular spasms. It strengthens the tendons, ligaments and bones.
Precautions: Because of its circulating properties it should be used cautiously for those with wasting and deficient heat symptoms.
Dosage: 3-15 gms. in decoction
(see *Eleutherococcus senticosus* under chi tonics, pg. 290)

SNAKE (Rattlesnake)

Energetics: sweet, salty, poisonous
Meridians/Organs affected: liver, spleen
Properties: antirheumatic, antispasmodic, analgesic, alterative
Uses: It increases flexibility of the sinews and treats various kind of rashes, stroke, spasms, tremors, seizures and facial paralysis.

Some acupuncturists and Chinese herbalists keep snakes pickled in alcohol. They will keep indefinitely in a covered wide-mouthed jar. A good quality vodka may be used, in the amount required to fully cover the freshly killed animal. When pickling the rattlesnake it might be safer to remove the head where the poisonous venom is held. There is reason to believe that a small amount of this venom enhances the therapeutic properties of the remedy, but until this is demonstrated conclusively removing the head is recommended. Non-poisonous snakes are considered to have similar but milder properties, so larger amounts may be taken. The non-poisonous snakes have a more neutral energy.

Dosage: tincture is administered in teaspoonful doses two or three times a day.

STIMULANTS
(Herbs for Warming the Interior and Eliminating Cold)

Herbal stimulants are used to raise the general vitality of the body. They disperse internal congestion, relieve coldness and aid circulation of blood and energy. These actions make them a good first treatment for many acute ailments in which raising vitality might be useful for overcoming the disease.

While coffee, tea and other substances containing caffeine may be used as stimulants to overcome the toxic effects of sedative drug poisoning, they tend to charge the adrenals and thus deplete the body's reserves. Spicy warm food-like stimulants, like ginger and cayenne, contain some nutritive properties, so their tendency to deplete reserves is less. Yet overuse of them, too, can be depleting.

The herbs in this category are said to *warm the yang*. They revive weakened organic functions and are particularly good for conditions of shock, collapse and pallor. They are used to revive the the heart and the pulse, as well as to rekindle the digestive fire. For upper warmer (lungs and heart) we would use herbs such as cayenne and ginger; for middle warmer (digestion) we would use herbs like ginger, red and black peppers, fennel seed and anise; for lower warmer organs we would use aconite, cinnamon and cayenne; for improving circulation any of the above might be used, but most often prickly ash.

In Ayurvedic *tridosha* theory, the stimulant herbs in this category are pro-pitta (fire) and therefore anti-kapha (mucus). Many have expectorant properties and are good for burning up phlegm and toxins. They should be used carefully in vata conditions, as they can create feelings of nervousness and anxiety. They are considered to be the hottest of all herbs, with the nature of fire; and like fire they can burn as well as give us warmth. They aid the digestive fire, agni, or digest food for us when our agni is weak.

They are contraindicated in conditions of yin deficiency, wasting diseases and symptoms of dryness and heat.

(See also section on warming therapy, pg. 99)

CAYENNE PEPPER   *Capsicum frutescens; Solanaceae*

Energetics: spicy, hot
Meridians/Organs affected: kidney, lungs, spleen, stomach, heart
Part used: the ripe fruits
Active constituents: a pungent alkaloid called capsaicine, a red carotenoid pigment, capsanthine, several vitamins including vitamins A and C
Properties: stimulant, expectorant, astringent, hemostatic
Uses: It warms the center, aids digestion, decongests the lungs, circulates chi and blood, stops bleeding and stimulates kidney yang (sympathetic immune system). Begin with small to moderate doses, gradually increasing the amount used. Thus the gastrointestinal tract will be able to adjust by increasing the amount of mucus coating the stomach lining. If used carefully in this way, cayenne pepper can heal stomach ulcers.
Dosage: 1-3 grams in decoction; powder, 500 mg.

BLACK PEPPER   *Piper nigrum; Piperaceae*

Energetics: spicy, hot
Meridians/Organs affected: kidneys, spleen, stomach
Part used: the fruits
Active constituents: essential oil that contains phellandrene, two acrid

resins, hot tasting amides, 5-9% piperine; piperidine and aromatic acids
Properties: stimulant, digestive
Uses: It is used for food congestion, weak digestion, coldness, poor circulation, and to dry mucus. It is an herb which, like pippli long pepper, is of singular importance as a metabolic stimulant in Ayurvedic medicine. Black pepper, pippli long pepper and ginger root are the three basic Trikatu herbs which are ground into a powder and mixed with honey to form a paste. This paste is taken in quarter to full teaspoon doses with a little hot water three times a day. It is used to counteract cold, damp symptoms and to stimulate digestion and warmth. Black pepper has the ability to recirculate vital nutrients. When fasting, grind seven peppercorns and take them mixed with a little honey each morning. Black pepper is a stimulant to the gastric mucosa and is less irritating than cayenne. While Traditional Chinese Medicine does not consider it to work on the kidney meridian, this action may be inferred from its Ayurvedic use.
Dosage: 2-5 gms.

PIPPLI LONG PEPPER   *Piper longum; Piperaceae*

Energetics: spicy, hot
Meridians/Organs affected: spleen, stomach, lungs, kidney
Part used: the fruits
Active constituents: 0.9% volatile oil which is very similar to piper nigrum, 0.19% piperine (an alkaloid)
Properties: stimulant, digestive, analgesic, decongestant
Uses: It counteracts coldness, aids circulation of chi and blood, relieves pain from swelling, aids digestion, dries mucus, treats vomiting, headache, toothache (applied locally) and rhinitis (inflamation of the nasal mucosa). Its drying action makes it of particular value in drying up clear discharges. In Ayurveda it is considered to be rejuvenative to the lungs (prepared in milk) and for kapha (water) types generally.
Dosage: 2-5 gms.

FENNEL SEED   *Foeniculum vulgare; Umbelliferae*

Energetics: spicy, sweet, warm
Meridians/Organs affected: spleen, stomach, liver, kidney
Part used: fruit
Active constituents: 3-4% volatile oil including 50-60% anethole, 20% fenchone, pinene, phellandrene, camphene cymene, limonene, dipentene, fatty oil (oleic acid, petroselinic acid), stigmasterol, 7-hydrozycoumarin
Properties: stimulant, carminative, antispasmodic, expectorant
Uses: It is used in treating indigestion, gas and flatulence, spasms of the gastrointestinal tract and abdominal pains; increases peristalsis of the stomach and intestines; and helps bring up phlegm from the lungs. It is very effective for cancer patients after radiation and chemotherapy. Dry-roasted it relieves pain of the testes and urinary bladder. Mixed with salt it lowers chi and with wine raises it. It is perhaps the mildest and safest of the herbs in this category to use.
Dosage: 3-9 gms.

PRICKLY ASH   *Xanthoxylum americanum; Rutaceae*

Energetics: spicy, warm and diffusing
Meridians/Organs affected: spleen, stomach, kidney
Part used: the bark
Active constituents: volatile oil, fat, sugar, gum acrid resin, a bitter alkaloid which may be berberine and a xanthoxylin
Properties: stimulant, analgesic, alterative, anthelmintic, astringent
Uses: It promotes capillary circulation, warms the body and circulation, relieves gastralgia (stomach pain) and dyspepsia caused by coldness and vomiting, stops diarrhea; treats rheumatic complaints, toothaches, swellings and injuries, applied internally or externally. The berries of the Chinese variety are called brown peppercorns or Sichuan pepper and used in Sichuan cooking. As the berries have a higher percentage of volatile oils, their properties are considered to be stronger. Western herbalists usually use the bark.
Dosage: 2-5 gms.

GINGER (dried)   *Zingiberis officinale; Zingiberaceae*

Energetics: spicy, hot
Meridians/Organs affected: heart, lung, spleen, stomach, kidney
Part used: the rhizome
Active constituents: volatile oil (1-3%) called zingerone, camphene, phellandrene, cineol, borneol, citral, gingerol and an acrid resin
Properties: stimulant, antispasmodic, carminative, emmenagogue
Uses: Dried ginger is considered to be more of an internal warming stimulant while fresh ginger is used more as a warming diaphoretic. It is one of the best herbs to use for nausea and vomiting and is said to warm the center (stomach), aid digestion and assimilation, relieve cold spasms and cramps, and promote menses. it is one of the most widely beneficial warming stimulants.
Dosage: 3-9 gms.

ANISE SEED   *Pimpinella anisum; Umbelliferae*

Energetics: spicy, warm
Meridians/Organs affected: stomach, liver, spleen, kidney
Part used: the seeds
Active constituents: essential oil with anethole, choline, fatty oil
Properties: stimulant, carminative, antispasmodic, expectorant
Uses: Its uses are very similar to those of fennel seed (see above). It also is useful as an expectorant for coughs.
Dosage: 3-9 gms.

STAR ANISE   *Illicium anisatum; Magnoliaceae*

Energetics: spicy, warm
Meridians/Organs affected: stomach, spleen, kidney
Part used: the fruit
Active constituents: anethole, anisaldehyde, methychavicol, anisic acid, anisyl acetone, phellandrene, pinene, cineole, limonene, safrole
Properties: stimulant, carminative, analgesic, upward rising energy
Uses: It warms the abdomen, dispels gas, regulates energy, treats belching, vomiting, abdominal pains, and hernia.
Dosage: 3 to 9 gms.

CLOVES   *Caryophyllus aromaticus; Myrtaceae*

Energetics: spicy, warm
Meridians/Organs affected: kidney, spleen and stomach
Part used: the flower-bud
Active constituents: clove oil is comprised of eugenol, caryophyllene, acetyl eugenol, tannin, wax and fat
Properties: stimulant, anti-nauseous, carminative, expectorant
Uses: It warms and aids digestion, allays nausea, helps chi descend, stops hiccoughs and vomiting caused by stomach coldness, and treats kidney-yang deficient impotence
Dosage: 2-5 gms.

CINNAMON BARK   *Cinnamomum cassia; Lauraceae*

Energetics: spicy, sweet, hot
Meridians/Organs affected: spleen, kidney, liver and urinary bladder
Part used: the bark
Active constituents: essential oil including phellandrene, eugenol, cinnamic aldehyde, methuleugenol; mucilage, tannin, sucrose and starch
Properties: stimulant, analgesic, astringent, carminative
Uses: It raises vitality, warms and stimulates all the vital functions of the body, counteracts congestion, is antirheumatic, stops diarrhea, improves digestion, relieves abdominal spasms, aids the peripheral circulation of the blood. Cinnamon is the second most widely used warming stimulant in Chinese medicine, used by Chinese herbalists much as Western herbalists have used cayenne.
Precautions: It is contraindicated for pregnant women or individuals with wasting and dryness, and signs of heat and fire.
Dosage: 3-9 gms.

BAYBERRY   *Myrica cerifera; Myricaceae*

Energetics: spicy, astringent, warm
Meridians/Organs affected: spleen, lungs, liver
Part used: the bark
Active constituents: volatile oil, starch, lignin, albumen, gum, tannic and gallic acids, acrid and astringent resins, an acid resembling saponin

Properties: stimulant, astringent, expectorant
Uses: It warms and aids circulation of chi and blood, dissolves and inhibits discharges, is good for treating fevers, colds and flu, diarrhea, bowel inflammation, excessive menstrual bleeding and uterine discharge. Bayberry bark powder makes an excellent toothpowder, combined with cinnamon bark powder, myrrh, salt, and echinacea root
Dosage: 3-9 gms.

ACONITE (Monkshood)   *Aconitum napellus;*
Ranunculaceae

Energetics: pungent, sweet, very hot, toxic
Meridians/Organs affected: heart, spleen, kidney
Part used: specially prepared root
Active constituents: aconitine, one of the fastest acting and deadliest alkaloids known
Properties: stimulant, cardiotonic, analgesic
Uses: The root was formerly much used in minute dosage of from $\frac{1}{30}$th to ½ drop of 10% tincture. It is much safer for the lay person to use in homeopathic doses. Aconite is a fine remedy to be taken at the first sign of acute diseases every 15 minutes until symptoms show improvement. It also is used for extreme fear and shock. It is one of the finest metabolic stimulants known. The homeopathic dose should be about 6X to 30X potency.

Chinese herbalism uses it as their most potent metabolic stimulant. They first render it relatively harmless by soaking the whole roots in vinegar for a month, then in salt water for another month, alternating and repeating the process three times. This is said to diminish the effect of the toxic alkaloids in aconite. If aconite tea causes a numbing sensation in the mouth, this is an indication that its toxicity has not been neutralized and that it should not be used.

In the prepared form, aconite is sold as *Aconitum praeparata* (fu zi). As the most yang herb, it is one of the most important of all Chinese herbs. It is frequently combined with ginger, cinnamon bark and *Atractylodes alba* to make a powerful internally warming formula for raising the metabolism in yin-cold conditions.

Ayurveda also prepares a similar form of aconite and uses it in much the same way.

Dosage: In minute homeopathic dosage or 3-9 gms. of specially prepared aconite.

HORSERADISH   *Amoracia lapathifolia; Cruciferae*

Energetics: spicy, hot
Meridians/Organs affected: lungs, colon, kidney
Part used: the root
Active constituents: essential oil with mustard oil, enzymes, glycosides, vitamin B, asparagin, thiocyanogen compounds and vitamin B
Properties: stimulant, diuretic, rubefacient, expectorant, laxative
Uses: It is used in treating gout, rheumatic diseases, bladder infections, colitis, phlegm, damp lung problems, sinus congestion, asthma, and added to baths for chilblains. For rheumatism take 3-4 tablespoons of horseradish daily with apple cider vinegar and honey. For colitis caused by putrefaction, take 15-20 drops of horseradish juice between meals. To decongest the sinuses chew one teaspoon of grated horseradish root that has been mixed with a tablespoon of apple cider vinegar until all the flavor is gone. Grated horseradish root topically applied acts as a counterirritant for injuries and bruises.

Since horseradish is only effective in its fresh state, various preparations are typically made to preserve its medicinal properties. A simple preparation is made by macerating grated horseradish in equal parts of apple cider vinegar and honey for a couple of weeks. This may be taken internally as a tincture or rubbed on externally as a liniment.

Without having its odor, horseradish has most of the advantages of garlic, including being high in sulphur (the antibiotic principle) and good for digestion, rheumatism and circulation. Syrup of horseradish is made by steeping a tablespoon of grated horseradish root in a cup of boiling water and covering it for two hours. The horseradish is then strained out and either sugar or honey is added. Heat until a thick syrupy consistency is achieved. Bottle for use.

Precautions: As horseradish is very hot, it is contraindicated for heat and dryness syndromes.

Dosage: Take a tablespoon every two hours at the first sign of a cold or flu or for any of the above conditions

GALANGAL   *Alpinia officinarum; Zingiberaceae*

Energetics: pungent, hot

Meridians/Organs affected: spleen, stomach

Part used: rhizome

Active constituents: essential oil including cineole, methyl cinnamate, eucalyptol, eugenol, pinene, cadinene; flavonoid comprised of galangin, kaempferide, alpinin; galangol

Properties: stimulant, carminative

Uses: It is regarded by the Chinese as the best herb for relieving cold stomach pains, cold-type vomiting, dyspepsia, gastralgia and chronic enteritis. The medieval mystic, saint and herbalist, Hildegarde of Bingen, recommended it as a heart tonic. It has been used traditionally in both East and West. It is used much like its relative, ginger.

Dosage: 3-6 gms.

AROMATIC STOMACHICS
(Aromatic Herbs that Resolve Dampness)

This category treats digestive disturbances associated with phlegm and fluid congestion in the abdomen. The symptoms of this condition include abdominal distension, bloating, nausea, vomiting, sour eructations (belches), thirst, diarrhea, greasy tongue with white or yellow fur, slippery pulse and bodily aches.

The herbs in this category have certain common characteristics that distinguish them from other types of digestion-promoting herbs. Digestives proper are enzymatic agents. Chi-moving herbs or carminatives affect the liver, and internal warming stimulants have a hotter nature. Aromatic dampness-resolving herbs are particularly fragrant, and are spicy, warming and uniquely drying in nature. They specifically strengthen spleen function. In Ayurvedic medical theory, the herbs in this category are pro-pitta (fire), anti-kapha (water) and anti-vata (air). They are milder and safer digestive stimulants than those in the previous category.

In Traditional Chinese Medicine, spleen-pancreas refers to the process of deep assimilation and transportation of nutrients in the form of food and water. In Western medicine, the pancreas secretes important enzymes as well as insulin for the digestion and utilization of food. The

spleen governs the lymphatic system which is important for the circulation of food and fluid throughout the body. Lymphatic congestion can
cause edema throughout the body and abdominal bloating. The herbs in
this category, through their warm, circulating and drying action, relate
directly to the lymphatic digestion and circulation which in Chinese traditional medicine is called *spleen yang*. Since the indications of spleen
yang deficiency are poor digestion, fluid retention and tendency towards
mucus, and mucus is often considered a secretion of the lungs, many of
the herbs in this category also act on the lungs.

There is much similarity between this category and warming
stimulants, carminative herbs and digestants. Because of their warming
nature, in all of these categories one must be cautious in giving these to
individuals with wasting disease, with excess heat signs caused by deficiency.

CARDAMON   *Eletarria cardamomum; Zingiberaceae*

Energetics: spicy, warm
Meridians/Organs affected: spleen, stomach, lungs, kidney
Part used: the fruit
Active constituents: essential oil including D-borneol, bornylacetate,
d-camphor, nerolidol, linalool
Properties: stomachic, carminative, expectorant, tonic
Uses: Cardamon treats gastralgia, enuresis (involuntary urination),
spermatorrhea, phlegm, indigestion and gas. This herb is an excellent
warming, antimucus stimulant to add to lung tonics. It is commonly
added to fruits such as baked pears to counteract mucus forming aspects
and heighten the lung tonifying effects. A good recipe for a delicious
lung tonic is to core a hard winter pear, stuff it with a combination of
brown sugar or honey and a ½ to 1 teaspoon of cardamon powder and
bake. According to the Chinese, the small green cardamons (sha ren) are
better for the kidneys, while the large white cardamons (bai dou kou)
are better for the lungs.
Dosage: Take directly in a powder of from ¼-1 teaspoon at a time. In
formulas 3-6 grams (do not boil for more than a few minutes).

CARAWAY   *Carum carvi; Umbelliferae*

Energetics: spicy, warm
Meridians/Organs affected: stomach, colon, lungs
Part used: the seeds
Active constituents: essential oil with arvene and limonene, fatty oil with linoleic, oleic and petroselinic acids, nitrogenous materials, tannins, coumarins, resin
Properties: carminative, antispasmodic, stomachic, appetizer, expectorant, galactagogue, emmenagogue
Uses: Caraway aids digestion, counteracts gas, relieves uterine cramps, promotes menses, increases mother's milk, acts as a mild expectorant.
Dosage: Take directly as a powder ¼-1 teaspoon at a time; standard dosage in formulas, 3-9 gms.

PATCHOULI   *Agastache rugosa or Pogostemon cablin; Labiatae*

Energetics: spicy, slightly warm
Meridians/Organs affected: spleen, lung, stomach
Part used: the aerial portions
Active constituents: Methylchavicol, anethole, anisaldehyde, limonene, pinene, p-methoxycinnamaldehyde, a-pinene, 3-octanone, etc.; Pogostemon contains patchouli alcohol, eugenol cinnamic aldehyde, pogostol, patchoulipyridine, epiguapyridine, caryophyllen, etc.
Properties: carminative, diaphoretic, alterative, astringent, antiemetic
Uses: It is used to treat dysentery, diarrhea, nausea, vomiting, colds with a tendency towards mucus without fevers (deficient spleen and lung yang)
Dosage: standard dosage or 3-9 gms.

DILL
Anethum graveolens; Umbelliferae

Energetics: spicy, warm
Meridians/Organs affected: stomach, spleen, liver
Part used: the seeds
Active constituents: essential oil, fatty oil, some acids
Properties: carminative, antispasmodic, stomachic, emmenagogue, diuretic, galactagogue, calmative
Uses: Dill is used to treat colic, gastralgia, gas, indigestion, and insomnia due to indigestion. It promotes the flow of breast milk. For infant's colic, steep an ounce of the powdered seeds in a pint of rice wine with some chamomile flowers for two weeks. Strain and bottle for use.
 Dosage: 2-10 drops two or three times a day as needed. The powder may be mixed with heated honey to make a paste. Standard dosage in formulas.

MAGNOLIA BARK
Magnolia officinalis;
Magnoliaceae

Energetics: bitter, pungent, aromatic, warm
Meridians/Organs affected: spleen, stomach, lungs, colon
Part used: the bark
Active constituents: magnolol, isomagnolol, essential oil (eudesmol, machilol), alkaloids (magnoflorine, salicifoline, magnocurarine). This herb contains a substance whose muscle-paralyzing action is similar to that of the South american curare.
Properties: stomachic, expectorant, carminative, emmenagogue
Uses: This is perhaps one of the very best substances to use for chronic digestive disturbances including gas, gastralgia, colic, bloating, chest and abdominal fullness, loss of appetite, acid stomach, vomiting and diarrhea. It also is excellent for lung problems associated with excess mucus, wheezing and cough. Generally it is best combined with a lesser amount of a more warming stimulant such as ginger root and an antispasmodic such as peony root.
Dosage: standard dosage or 3-9 gms.

CARMINATIVES
Herbs that Move and Regulate Chi

Carminatives are used to aid digestion and relieve gas and distention. In Chinese medicine they are called *chi-moving* herbs, as they dispel blockages of energy or chi that may be causing these problems. They are related to other digestion-promoting herbs, from which they chiefly differ in their ability to affect the emotions, harmonize moods and regulate menstruation. Thus they aid the circulation of chi or energy generally. While aromatic herbs that resolve dampness work more on the pancreatic enzymes, herbs in this category that enter the liver meridian work more on aiding liver enzyme secretions, which are important for digestion and assimilation. Symptoms these herbs treat include epigastric pains, abdominal distension, belching, gas, sour eructations, nausea, vomiting, diarrhea and constipation (also alternating diarrhea and constipation).

In terms of Ayurveda they reduce kapha (water) and regulate vata (air; nervous energy, particularly as relating to the digestive nerves). Those that work on the spleen usually have a warming energy and increase pitta (fire) but those that act on the liver are usually cooling and reduce pitta. These herbs are usually spicy or bitter in taste. Many, like some herbs of the previous category, would be classified as aromatic bitters in Western herbalism. Conditions that indicate the combined use of carminative and antispasmodic properties are more characteristic of this specific category.

Stagnation and irregularity of liver chi is associated with the moodiness and depression characteristic of premenstrual syndrome. Swollen and tender breasts and irregular menses are thus signs of irregular and stagnant chi. More chronic manifestations can be abdominal and ovarian cysts, breast lumps and cancer. Liver chi stagnation often manifests as subcostal or hypochondriac pain and distention and may also be associated with hepatitis, gall stones or intercostal neuralgia. Bupleurum, traditionally classified by the Chinese under cooling diaphoretics, is used as a carminative and as the primary herb for moving liver chi. It is the major herb in several harmonizing formulas that have been in use for nearly two thousand years (see also section on harmonizing therapy, pg. 96).

Another kind of chi or energy stagnation treated by some of the herbs in this category is stagnant lung conditions with wheezing cough, shortness of breath and a feeling of chest tightness.

Like other digestion-promoting herbs these are often aromatic and drying, and therefore not to be used in dry or heat conditions. Most of the herbs in this category should not be used in substantial doses during pregnancy, as moving the chi may move the blood (i.e. promote menstruation).

The Three Citrus

Traditional Chinese Medicine distinguishes three types of citrus and their actions as follows: ripe mandarin orange peel is for digestion; unripe mandarin orange peel or green citrus is more specifically for bile congestion in the liver; bitter orange is used for abdominal distension, gas and pains with lumps and accumulations.

Most if not all citrus peels have carminative and chi-regulating properties. Lemon peel moves both liver and spleen chi; lime is specific for the liver and grapefruit peel is more for the spleen. Common orange peels have a cooler energy and milder action than those of the mandarin orange. The seeds of mandarin orange are good to use for phlegm and pain in swollen testicles. The inner threads of the mandarin orange are specifically used as a carminative and antiemetic for abdominal distension, bloat, vomiting and hiccoughs.

MANDARIN ORANGE PEEL   *Citrus reticulata; Rutaceae*
(Chen pi)

Energetics: spicy, bitter, warm
Meridians/Organs affected: spleen, stomach, lungs
Part used: the peel of the ripe fruit
Active constituents: essential oil which includes limonen, linalool, perpineol; hesperidin, carotene, cryptosanthin, vitamins B[1] and C
Properties: carminative, aromatic, expectorant, tonic
Uses: It is used to treat indigestion, gas and lung mucus. It is a mild digestive stimulant with tonic properties for the spleen that make it useful to use with other chi tonics like ginseng. The more aged it is, the better the quality.
Dosage: standard dosage or 3-9 gms.

GREEN CITRUS   *Citrus reticulata; Rutaceae*
(Qing pi or unripe Mandarin orange peel)

Energetics: pungent, bitter, warm
Meridians/Organs affected: liver, gall bladder
Part used: the immature peel
Active constituents: flavonoids and other ingredients similar to the ripe peel
Properties: carminative, cholagogue, analgesic for hernia-like pains
Uses: It is used in treating liver, gall bladder, bile congestion, chest fullness and pains, hernia-like pains, food stagnation, belching, abdominal distention, mucus and lymphatic congestion with lung mucus, intermittent fevers and chills, breast cancers and abscesses
Dosage: 3 to 9gms.

BITTER ORANGE   *Citrus aurantium or Poncirus*
trifolata; Rutaceae

Energetics: bitter, slightly cold
Meridians/Organs affected: spleen, stomach
Part used: the immature fruit
Active constituents: neohesperidin, naringin, rhoifolin, lonicerin, vitamin C and flavonoids
Properties: carminative, expectorant, laxative
Uses: It is used for epigastric or abdominal pains and distention, food stagnation, indigestion with gas and constipation. Bitter orange is considered one of the strongest chi-moving herbs, with the power to help break tumors and accumulated masses. The hardiest citrus, it is grown in this country as far north as Baltimore as an ornamental.
Dosage: 3-9 gms.

CYPERUS (Sedge root)   *Cyperus spp.; Cyperaceae*

Energetics: spicy, bitter, sweet, slightly warm
Meridians/Organs affected: liver, triple warmer
Part used: the rhizome
Active constituents: 0.5% essential oil comprised of cyperol, cyperene, cyperone, pinene and sesquiterpenes

Properties: carminative, antispasmodic, emmenagogue
Uses: It is used for digestive problems, gas, bloating, food stagnation, colds (some colds and cold symptoms are specifically caused by food congestion), irregular menses, depression and moodiness. It is like Bupleurum in its power to regulate liver chi. It is one of the best menstrual regulators (used also in this way in Ayurveda) and is especially good for cramps. Members of this genus are commonly found in marshy and river bottom areas throughout the country.
Dosage: 3-9 gms.

SANDALWOOD   *Santalum albus; Santalaceae*

Energetics: spicy, warm
Meridians/Organs affected: spleen, stomach
Part used: the heartwood
Active constituents: volatile oil with at least 90% total alcohols including alpha-santalol and beta-santalol; other constituents includes isovaleric aldehyde, santene, santenone, teresantol, santalone, and santalene
Properties: aromatic, stomachic, carminative, analgesic in nervous gastralgia
Uses: The heartwood is used to move chi, stagnant energy causing pain in the chest and abdomen. It is also used for genito-urinary tract inflammations and to help the passing of stones, for nephritis, prostatitis and as a urinary antiseptic. The oil massaged on the forehead and between the eyes is good for centering and calming the mind. Sandalwood oil is used in India for cooling the body down in summer or in heat (pitta) conditions. In Ayurveda it is regarded as cooling and is used for fevers and infections of all kinds.
Precautions: It is contraindicated for deficient wasting heat diseases.
Dosage: ½-6 gms.

CHINESE CHIVE   *Allium macrostemon; Liliaceae*

Energetics: acrid, bitter, warm
Meridians/Organs affected: lung, stomach, colon
Part used: the bulb
Active constituents: scorodose

Properties: carminative, antispasmodic, analgesic
Uses: It alleviates abdominal fullness and associated pains, pains of the chest, flank and upper back pain, dyspnea, coughing and wheezing from food congestion. It is an important herb for treating angina pain and cardiac diseases.
Dosage: 6-9 grams dried or 30-60 grams fresh

ROSE PETALS   *Rosae rugosa; Rosaceae*

Energetics: sweet, slightly bitter, warm
Meridians/Organs affected: liver, spleen
Part used: the young flower
Active constituents: citronellol, geraniol nerol, eugenol, linalool, L-p-menthene, cyanin, gallic acid, beta-carotene
Properties: carminative, stimulant, emmenagogue
Uses: It dries cold, clear mucous discharges, relieves constrictive feelings of the chest and abdomen (stuck liver chi) treats poor appetite, harmonizes blood and is used for irregular menstruation and pain caused by blood stagnation
Dosage: ½-6 gms.

PERSIMMON CALYX   *Calyx Diospyros kaki;*
Ebenaceae

Energetics: bitter, astringent, neutral
Meridians/Organs affected: lung, stomach
Part used: the calyx attached to the fruit
Active constituents: sugar, tannin, malic acid, trioxybenzoic acid, arabinose, lycopene, carotene, zeaxanthin, oxidase, pentosans, vitamins A, B and C
Properties: carminative, astringent
Uses: It is used primarily to treat hiccoughs and bleeding hemorrhoids. Uncooked in powder form it is good for constipation. When dry roasted and cooked it is good for diarrhea and dysentery.
Dosage: 6-15 gms.

CUMIN   *Cuminum cyminum; Umbelliferae*

Energetics: spicy, cool
Meridians/Organs affected: liver, spleen
Part used: seeds
Active constituents: volatile oil comprised of cymol, cymene and cuminic aldehyde
Properties: carminative, stimulant, antispasmodic
Uses: Cumin treats digestive weakness with accompanying gas, bloat, colic, headache. It also may be used as a fomentation to hasten the healing of painful bruises and injuries.
Dosage: standard dosage or 3-9 gms.

DIGESTANTS
(Herbs that Relieve Food Stagnation)

The herbs in this category aid the passage of food through the gastrointestinal tract and its assimilation. They increase gastrointestinal secretions, enhance enzymatic functions and aid peristalsis.

One of the causes of indigestion is a lack of stomach and spleen chi with coldness, that causes feelings of heaviness and mental dullness. Symptomatic of cold food stagnation is a greasy whitish tongue fur, weak, thin pulse, and an aversion to cold foods and drinks. Hot food stagnation, on the other hand, is characterised by bad breath, greasy yellow tongue coating and a strong slippery pulse.

The main distinction between most of the herbs in this category and other herbs for digestion is in the use of various grain sprouts and yeast. This suggests strongly that these substances are specifically involved with the enzymatic aspects of digestion and are almost food supplements.

It is usually necessary to combine herbs from this category with herbs that counteract coldness or heat, carminatives, and purgatives, if stagnation is more severe. As this is a mildly attacking therapy it should be used with caution in cases of deficiency.

HAWTHORN BERRY   *Crataegus spp.; Rosaceae*

Energetics: sour, sweet, slightly warm
Meridians/Organs affected: heart, spleen, stomach, liver
Part used: the berries, as well as the young leaves have been shown to be effective for treating valvular heart diseases.
Active constituents: crategolic acid, citric acid, tartaric acid, glavone, sugars, glycosides, vitamin C
Properties: digestant, antidiarrheic, cardiac tonic, emmenagogue
Uses: East and West have had different uses for this herb. Usually Western herbalists learn from traditional Chinese practice, but this is an instance of the opposite happening.

Western herbalists have long recognized the value of hawthorn berry and, recently the superior virtues of the fruit in the treatment of heart diseases. The Chinese, on the other hand, have used hawthorn berries to control appetite, and aid digestion and assimilation. The older classification is followed here to conform with traditional Chinese usage, but the Chinese recently learned from the West the value of this herb as a cardiac tonic. They now add it to many classical Chinese formulas for moving the blood and treating cardiac diseases, even though they still classify it as a digestive herb.

Hawthorn berries are one of the most reliable herbs for heart problems including cholesterol and valvular heart diseases.

They stimulate a failing appetite and as a digestant, are especially helpful as an aid in the digestion of meat. They also are useful for abdominal distention. The green fruit is good for diarrhea and the roasted and charred fruits are excellent to use both for diarrhea and chronic dysentery-like disorders.
Dosage: 6-12 gms.

BARLEY SPROUTS   *Hordeum vulgaris; Graminaceae*

Energetics: sweet, slightly warm
Meridians/Organs affected: spleen, stomach
Part used: the germinated seed
Active constituents: amylase, invertase, dextrin, phospholipid, maltose, glucose, vitamin B

Properties: digestant, carminative
Uses: It is used to help dry mother's milk, and to treat food stagnation, weak stomach, weak digestion, stagnated and undigested starchy foods and loss of appetite. It is also used to assist infants in the digestion of milk. In helping to dry mother's milk, it relieves painful and distended breasts. It regulates energy and relieves distention and tightness of the chest with belching and loss of appetite.

Barley sprouts are a valuable aid to digestion for patients with digestive disturbances associated with Candida albicans overgrowth and hepatitis.
Precautions: It is contraindicated for nursing mothers.
Dosage: 5-15 grams taken directly as a powder, 12-30 grams in decoction (up to 60 grams to inhibit lactation). It is neutral raw; toasted it is warming and helps the spleen yang.

RICE SPROUTS   *Oryzae sativa; Graminaceae*

Energetics: sweet, neutral
Meridians/Organs affected: spleen, stomach
Part used: the sprouted rice seed
Active constituents: Amylase and vitamin B
Properties: digestant, carminative
Uses: It is used to dry mother's milk and for weak digestion, with a stagnation and accumulation of starchy foods. It is effective in treating loss of appetite. Indications and contraindications are similar to those for barley sprouts. The germinated seed of millet also has similar uses.
Dosage: same as barley sprouts

LIVE YEAST Fermented yeast

Energetics: sweet, acrid, warm
Meridians/Organs affected: spleen, stomach
Properties: digestant, carminative
Uses: It is used for weak digestion, removing stagnant starch and food from the stomach, cold stomach with food stagnation accompanied with diarrhea, fullness and distention of the chest and abdomen.

The Chinese make a fermented mixture with wheat flour, bran and

various herbs including wormwood, apricot seed and cocklebur *(Xanthium)*. This mass is pressed into small cakes and cubes and sold under the name of *Shen Chu*. It is an excellent remedy for the initial stages of colds and flu. Other live yeast preparations possess similar properties.
Dosage: 6-15 gms.

RADISH SEEDS   *Raphanus sativus; Cruciferae*

Energetics: spicy, sweet, neutral
Meridians/Organs affected: lung, stomach, spleen
Part used: seed
Active constituents: erucic acid, oleic, linolenic and linoleic acids; glycerol sinapate, raphinin
Properties: digestant, carminative, expectorant
Uses: It is used to treat abdominal fullness, sour eructations, diarrhea caused by food congestion, phlegm with productive cough and wheezing. Because of its neutral energy, it is very effective in breaking up congestion in patients with extreme heat. Turnip seeds have similar properties.
Precautions: Since it is stimulating it should be used with caution for patients with weak chi.
Dosage: 6-12 gms.

ASAFOETIDA   *Ferula asafoetida; Umbelliferae*

Energetics: spicy, bitter, hot
Meridians/Organs affected: liver, spleen, stomach
Part used: the resin
Active constituents: essential oil, resin, ferulic acid, glue, sec-butyl-propenyl disulfide, farnesiferol
Properties: digestant, aromatic, carminative, expectorant
Uses: It is used to treat indigestion, bloat and gas, and to calm hysteria. This is the major component in the famous Ayurvedic herbal formula *Hingashtak,* (its Sanskrit name is *hing)*. To prevent gas and bloating, add a pinch when cooking beans. It is very helpful for damp cold spleen conditions associated with Candida albicans overgrowth.
Dosage: 100 mg.-1 gm.

HEMOSTATICS
(Herbs for regulating blood)

This category of herbs is used to inhibit bleeding. They are used most commonly in gynecology, but they are effective for any bleeding, including nose bleeds, coughing of blood, blood in the urine and stool, and bleeding from trauma.

Chinese medicine considers bleeding to indicate heat in the blood. Therefore most of the herbs in this category have a cool energy and are usually combined with heat-clearing herbs. These herbs are used symptomatically for any kind of acute bleeding.

In Western herbalism, bleeding is regarded as a kind of blood congestion, and therefore circulatory stimulants such as cayenne pepper are used to stop bleeding. This, too, is effective treatment. The art of herbalism, as may be seen from these examples, offers varying strategies.

Since the time of the early nineteenth century herbalists Samuel Thompson and the late Dr. Christopher, cayenne has been extolled as a near panacea. This exaggerates its usefulness, especially for yin or essence deficient conditions. The principle of using cayenne, which is a warming herb, is that it disperses stagnation and congestion. Since dispersing, warming stimulants are contraindicated for wasting deficient heat conditions, it may be better to use cooling-hemostatics for most chronic bleeding patterns. However, cayenne is quite effective for many acute bleeding conditions such as cuts and injuries when directly applied and sometimes when taken internally.

The hemostatic principle of these herbs varies. Some are more astringent-hemostatic, others are cooling-hemostatic, still others are moving blood-hemostatic and finally a few are warming-hemostatic.

For this reason, one cannot define specifically, according to Ayurvedic theory, the humoral predominance of hemostatic herbs. Most would be anti-pitta (fire), as bleeding usually is regarded in Ayurveda as a condition of heated blood. These herbs generally decrease kapha (fluids) but increase vata (dryness).

The ability of hemostatic herbs to inhibit bleeding intensifies when they are charred or carbonized into ashes, in which form they may be taken as a powder in capsules. Perhaps one of the most effective is calcined human hair, but any hemostatic herb that has been calcined will be more effective, whether taken internally or locally applied. The great Chinese herbalist, Li Shi Shen stated in his Materia Medica that "when red (blood) sees the black (ashes), it will cease to flow." In the Chinese five element theory red stands for the fire element and blood, while black is the water element (which controls fire).

It is important to consider the administration of a tonic (such as ginseng) to support the essential energy of the body when there has been significant blood loss. Hemostatic herbs are rarely used alone. More often they are combined with other herbs in a formula to help treat the underlying cause of the bleeding. Since they often are used for acute conditions, it is important that they be used externally as appropriate to the site and condition being treated.

RASPBERRY LEAVES   *Rubus ideaus; Rosaceae*

Energetics: mild, bitter, cool
Meridians/Organs affected: spleen, liver, kidneys
Part used: the leaves
Active constituents: 1 to 2% organic acids of which 90% is citric acid; vitamin C, pectins and sugar
Properties: hemostatic, astringent, mild alterative, parturient
Uses: It is used to treat irregular and excessive menstruation, diarrhea and dysentery, is a general hemostatic for bleeding, and commonly is used before childbirth to prepare the womb for birthing
Dosage: 6-15 gms.

AGRIMONY   *Agrimonia eupatori; Rosaceae*

Energetics: slightly bitter, astringent, warm
Meridians/Organs affected: lung, liver, spleen
Part used: the aerial portions
Active constituents: tannins, bitter glycosides, nicotinic acid amide, silicic acid, vitamins B and K, iron and essential oil
Properties: astringent, hemostatic, anti-inflammatory, analgesic
Uses: Agrimony is used for bleeding from any part of the body, caused by either an underlying cold or hot condition. It also may be used as a suppository, combining the extract with cocoa butter and inserting into the rectum for hemorrhoids, tapeworms, and diarrhea. Because of its bitter taste, it is a specific for childhood diarrhea, appendicitis, mucous colitis and urinary incontinence, and is a digestive bitter tonic remedy.
Dosage: 6-15 gms.

MUGWORT   *Artemisia vulgaris; Compositae*

Energetics: bitter, acrid, slightly warm
Meridians/Organs affected: spleen, liver, kidney
Part used: the leaves
Active constituents: essential oil: cineole, thujone, bitter principle
Properties: emmenagogue, hemostatic, antispasmodic, mild narcotic, bitter tonic
Uses: Mugwort stops excessive menstrual bleeding caused by deficiency and coldness, circulates the blood, warms the womb, pacifies the fetus, arrests threatened miscarriages, and alleviates abdominal pains caused by coldness. It also is used as a bitter tonic for the liver and stomach. It can be topically applied as a liniment or wash to relieve itching. Internally and externally it is effective both as a curative and preventive of parasites and worms. The dried, aged and powdered herb, which has a cottony consistency, can be rolled into a cigar using tissue paper. One end is burned and held near the site of a painful area to increase blood circulation and give relief from pain. This is particularly effective for injuries and bruises. Called *moxibustion,* this is a standard method of treatment used by acupuncturists: instead of needles, the burning cylin-

der is held over certain acupuncture points.

Dried mugwort alone, or mixed with other herbs like sage, thuja leaves or osha root, may be burned over a piece of charcoal in a sea shell (or other suitable container) and the smoke used to purify the spiritual and physical environment. This is a Native American practice called "smudging."

Dosage: 3-9 gms.

THUJA (Cedar tree leaves)   *Thuja occidentalis;*
                                                            Pinaceae

Energetics: bitter, spicy, astringent, slightly cold
Meridians/Organs affected: lung, liver, colon
Parts used: the leaves and seeds
Active constituents: volatile oil comprised of pinene and caryophyllene; pinipicrin, a bitter principle; tannin and resin
Properties: astringent, hemostatic, antipyretic, emmenagogue
Uses: It cools the blood, stops bleeding, and may be used for heated blood syndrome, or with warm herbs for cold and stagnant blood circulation. It also is used internally to treat dysentery, alleviate cough and as an expectorant, especially when the phlegm is streaked with blood. Topically, it can be applied in powder form to promote the healing of burns. The young twigs of thuja may be made into an infusion and taken as a tea for bronchial catarrh and for dry irritable coughs. It also is beneficial for heart weakness. Thuja twig tea may be used to treat delayed menstruation.

It also is helpful in treating frequent urination caused by loss of muscle tone. For its alterative antifungal properties it may be taken internally or applied externally in the form of a liniment. It is used externally for rheumatic pains and psoriases. A few drops of the tincture may be taken internally to counteract negative side effects of inoculations or vaccines. Take about ten drops four times a day for four days. The dried twigs may be crumbled and burnt over charcoal as a smudging herb (see mugwort above).

Precautions: Thuja is contraindicated during pregnancy.
Dosage: 6-15 gms.

CATTAIL POLLEN   *Typhus spp.; Typhaceae*

Energetics: sweet, acrid, neutral
Meridians/Organs affected: liver, heart, spleen
Part used: the yellow pollen
Active constituents: iso-rhamnetic, fatty oil and a sitosterol.
Properties: hemostatic, diuretic, astringent, nutritive, vulnerary, emmenagogue
Uses: It may be dusted on externally or taken internally to stop bleeding. At the same time it benefits blood circulation, relieving conditions of blood stagnation such as abdominal pains and menstrual pains. It also is very effective for heart pains (angina pectoris). For external use, the pollen is mixed with honey and directly applied to painful swellings and sores to promote healing. For an external treatment of bleeding caused by traumatic injuries, it is combined with powdered cuttlefish bones.
Precautions: Because of its emmenagogic properties, it should be used with caution during pregnancy.
Dosage: 5-10gms.

THISTLES   Various thistle species; *Compositae*

Energetics: sweet, bitter, cool
Meridians/Organs affected: liver, spleen
Part used: the aerial portions
Active constituents: Blessed thistle *(Carbenia benedicta)*, which is the most commonly used, contains tannin, a bitter principle (cnicine); a sesquiterpenoid lactone, mucilage and a trace of essential oil. Milk thistle *(Silybum marianum)*, which recently has received considerable attention as a liver tonic, has a flavanoid (silymarine), amines (thyramine and histamine), a bitter principle and an oil.
Properties: astringent, alterative, hemostatic
Uses: It resolves blood clots, stops bleeding, lowers fevers, cures liver disorders and jaundice, and purifies the blood. It is used in the treatment of boils, sores, swellings and menstrual problems.

The seeds of milk thistle *(Silybum marianum)* make one of the best liver tonics in the vegetable kingdom, effective even against the most virulent hepato-toxin, the *Amanita phalloides* mushroom. Injections of extract of silybum seeds were given to a number of patients in Europe who had been poisoned with this deadly mushroom. The rate of recovery was nearly 100%.

Blessed or holy thistle, of which the leaves usually are the part used, is, similarly, a liver tonic, circulatory stimulant, diaphoretic, emetic and emmenagogue.
Dosage: 5-15 gms.; 30-60 gms. if used fresh

SHEPHERD'S PURSE   *Capsella bursa-pastoris; Cruciferae*

Energetics: pungent, sweet, neutral
Meridians/Organs affected: liver, stomach
Part used: the aerial portions
Active constituents: amino-alcohols: choline, acetylcholine, aminophenol and tyramine; also diosmin, a flavonoid
Properties: astringent, hemostatic, alterative, diuretic
Uses: A tincture made from the fresh herb and taken every hour or two is one of the most effective hemostatics. It is used for excessive menstrual bleeding, genito-urinary problems, difficult urination, postpartum bleeding.
Dosage: 5-15 gms.

BURNET ROOT   *Sanguisorba officinalis; Rosaceae*

Energetics: bitter, sour, cold
Meridians/Organs affected: liver, colon, stomach
Parts used: the root primarily, and the leaves
Active constituents: tannin; the leaves contain a sapanoside and flavones
Properties: hemostatic, astringent, alterative
Uses: It stops bleeding, and also is used internally for acute bacillary dysentery
Dosage: 5-15 gms.

LOTUS NODES   *Nelumbo nucifera; Nymphaceae*

Energetics: sweet, astringent, neutral
Meridians/Organs affected: lung, stomach, liver
Part used: the nodes of the root
Active constituents: asparagine and tannin in the nodes; nelumbine, carotene, thiamine, nicotinic acid, riboflavin, ascorbic acid in the receptacle
Properties: hemostatic, astringent, emmenagogue
Uses: It stops bleeding and at the same time removes stagnant blood (clots). It is used to treat many kinds of bleeding, including bleeding in the stomach and lungs, uterine bleeding, blood in the urine and bleeding associated with threatened miscarriage. The root of the lotus has similar but weaker properties.
Dosage: 5-15 gms.

DRAGON'S BLOOD   *Daemonorops draco; Palmae*

Energetics: pleasant but salty taste, neutral
Meridians/Organs affected: liver
Part used: the resin
Active constituents: a resinous principle, benzoic and cinnamic acids
Properties: astringent, emmenagogue, hemostatic, vulnerary
Uses: It is applied externally as a wash or liniment to stop bleeding and promote healing. Internally it is used for menstrual irregularities, chest pains, post-partum bleeding and traumatic injuries.
Dosage: 1-3 grams taken in wine or alcoholic tincture form

TRILLIUM   *Trillium pendulum; Liliaceae*

Energetics: pungent, bitter, warm
Meridians/Organs affected: spleen, heart, lungs
Part used: the root
Active constituents: tannin, resin, glycosides trillin and trillarin, traces of essential oil, saponin, fatty oil and starch
Properties: astringent, parturient, antispasmodic, expectorant, emmenagogue, antiseptic, alterative

Uses: It ameliorates the process of childbirth, stops excessive bleeding, regulates menses, aids in bringing up phlegm from the lungs
Dosage: 3-9 gms.

MADDER ROOT

Rubiae cordifoliae and R. tinctoria; Rubiaceae

Energetics: bitter, sweet, cold
Meridians/Organs affected: heart, liver
Part used: the root
Active constituents: purpurin, pseudopurpurin, manjistin, alizarin
Properties: alterative, astringent, deobstruent, emmenagogue
Uses: It stops bleeding and counteracts inflammations, and is considered one of the best blood purifying herbs. In Ayurvedic medicine it is used for many pitta-type bleeding conditions (rakta pitta).
Dosage: 5-10 gms.

CALCINED HUMAN HAIR

Crinis carbonisatus

Energetics: bitter, neutral
Meridians/Organs affected: heart, liver, kidney
Active constituents: eukeratin, sulfur
Properties: astringent, hemostatic
Uses: It is used for hematemesis, hematuria, menorrhagia, leucorrhea. It is applied externally for bloody nose and bleeding gums.
Dosage: 2-15gms.

TIENCHI GINSENG

Panax pseudoginseng; Araliaceae

Energetics: sweet, slightly bitter, slightly warm
Meridians/Organs affected: liver, stomach, colon
Part used: the root
Active constituents: arasopanin A and B
Properties: tonic, hemostatic, emmenagogue
Uses: This is one of the most valuable Chinese herbs for traumas and injuries because of its ginseng-like tonic properties and its strong

hemostatic action in acute conditions. It is used externally as a trauma liniment for swelling and pain from falls, injuries, contusions and sprains. It is taken internally, alone or with other herbs, for injuries, cuts and even gunshot wounds. It will effectively dissolve blood clots when taken internally. It works very well for most abnormal bleeding when combined with the ashes of human hair. Its healing, astringent properties increase when combined with comfrey root. Like *Panax ginseng*, it also may be taken as a blood and energy tonic, and is regarded by some as equally effective. It is considered preferable for younger people, because it moves the chi more than the common American or Oriental ginsengs. It also strengthens the heart and improves athletic performance, making it a preferred tonic for the purposes of sports medicine. **Dosage:** ½-3 gms.

EMMENAGOGUES
(Herbs that vitalize blood)

In this category the traditional Chinese indicated use and application is much broader than that of Western herbalism. The term "emmenagogue" tends to restrict the use of these herbs to women and to the regulation of menstruation, whereas the Chinese concept of moving blood indicates their therapeutic value for men and women of all ages. For these herbs can treat injuries, heart disease, pain caused by blood clots, and tumors and cancer, as well as gynecological disorders. Most of these herbs have been shown to have vasodilatory, antihypertensive and analgesic properties.

Throughout history, people have recognized the value of bloodletting as a valid and important part of natural healing practice. This technique has been abused, but it has a therapeutic effectiveness for a number of conditions when properly used. Blood-letting is an important technique for both Ayurvedic and Traditional Chinese Medicine. Some styles of traditional Chinese acupuncture use it almost as much as needling.

A simple way of relieving a severe headache is to prick the vein at the forehead or temple and draw out a few drops of blood. The headache will quickly disappear. Blood pressure can be lowered by taking a few drops from the apex of the outer tip of the ear. A drop or so of blood taken from the thumbside corner of the index finger relieves sore throat. A properly sterilized needle always is used.

In Ayurvedic medicine live leeches are applied to chronic sores and rashes to suck out the "bad blood" which causes them. The leech gluts itself on the bad blood and then releases its hold, leaving the area clean and well on the way to being healed. This is an ideal method for conditions such as psoriasis and leprosy. In Traditional Chinese Medicine, a decoction to dissolve blood clots is made from dried leeches, cockroaches and gadflys. It is used to treat a variety of gynecological and other internal disorders.

Between blood and energy there is a reciprocal action: blood needs energy for movement while energy needs blood for nourishment. A stagnation of blood therefore can also give rise to a stagnation of energy. Either of these can cause many disease symptoms including pain. Blood stagnation pain is fixed and sharp, while energy stagnation pain is intermittent, dull and migratory. Blood stagnation can cause amenorrhea, dysmenorrhea, puerpural pain, tumors, abdominal masses, blockage syndromes as in arthritis, muscle and joint pains, and sciatica and coronary angina. External pains of traumas and injuries also involve blood stagnation.

Some of the herbs in this category are spicy or pungent in flavor and warm in energy. In Ayurvedic herbal medicine they are considered pro-pitta (fire) and anti-vata (air). Others are cooling and alterative, lowering pitta and increasing vata. These herbs usually decrease kapha (fluids) and have a thinning effect upon the blood.

There may be associated causes of pain, requiring the addition of herbs from other categories. These include excess cold obstructing, which requires the combination of internal warming and dispersing diaphoretic herbs. Chi or energy stagnation pain requires the addition of energy regulating herbs. Yang deficiency pain requires the addition of yang tonics. Fluid obstruction pain requires diuretics. Energy deficiency and blood deficiency pain require appropriate tonics. Excess heat pain requires heat clearing or alterative herbs. The herbalist seeks to discover the underlying cause of pain and to treat it, rather than simply giving drugs that anaesthetize sensation.

Emmenagogues are contraindicated during pregnancy, especially the earlier stages, during menstruation, for women who have a tendency towards excessive menstrual bleeding, and for individuals who bleed easily.

ANGELICA (see warming diaphoretics, pg. 148)

LOVAGE (see warming diaphoretics, pg.149)

VERVAIN   *Verbena officinalis; Verbenaceae*

Energetics: cold, bitter
Meridians/Organs affected: liver, spleen
Part used: the aerial portions
Active constituents: two glycosides (verbenaline and verbenine) and essential oil, tannin, bitter principle and mucilage
Properties: emmenagogue, astringent, antispasmodic, diaphoretic, alterative, diuretic, galactogogue, cholagogue
Uses: It is used for delayed and painful menses, nervousness, hemorrhage, fevers, urinary problems, hepatis, jaundice, insufficient mother's milk, liver congestion, cirrhosis, ascites and mastitis. During the middle ages is was used to make an ointment that was regarded as useful for sorcery.
Dosage: standard dosage or 3-9 gms.

CORYDALIS (Turkey corn)   *Corydalis formosa and spp.;*
                                                              Papaveraceae

Energetics: acrid, bitter, warm
Meridians/Organs affected: lungs, liver, heart
Part used: the root
Active constituents: a wide variety of alkaloids including bulbocapnine, and corydaline
Properties: emmenagogue, analgesic, antispasmodic, diuretic, bitter tonic
Uses: This is one of the best herbs for relieving internal, menstrual, abdominal, heart and deficiency pains. It may be used with other appropriate guiding herbs for almost any kind of pain, including the pain of rheumatism and arthritis. This is the most valued herb for pain in Traditional Chinese Medicine. It is an herbal morphine that does not have the addictive, toxic side effects of the chemical drugs. Combined with other herbs, it is used as a bitter tonic for stomach and urinary

problems. Corydalis deserves wider appreciation from Western herbalists.

Dosage: 3-20 gms.

TURMERIC   *Curcumae longa; Zingiberaceae*

Energetics: spicy, bitter, warm
Meridians/Organs affected: heart, liver, lung
Part used: rhizome
Active constituents: essential oil, valepotriates, alkaloids
Properties: emmenagogue, aromatic stimulant, cholagogue, alterative, analgesic, astringent, antiseptic
Uses: It regulates the menses, aids digestion, dissolves gallstones, decongests the liver, may be combined with barberry or Oregon grape root for releasing the liver as effective as Chinese bupleurum. It relieves menstrual pains and helps reduce uterine tumors. Used externally or internally, turmeric promotes healing in cases of trauma or injury. A condiment for cooking, it is the main ingredient in curries. The Chinese prefer the smaller, less aromatic roots (yu jin), which they consider to be cooling, for medicinal usage.
Dosage: standard dosage or 3-9 gms.

MOTHERWORT   *Leonorus cardiaca; Labiatae*

Energetics: bitter, spicy, slightly cold
Meridians/Organs affected: pericardium, liver
Part used: the aerial portion
Active constituents: bitter principle, and bitter glycosides, leonurin, alkaloids, tannin, essential oil, resin, organic acids
Properties: emmenagogue, astringent, carminative, cardiac tonic, diuretic, antispasmodic, antirheumatic
Uses: It is used to treat menstrual disorders, (delayed or stopped menses), menopause, as a uterine stimulant, for cramps, gas, nervous heart problems, cardiac edema, swollen thyroid, neuralgia and rheumatic complaints. Chinese women often use it combined with dong quai as a menstrual regulator. This is an important heart herb in Western herbalism.
Dosage: 10-30 gms.

BUGLEWEED
Lycopus virginicus; Labiatae

Energetics: bitter, spicy, warm
Meridians/Organs affected: spleen, liver
Part used: the aerial portions
Active constituents: tannin, lithospermic acid, phenolic substances and traces of essential oil
Properties and uses: Western bugleweed is noted for its sedative, astringent and mildly narcotic properties. It should be used only in its fresh state (or freshly tinctured), not dried. It is different from the Chinese species *(Lycopi lucidus)*, which it closely resembles, although both grow in damp or marshy environments. The Chinese variety has emmenagogue and diuretic properties and is used for delayed menstruation and urinary problems. For treating traumatic bruises and injuries, it is combined with other herbs in a liniment, and also taken internally. Both varieties are good for cardiac problems. B. virginicus has been shown to be effective for sedating high thyroid, especially when combined with motherwort. Effects are only noted after taking the combinations for two weeks.

Precautions: Generally contraindicated in pregnancy, as are most herbs in this category.
Dosage: 3-9 gms.

PEACH SEED
Prunus persica; Rosaceae

Energetics: bitter, sweet, neutral
Meridians/Organs affected: heart, liver, colon
Part used: inner kernel of the seed
Active constituents: amygdalin, emulsin, oleic acid, glyceric and linoleic acids
Properties: emmenagogue, demulcent, laxative
Uses: It is used to treat delayed menses and congested blood (especially in the lower pelvic cavity) and abdominal pains. For traumatic injuries it is both taken internally and used externally in a liniment. It is one of the stronger blood-moving herbs, and therefore useful in reducing tumors. It is an important demulcent laxative, especially when combined with other laxative herbs.

Precautions: Contraindicated during pregnancy.
Dosage: 3-9 gms.

SAFFLOWER   *Carthamus tinctorius; Compositae*

Energetics: spicy, bitter, warm
Meridians/Organs affected: spleen, liver, heart
Part used: flowers
Active constituents: carthamin, palmitic acid, stearic acid, arachic acid, oleic acid, linoleic and linolenic acids, safflower yellow
Properties: emmenagogue, analgesic, carminative, mild diaphoretic
Uses: It is used for delayed menses, congested and stagnant blood, poor blood circulation, blood clots, lower abdominal pains caused by blood congestion (especially in women); both internally and externally for bruises and injuries (used in liniments); and for eruptive diseases such as measles.
Dosage: 3-6 gms.

SAFFRON   *Crocus sativus; Iridaceae*

Because it is much cheaper, safflower has been used as a substitute for saffron, sometimes under the misleading name of American or Mexican "saffron".

Energetics: spicy, sweet, bitter, neutral
Meridians/Organs affected: spleen, heart, liver, kidney
Part used: the yellow stigmas
Active constituents: When dried, the stigmas produce a glycoside called picrocine which then forms safranal. This has the characteristic smell and the carotenoid pigment of crocine.
Properties: emmenagogue, stimulant, carminative, antispasmodic, rejuvenative, aphrodisiac, alterative, abortive
Uses: It is very expensive, but is one of the finest blood vitalizers known. It counteracts inflammatory conditions associated with excess pitta (fire), while at the same time powerfully stimulating the circulation and regulating the spleen, liver and heart. According to David Frawley, "It is not a tonic in itself but when used together with other tonics like dong quai, it will catalyze them to promote tissue growth in the reproductive organs and in the entire body." He further states that it is very *sattvic* or spiritually balancing and gives "the energy of love,

devotion and compassion". This makes it excellent for those practicing *bhakti* or a devotional religious path.

It is used for a wide variety of problems including menstrual pains and irregularities, menopause, impotence, infertility, anemia, hysteria, depression, enlarged spleen and liver, neuralgic and rheumatic pains, chronic cough, asthma and chronic diarrhea.

Crocine is a very powerful yellow pigment and is highly valued in the Middle East for the fine quality of yellow dye it yields. Even in one part per 100,000, it will color water yellow. Generally it is used to make saffron rice, to which it imparts its beautiful yellow color.

Combined with food, saffron will aid assimilation into the deeper tissues. It is used as a tonic with other herbs and teas, in medicated oils, in medicated ghees, or in milk with honey, mixing 100 to 500 milligrams in heated milk.

Precautions: In large doses it can be narcotic, toxic and even lethal, causing violent hemorrhages. Definitely contraindicated during pregnancy.

Dosage: 100-500 mg.

CALENDULA   *Calendula officinalis; Compositae*

Energetics: spicy, bitter, neutral
Meridians/Organs affected: liver, heart, lungs
Part used: the petals
Active constituents: essential oil containing carotenoids (carotene, calenduline and lycopine), also a saponin, resin and bitter principle
Properties: emmenagogue, diaphoretic, alterative, astringent
Uses: When taken internally it will act very similarly to safflower in regulating the menses. It also is used to ripen eruptive diseases such as measles; and promotes diaphoresis, making it useful for fevers. It is most commonly used externally, as an ointment or oil for burns, bruises and injuries.
Dosage: 3-6 gms.

FRANKINCENSE   *Boswellia carterii; Burseraceae*

Energetics: spicy, bitter, warm
Meridians/Organs affected: heart, liver, spleen
Part used: the resinous exudate
Active constituents: boswellic acid A and B, olibanoresene, arabic acid, bassorin, pinene, dipentene, A and B phellandrene
Properties: emmenagogue, antiseptic, antispasmodic, nervine
Uses: It relieves menstrual pains, promotes menstruation, treats rheumatic aches and pains, and ripens carbuncles, sores and abscesses. Externally it is used in liniments for bruises and injuries, and for its antiseptic properties. It is widely used as an incense in the orient and occident, and is thought to calm the mind and clear the cerebral circulation.
Dosage: 3-6 gms.

MYRRH   *Commiphora myrrha; Burseraceae*

Energetics: bitter, spicy, neutral
Meridians/Organs affected: heart, liver, spleen
Part used: the gum resin
Active constituents: an essential oil, resins and gums
Properties: emmenagogue, expectorant, antispasmodic, disinfectant, stimulant, carminative
Uses: Its uses are similar to those of frankincense, with which it is often combined in liniments and incense. Myrrh is more blood-moving while frankincense tends to move the chi more and is better for arthritic conditions. Myrrh is one of the most effective of all known disinfectants and is widely used medically for this purpose. It increases circulation and heart rate and power. It is useful for amenorrhea, dysmenorrhea, menopause and uterine tumors, as it purges stagnant blood out of the uterus. Myrrh is good for many chronic diseases, including obesity and diabetes. It helps toothache pain applied externally.

For inner ear infections, combine equal parts of echinacea and mullein with one-quarter part myrrh to make a tea. The alcoholic extracts of these herbs are combined to make a medicated oil. An excellent liniment for bruises, aches and sprains is made from a combination of equal parts of myrrh, golden seal and cayenne, macerated in rubbing alcohol for about two weeks. Combined with peach seeds and safflower, myrrh is good for stomatitis, gingivitis and laryngitis.

Myrrh is most commonly used in Chinese medicine for rheumatic, arthritic and circulatory problems. It is combined with such herbs as tienchi ginseng, safflower, dong quai, cinnamon and *Salvia miltorrhiza (dan shen)*, usually in rice wine, and used both internally and externally. However, myrrh is not as important in Chinese medicine as it is in the systems of India, the Middle East and the West, which ascribe to it tonic and rejuvenative properties.

A related species known as *guggul* in Ayurvedic medicine is considered one of the best substances for the treatment of circulatory problems, nervous system disorders and rheumatic complaints (see guggul in Planetary Formulas section, pg. 134). Pitch from pine trees and other bush and tree resins also are used as antirheumatics.

The preparation of guggul in traditional Ayurvedic medicine can serve as a model for the detoxification of various resins intended for internal use. Place the myrrh or other resinous material in a porous or muslin bag and suspend it from two crossed sticks into a simmering tea of Triphala or other alterative herbs (turmeric also is good for improving the blood-moving properties of myrrh). After simmering for a period of time, remove the sack with the residue and continue to cook the tea down to a thick moist mat at the bottom of the pot. This is spread out in the open air to dry into solid chunks; or the residue is further prepared and softened with ghee and rolled into little pills. The dose is two or three pills the size of a mung bean two or three times a day.

Precautions: Any resins tend to be difficult to eliminate and can cause minor damage to the kidneys if taken internally over an extended period.

Dosage: of the powder 1-15 grains for limited periods. In formulas (also for limited periods) 3-12 gms.

WILD GINGER   *Asarum canadensis; Aristolochiaceae*

Energetics: spicy, bitter,warm
Meridians/Organs affected: liver, heart, lungs
Part used: the whole plant
Active constituents: essential oil including asarone, acids, tannin, flavonoids and resin
Properties: emmenagogue, stimulant, diuretic, carminative, diaphoretic. The Chinese variety is classified as a stimulating diaphoretic.
Uses: It promotes menses, stimulates the circulation of blood and chi, opens the meridians, aids digestion, and counteracts and eliminates gas. It also is used as a stimulating diaphoretic to promote perspiration for the treatment of colds, coughs and flu. The Pomo Indian women of California used to drink it each month the week before their period was due to regulate childbirth. The Chinese use their variety as a primary herb for headaches, facial nerve pain and sinus congestion.
Dosage: 2-5 gms.

PENNYROYAL   *Hedeoma pulegiodes or*
Mentha pulegium; Labiatae

Energetics: spicy, bitter, warm
Meridians/Organs affected: liver, lung
Part used: The aerial portions
Active constituents: The major constituent is ketone puylegone. It also contains about 1 percent volatile oil
Properties: emmenagogue, diaphoretic, carminative, antispasmodic, mild sedative
Uses: It promotes menstruation, induces perspiration, and is used for the treatment of colds and flu. It eliminates gas, calms nausea and relieves nervous tension. A strong infusion of the tea with brewer's yeast treats delayed menses. The oil externally applied wards off mosquitoes. For this purpose it is used alone or combined with citronella.

Precautions: To take the oil internally to terminate an unwanted pregnancy is very dangerous and in a few cases has resulted in death. All essential oils are life-threatening if taken internally. There is a possibility of fetal damage from the use of pennyroyal to induce abortion, but this may be true only of the undiluted oil and not the infusion.
Dosage: 3-6 gms.

TANSY
Tanecetum vulgare or Chrysanthemum vulgare; Compositae

Energetics: bitter, acrid, warm
Meridians/Organs affected: liver, pericardium
Part used: the flower heads
Active constituents: essential oil, possibly thujone, bitter principles, glycosides, tanacetin 1 and 11, acid, resin, sugar, fat and carotenoids
Properties: emmenagogue, carminative, vermifuge
Uses: Tansy is a strong remedy to promote delayed or stopped menstruation. It also is used to eliminate worms (ascaris and pinworms). The oil is externally applied to treat injuries, bruises and rheumatic complaints.
Precautions: Overdose can be toxic.
Dosage: 1 teaspoon steeped in a cup of boiling water for 20 minutes, one cup two to three times daily. In formulas 1-3 gms.

BLUE COHOSH
Caulophyllum thalictroides; Berberidaceae

Energetics: acrid, bitter, warm, mildly toxic
Meridians/Organs affected: liver
Part used: the root
Active constituents: gum, starch, salts, phosphoric acid, soluble resin, a substance similar to saponin
Properties: emmenagogue, antispasmodic, diuretic, diaphoretic, anthelmintic
Uses: It regulates the menses and relieves cramping pains. It is taken during the last month of pregnancy to facilitate labor. Native American women used it when delivering babies fathered by whites, because it

helped dilate the uterus and vaginal canal to accommodate the larger heads. It also is used for rheumatic problems, edema and swelling, epilepsy, hysteria, and chronic cases of uterine inflammation.
Dosage: standard dose or 3-9 gms.

ROSE FLOWERS   *Rosa chinensis and spp.; Rosaceae*

Energetics: sweet, warm
Meridians/Organs affected: liver, heart
Part used: the partially opened tea rose flower
Active constituents: terpene alcohol
Properties: emmenagogue, mildly carminative, aperient
Uses: It promotes blood circulation, and treats painful, delayed or stopped menses. Add brown sugar when treating stopped or light menses accompanied by pain, emotional tension and possible constipation.
Dosage: 3-6 gms. in infusion

CHASTE BERRIES   *Vitex agnus-castus; Verbenaceae*

Energetics: acrid, spicy, warm
Meridians/Organs affected: liver, spleen
Part used: the berries
Active constituents: essential oil, fatty oil, flavonoid casticin, iridoglycoside agnuside and aucubin
Properties: emmenagogue, vulnerary
Uses: It is a specific to counteract premenstrual syndrome. It also stimulates progesterone production and regulates the menses. It is specifically useful menopause and long-term taken internally for the treatment of ovarian cysts and non-cancerous breast lumps. The pulp of the berries is applied externally to relieve paralysis and limb weakness and pains. In ancient Greece and Rome, the temple priestesses used it to lessen sexual desire.

Dosage: 3-6 gms.

RUE   *Ruta graveolens; Rutaceae*

Energetics: bitter, pungent, warm
Meridians/Organs affected: liver, spleen
Part used: the aerial portions

Active constituents: essential oil, flavonoids, hyperine, rutin, hypericin, tannin, pectin, choline
Properties: emmenagogue, antispasmodic, sedative
Uses: Rue is used to regulate delayed or scanty menses, to treat cramping, strengthen the capillaries and vessels, and to lower arterial blood pressure. The tincture is taken internally to promote flexibility of the ligaments, relieve muscular spasms and rheumatic aches and pains. The oil is topically applied to relieve spasmodic pains. Oil of rue is made by macerating the leaves in olive oil and may be used as ear drops to relieve earache.

The homeopathic juice of the fresh plant extract applied directly strengthens the eyes. Fresh rue juice for the eyes can be preserved and applied with honey. One drop of rue honey is administered to each eye two or three times daily. The infusion of the leaves is a gargle for sore throat. Taken internally the infusion is a carminative and diaphoretic for the treatment of stomach disorders, colds, flu and similar acute problems.

Precautions: Rue should not be taken in large doses. It can have mildly toxic effects and the juice of the leaves can be a local irritant.
Dosage: Steep one teaspoon of the dried leaves in ½ cup of water and take over the period of a day. A cold extract is made by soaking a teaspoon of the dried herb in a cup of cold water for ten hours. This can be strained and taken in one or two doses during the day. Tincture of rue should be used only in doses of 5-20 drops at a time. Dose in formulas 1-3 gms.

COLLINSONIA   *Collinsonia canadensis; Labiatae*

Energetics: spicy, sour, warm
Meridians/Organs affected: liver, pericardium, lung, colon
Part used: the root
Active constituents: resin, starch, tannin, mucilage and a wax-like substance
Properties: emmenagogue, astringent, diuretic, alterative
Uses: It is used for various female disorders, including excessive, insufficient and painful menstruation. It has mild regulatory function, and is

used internally for gastro-intestinal diseases such as gastritis, diarrhea, dysentery and colitis. It also is helpful for sore throat, bronchitis, asthma, chronic laryngitis and tracheitis, for which it is given in a honey syrup.

It relieves both chi and blood congestion making it helpful for neural irritations, especially of the pneumogastric nerve regulating the heart and lungs.

It has a tonic action upon the bowels and is nearly specific for hemorrhoids caused by constipation with vascular blockage. This herb is known to have a near specific affinity for problems of the rectum and anus. It is given for rectal pains and inflammation; and for dysentery with accompanying rectal problems. It treats anal fistulae, rectal ulcers and pockets, and nervous conditions affecting the rectum. Its specific indications seem to be a bearing-down sensation with accompanying heat, constriction and dryness. For rectal problems small doses are preferred: 1 to 2 drops of the tincture in water three or four times daily. It seems to be safe for use by pregnant women. It may be taken internally and directly applied to the rectum nightly in the form of an ointment or bolus. Applications of the green portions of the plant have been found to be very effective for the relief of poison oak and ivy dermatitis.

Dosage: 1-15 drops of the tincture 3 or 4 times daily. For bronchial and heart problems use 10-30 drops 3 or 4 times daily. In formulas 2-5 gms.

TONICS

Herbal tonification is the most developed and singular contribution of Oriental herbalism, because in the East the cause of illness is seen in terms of deficiencies. Because the West tends to view sickness as a condition of stagnation and excess, the emphasis here has been on elimination and detoxification.

Thus the Western tonics are often "bitters" taken in small alcoholic doses before meals to stimulate digestive secretions so that food, assimilated more efficiently, itself becomes a tonic. Many of the herbs, such as gentian and golden seal, seen as tonics in Western herbalism, would be classified as alterative or toxic heat-clearing herbs by the Chinese. Western herbalism also uses them in higher dose for treating fevers, particularly malaria.

A tonic is traditionally defined as a substance that supplements or supports general or specific physiological functions and is used in cases of deficiency and weakness. In Ayurvedic medicine, the class of tonics includes those substances nourishing to the seven *dhatus* or bodily tissues of 1. plasma *(rasa)*, 2. blood *(rakta)*, 3. muscle *(mamsa)*, 4. adipose tissue *(meda)*, 5. bone *(asthi)*, 6. bone marrow and nerve tissue *(majja)*, and 7. reproductive secretions *(shukra)*. Each of these in turn nourishes the others and all promote *ojas*, which is the glow of radiant health and vitality deriving from good digestion. Excess worry and stress, malnourishment, and overindulgence in sex are all considered detrimental to *ojas* and to shorten the lifespan.

From the Chinese perspective, tonics are subdivided into chi or energy tonics, yang or sympathetic adrenal tonics, blood tonics, and yin or parasympathetic adrenal tonics. Since chi is a part of yang, and blood is a part of yin, there is a strong connection between herbs that tonify chi and yang, as well as those that tonify blood and yin. The term "yang" includes both chi and warming functions, while that of "yin" includes both blood and fluids. Thus, chi deficiency often includes or directly leads to yang deficiency, with accompanying coldness and fluid retention; while blood deficiency often includes or leads to yin deficiency, with accompanying inflammatory conditions resulting from strumous or wasting diseases.

Just as in Ayurveda tonification of one of the seven *dhatus* begins a cycle of supporting and nourishing each of the succeeding tissues, in Chinese herbalism, yin and yang are said to be rooted in each other, so that to benefit one, it may be necessary to strengthen the other. Further, chi is considered the *commander of blood* and is thus the motivating factor of blood, while blood is considered the *mother of chi,* nourishing the chi.

This means that to tonify yang, one may have to include some degree of yin tonification, and vice versa. This shows the mutual attraction of yin and yang. Thus to tonify chi or yang one may have to tonify blood or yin. This strategy is found in various traditional kidney yang herbal formulas, to which yin tonic herbs (such as prepared rehmannia or lycium berries) are added. An important traditional Chinese herbal formula for treating anemia uses a preponderant amount of astragalus, a chi tonic, and a smaller amount of dong quai, the actual blood tonic.

Another principle of tonification is to first prepare the body with a preliminary clearing and detoxification therapy, using purgative and alterative herbs for a period of a day to a month. The principle is to make weak before making strong. In using a wild ginseng root, costing three hundred dollars or more for a single root, it makes sense to first administer a detoxification tea so that the benefits of the tonic will be fully utilized.

Stagnation is one of the possible side effects of the inappropriate use of tonics. Stagnation of chi can occur with the overuse of chi tonics like ginseng, causing gastrointestinal fullness, chest pains and tightness, spasms and headaches. This is avoided by using the tonics in moderate doses according to the needs of the individual and the seasonal requirements, and possibly with preliminary detoxification. Another practice is to combine them with *moving* type herbs. Thus chi tonics are often combined with a small amount of chi-regulating or carminative herbs, such as citrus, ginger and cardamon. Yang tonics are often combined with warming stimulants like aconite or cinnamon. Blood tonics are combined with a small amount of blood-moving or emmenagogue herbs, like ligusticum or wild ginger. Yin tonics are combined with a small amount of chi-moving or carminative herbs. With small additional amounts of these circulating herbs, the tonic properties are better utilized and symptoms of stagnation prevented.

Oriental tonic herbs are generally classified as having a sweet flavor. If the right herb or combination is chosen, the flavor and aroma may seem particularly intriguing or appealing to the person being treated. Since the Chinese and East Indians believe that food is the best tonic, tonic herbs are often combined with food. For those who are weak, the Chinese use rice porridge *(congee)*, slowly cooking the rice in a tea made of the tonic herbs. Another method is to combine the tonic herbs with a hearty meat soup. In India, the vegetarian Hindus add them to boiled warm milk to achieve a similar deeply nourishing effect. If flesh foods are used, then one would select those parts and organs of the animal corresponding to those one is trying to strengthen. Combining concentrated foods with tonic herbs allows them to mutually increase their effectiveness and utilization by the body and will produce stronger tonic effects then when either is used alone. (See chapter on principles of food therapy, pg. 73)

Tonification never should never be attempted during an acute phase of disease, when there is high fever and severe inflammation. To do so could cause a severe aggravation of the symptoms. It is, therefore, important to distinguish genuine from false yin or yang symptoms. A genuine yin condition may exhibit obvious signs of weakness and emaciation, with some accompanying false yang symptoms of ruddy complexion, red tongue with no coat, rapid thready pulse, feverish sensations or mild inflammation. Mistaking this condition for a genuine excess yang state, and giving purgative, eliminating therapies, could result in dangerously further weakening the individual and aggravating the symptoms.

Conversely, there are genuine excess yang conditions with various false yin signs. The individual may be heavy-set, with a condition of paleness, edema and tiredness caused by stagnation, with a deep slow pulse and an enlarged tongue with a thick white coat. Mistaking such a condition for deficiency and weakness and giving ginseng could result in an aggravation of the symptoms.

As stated, contrary to Western herbal tonics which are bitter, Oriental tonics are largely sweet. This reflects the fundamental life-supporting effects of the sweet taste, which is the anabolic flavor that builds up all the bodily tissues and represents fundamental nourishment. From this, one can create a powerful tonic using concentrated foods and herbs.

A combination of herbs is more than the sum of its parts. One may make a combination of 20 or more apparently non-tonic herbs and, with the addition of raw, unrefined sugar, honey, clarified butter, sesame oil, salt and boiled down whole milk, create a powerful tonic action that may not be present in any one of the individual herbs. This is commonly achieved in Ayurveda.

HERBAL TONICS AND THE IMMUNE SYSTEM

Tonics are used specifically to strengthen the immune system. A deficiency of chi will cause one to feel tired, run-down, and to be subject to frequent disease and sickness. A deficiency of yang will cause one to be susceptible to cold diseases, with lack of motivation and sexual libido. A deficiency of yin will cause one to have inflammatory symptoms and wasting diseases associated with a loss of bodily essence. A deficiency of blood causes tiredness, weakness and low vitality.

Ginseng is considered the father of all tonics. Although classified as a chi tonic by the Chinese, it can be used to tonify any genuine deficiency, whether chi, yang, yin or blood. It is used for wasting of bodily fluids and is one of the best herbs to satisfy thirst. *Astragalus mongolicus* is probably the most powerful herb for the *Wei chi* or immune system. Besides its use for this purpose and to aid digestion, it has proven effective in counteracting the effects of radiation and chemotherapy, for which purpose it it also is used by the Chinese.

The immune system is very complex. Its processes extend far beyond our simple understanding of phagocytosis or the function of various antibodies, such as white blood cells, in overcoming invading pathogens. The immune system is intimately connected with digestion, the liver and the hormonal system, and is affected either positively or negatively by the emotions. Only tonic foods and herbs, with their broad and holistic action, have the ability to build the immune system.

A principle of Oriental herbal therapy is to "preserve the righteous chi". This is done by adding a small amount of an appropriate tonic when giving a detoxifying herbal therapy. (This is especially necessary if there is a combination of excesses that need to be cleansed, in addition to underlying deficiencies.) By so doing, one can effect a smoother elimination of toxins and largely avoid the so-called healing crises. Western approaches to natural treatment often seem to provoke the healing crisis. Oriental approaches try to avoid these reactions by using a more balanced therapy and through a more precise understanding of what needs to be eliminated (as distinguished from what should be preserved and strengthened). In actual practice, however, healing crises often occur with Oriental herbal therapy, too.

Still another important consideration is the amount of tonics to be given. Too much or too little may produce side effects, either because the individual was unable to handle the too high dose or because not enough was given to stimulate a positive reaction. Generally, it is better to underprescribe, so that the dose, if reasonably accepted, may be gradually increased as needed.

Most wild foods are considered tonic. It is considered that they may be able to impart to those who ingest them their abilities to adapt to their natural environments, thus helping us to counteract various physiological as well as psychological stresses. Herbs that have adapted themselves to grow in harsh, rugged environments tend to impart their acquired strength to one who uses them. For this reason, perhaps, aboriginal peoples tended to ignore the process of tonification, since almost everything they ate was wild and strength giving. However, this made them easy prey to various plagues and diseases, brought in by the white invaders, that were previously foreign to their environment. Most of North American Western herbalism is based upon Native American herbs, but the native peoples had very little use for such tonics as American ginseng, except as a treatment for chronic cough and as a charm.

The traditional Oriental cultures, such as the Chinese and East Indians, have given us immune-potentiating tonics—such as ginseng and astragalus or the Ayurvedic ashwagandha—that can afford protection against life in an overcrowded environment, with its attendant pollution. What we have inherited from the Native Americans are highly effective herbal treatments for their most common ills before the coming of the white man: some acute diseases, injuries, wounds, and such. Thus, we have yet to discover the tonic potential in many of our native plants. It is hoped that this will be accomplished before the natural environment is irreparably damaged.

Ayurvedic medicine classifies most tonics as kapha or water predominant, because of their building properties. Generally, they tend to reduce vata (air), as air-types tend towards deficiency (lightness). Yang and some chi tonics may reduce kapha by their fiery nature, while yin and blood tonics tend to decrease pitta (fire) by their fluid-promoting action. Ayurveda, even more than Chinese medicine, prescribes tonics only after toxins or excesses are removed or reduced.

(For further discussion of tonics, see also section on supplementing therapy, pg. 103)

CHI OR ENERGY TONICS

Herbs that directly increase energy and stamina are called *chi tonics*. According to traditional Chinese medical theory, they work primarily on the major organs that increase energy: the lungs that derive energy directly from the air, the heart that is the seat of divine consciouness, the spleen-stomach that derives energy from food and drink, and the kidney-adrenals that house the root or ancestral energy.

If the body is weak it functions poorly, resulting in sluggishness, lack of motivation, prolapse of the organs, spontaneous sweating, chronic diarrhea and related symptoms. If there is deficient lung chi, there may be shortness of breath, lethargy, soft voice and spontaneous sweating. Spleen-stomach weakness produces a lack of appetite or excessive appetite with low energy, emaciation, chronic diarrhea, prolapse of organs, a tendency to bleed or bruise easily, and perhaps anemia. Chi deficiency of the heart causes palpitations, angina pains, coldness and a weak pulse. Kidney-adrenal deficiency causes frequent urination, premature ejaculation or seminal emission, impotence, and weakness of the lower back, knees and joints.

Chi tonics treat these organ weaknesses but particularly those of the spleen and lungs.

Clinical research in Russia, China and Japan has demonstrated that chi tonic herbs increase one's resistance to both physiological and emotional stress.

In terms of Ayurveda, these herbs primarily strengthen vata, the air humor, and are good for conditions of nervous and weak digestion. Yet some, like ginseng, may be too stimulating for extremely ennervated conditions. They increase pitta and most increase kapha (except those which are drying or diuretic like *Atractylodes*).

Chi or energy tonics are contraindicated for any excess or acute conditions or a more primary yin or blood deficiency.

The Issue of Ginseng

Various plants that are called ginsengs may not even belong to the same plant family. They have somewhat different potencies and therapeutic actions. These include the following:

American ginseng *(Panax quinquefolium)*: botanically the closest to Chinese ginseng and the other plant capable of cross-pollinating with it. The Chinese claim it is more bitter, cooler and generally inferior to their own. Nevertheless, they have purchased both the wild and cultivated varieties by the tons for several centuries. Spectrographic analysis reveals a higher content of ginsenosides in American ginseng than in the Oriental variety. Whether American ginseng is cool and Oriental ginseng is warm seems to be debatable.[1]

The Chinese sometimes regard white Chinese ginseng as neutral. The Koreans, who cultivate the major part of the world's ginseng, preserve their roots from insect infestation by steaming them. This causes them to turn out red, and they definitely are considered to have a warm energy.

Codonopsis *(Codonopsis pilosula):* Most often used as a mild substitute for *Panax ginseng,* but double the amount is required. Even so, is is considered safer for year round use. (see below).

Prince's Ginseng *(Pseudostellaria heterophylla):* is not in the ginseng family, but in the *Caryophyllaceae.* Nevertheless, Prince's ginseng is considered a chi tonic for spleen, heart and lung deficiencies, and treats loss of appetite and fatigue. It is especially therapeutic for wasting dryness of the lungs.

Tienchi ginseng *(Panax pseudoginseng):* is a member of the ginseng family and is cultivated in Hunan province, China. It is usually classified as a trauma herb and a hemostatic (see pg. 269) but often is used as a tonic. It is sometimes preferred to other varieties of ginseng for individuals under the age of 40 or those involved in sports. This is because it seems to greatly increase stamina, but without the danger of overtonification that can occur with regular ginseng.

The Russians have discovered ginseng-like properties in what is known as "Siberian ginseng" *(Eleutherococcus senticosus).* Its Chinese name is "si wu jia", one of the varieties of "wu jia" (mostly members of the *Acanthopanax* species). This herb, a close relative to ginseng is used in China primarily as an antirheumatic.

Two other North American plants in the ginseng family, with remarkable ginseng-like tonic properties, are devil's club *(Oplopanax horridum),* classified here as a blood tonic and specifically useful for regulating blood sugar, and spikenard *(Aralia racemosa* and *A. californica),* which seems to be especially beneficial as a hormone precursor for women.

The unrelated South American plant suma is called "Brazilian ginseng" by the Japanese who have studied it and found it to have ginseng-like properties. In India, *Withania somnifera,* called ashwagandha, has strengthening and immune potentiating ginseng properties especially valuable for counteracting weakness, diseases of aging and impotence (see yang tonics, pg. 309). It has been figuratively (not botanically) called "Indian ginseng", Since it is the principal strengthening tonic herb in the

Ayurvedic system, as ginseng is in the Chinese.

Some other Chinese herbs called *shen* (ginseng is *ren shen*) are sometimes known as "ginsengs". Various *shen* or spirit herbs treat the different organs. Ginseng is for the spleen; adenophora *(sha shen)* for the lungs; scrophularia *(xuan shen)* for the kidneys; and sophora *(ku shen)* for the liver. To call them "ginsengs", though, is not strictly accurate.

There is a tendency for any new and powerful herb to be compared to ginseng or called a kind of ginseng. In purchasing an herb represented as ginseng, examine it carefully to be sure it is not inexpensive quasi-ginseng herb rather than the expensive authentic Chinese or American variety.

GINSENG   *Panax ginseng; Araliaciae*

Energetics: sweet, slightly bitter, slightly warm
Meridians/Organs affected: spleen, lungs, heart
Part used: root
Active constituents: triterpenic saponosides, known as ginsenosides, and traces of essential oils. Ginseng also is known to contain trace amounts of germanium which may be partially responsible for its remarkable action.
Properties: chi tonic, demulcent, stimulant, rejuvenative
Uses: It treats all deficiency diseases, strengthens the lungs, nourishes body fluids, counteracts thirst, and calms the spirit. It may be used for shock, collapse, lung deficiency, chronic febrile diseases, and heart weakness. It is helpful for convalescence, debility and weakness in old age. Ginseng also increases wisdom, promotes longevity and increases resistance to disease.
Dosage: 3-9 gms. (up to 30 gms. for shock)

AMERICAN GINSENG   *Panax quinquefolium;*
                                                             Araliaceae

Energetics: sweet, bitter, neutral
Meridians/Organs affected: lungs, spleen
Part used: root

Active constituents: similar to Chinese ginseng
Properties: chi and yin tonic, demulcent, rejuvenative
Uses: Its uses are similar to those of Chinese ginseng. It is a little milder and safer for general use and may be taken in the summer or by those who find regular ginseng overly stimulating. It is particularly good for increasing body fluids
Dosage: 3-9 gms.

CODONOPSIS (Dang shen)   *Codonopsis pilosula;*
                                                                Campanulaceae

Energetics: sweet, slightly warm
Meridians/Organs affected: spleen, lung
Part used: root
Active constituents: saponin, starch, sugar
Properties: chi tonic, demulcent, expectorant
Uses: It increases vital energy. It is used as a substitute for ginseng and considered safer for both sexes and in all climates. It has a more demulcent or sticky property and, since it is more likely to aggravate chi stagnation, it might be advisable to combine it with carminative herbs.
Dosage: 6-20 gms.

ASTRAGALUS   *Astragalus mongolicus,*
(Yellow vetch)   *A. membranaceus* and *A. hoantchy; Leguminosae*

Energetics: sweet, slightly warm
Meridians/Organs affected: spleen, lung
Part used: the root
Active constituents: 2'4'-dihydroxy-5,6-dimethoxyisoflavane, choline, betaine, kumatakenin, sucrose, glucoronic acid, B-sitosterol
Properties: chi tonic, diuretic, anhydrotic (stops sweating)
Uses: It strengthens digestion, raises metabolism, strengthens the immune system, and promotes the healing of wounds and injuries. It treats chronic weakness of the lungs with shortness of breath, collapse of energy, prolapse of internal organs, spontaneous sweating, chronic lesions, and deficiency edema. It is very effective in cases of nephritis that do not respond to diuretics.
Dosage: 6-15 gms.

JUJUBE DATES   *Zizyphus sativa; Rhamnaceae*

Energetics: sweet, warm
Meridian/Organ affected: spleen
Part used: the fruit
Active constituents: mucilage, sugar, fat and zizyphic acid
Properties: chi tonic, expectorant, nutritive, mild sedative
Uses: It nourishes blood and chi, calms the spirit, increases weight, and harmonizes and sweetens herbal formulas.
Dosage: 3-12 gms.

ATRACTYLODES   *Atractylodes alba; Compositae*

Energetics: bitter, sweet, warm
Meridians/Organs affected: spleen, stomach
Part used: the root
Active constituents: essential comprised of atractylon (C14 H18 O) and atractylol (15 H26 O)
Properties: chi tonic, diuretic, carminative
Uses: It tonifies digestion, and counteracts fatigue, diarrhea, lack of appetite and vomiting. It is good for fluid retention accompanied by low energy, and involuntary sweating caused by low energy. It also treats chronic gastroenteritis.
Dosage: 3-12 gms.

LICORICE   *Glycyrrhiza glabra and spp.; Leguminosae*

Energetics: sweet, neutral
Meridians/Organs affected: spleen, lung (all 12 meridians)
Part used: the root
Active constituents: glycyrrhizic acid, glycyrrhetinic acid, glycyrrhizin. Substances in this herb seem to produce physiological reactions of desoxycorticosterone, with associated retention of sodium and water and the excretion of potassium.
Properties: chi tonic, expectorant, demulcent, aperient, mild sedative.
Uses: It strengthens digestion, treats stomach and duodenal ulcers, and improves energy (especially when honey-roasted in a wok which gives it a warmer energy). It is good for dryness of the lungs, coughs and

colds; it clears heat, detoxifies poisons, relieves abdominal pains and
spasms, and counteracts sore throat. It is used as a harmonizing and
flavoring agent in many herbal formulas.

Precautions: Its principal contraindication is in cases where there is a
tendency towards fluid retention, edema with high blood pressure. It
should be used moderately for women, who tend to retain water more
than men. It is fifty times sweeter than sugar and the smallest amount
will cut through a formula and prevent any uncomfortable side effects.

Dosage: 1-9 gms.

DIOSCOREA
Dioscorea batata, D. japonica;
Dioscoreaceae

Energetics: sweet, neutral
Meridians/Organs affected: lung, kidney, spleen
Part used: the tuberous root
Active constituents: 16% starch, mucilage, amylase, albuminoid mat-
ter, fat, sugar, amino acids including arginine, leucine, tyrosine, and
glutamine
Properties: chi tonic, nutrient, demulcent
Uses: It treats digestive weakness, enteritis, diarrhea, diabetes, weak-
ness of the lungs and kidneys, chronic cough, enuresis, spermatorrhea,
emotional instability and frailty.
Dosage: 6-15 gms.

BARLEY MALT or RICE SYRUP
Sacharum
granoram; Graminaceae

Energetics: sweet, warm
Meridians/Organs affected: spleen, stomach, lung
Part used: the malt sugar extract
Active constituents: maltose
Properties: chi tonic, demulcent, nutritive, antispasmodic
Uses: It imparts vitality and strength, moistens the lung, stops cough,
and treats weakness of digestion. It is good for abdominal pain, particu-
larly in children.
Dosage: 30-60 gms.

HONEY   *Mel*

Energetics: sweet, neutral
Meridians/Organs affected: stomach, spleen, lungs
Active constituents: vary according to the type of honey
Properties: tonic, demulcent, nutritive, laxative, expectorant
Uses: it is similar to sugar but better to use for kapha or overweight conditions with fluid retention, as it is more drying. However, since it is more astringent it is more difficult to digest and can be stagnating. It is good for sweetening and harmonizing most formulas and as an anti-dote for most natural poisons. It treats dryness of the bowels and also may be used to strengthen the eyes, introducing one drop directly into each eye. Other bee secretions, like propolis and royal jelly, also have chi tonic properties, the latter to a high degree.
Dosage: take as needed

SPIKENARD   *Aralia racemosa, A. califorica,*
                              A. nudicaulis and A. quinquefolia; Araliaceae

Energetics: sweet, acrid, warm
Meridians/Organs affected: lung, spleen
Part used: the root
Active constituents: essential oil, tannins, saponin, spogenins, diter-pene acids
Properties: chi tonic, diuretic, expectorant, carminative, alterative, stimulant, diaphoretic
Uses: It is used for chronic pulmonary diseases, digestive weakness, gynecological problems, blood purification, venereal diseases, and rheu-matic aches and pains. As a chi tonic it may be more effective when roasted with honey.
Dosage: 3-9 gms.

STARFLOWER   *Trientalis borealis; Primulaceae*

Energetics: acrid, sweet, warm
Meridians/Organs affected: lungs, spleen, heart
Part used: the root
Active constituents: not presently known

Properties: chi tonic, stimulant
Uses: It is used for weakness, fatigue, exhaustion
Dosage: 3-6 gms.

ELECAMPANE ROOT   *Inula helinum; Compositae*

Energetics: sweet, acrid, bitter, warm
Meridians/Organs affected: lung, spleen
Part used: the root
Active constituents: essential oil, bitter principles, resin, inulin
Properties: chi tonic, carminative, expectorant, diuretic, antiseptic, astringent, stimulant
Uses: It is used for chronic cold lung conditions with clear expectoration, cough, consumption, bronchitis and asthma. It strengthens digestion and inhibits the formation of mucus from weak digestion. The flowers alone are used to lower the chi and therefore stop coughs. To increase its tonic properties, roast in a wok with honey.
Dosage: 3-9 gms.

SUMA   *Pfaffia paniculata; Amarantheaceae*

Energetics: acrid, sweet, warm
Meridians/Organs affected: spleen, lung
Part used: the root
Active constituents: novel type of saponin called nortriterpenoid, in which pfaffic acid was identified as a hydrolysis product. Six kinds of saccharide derivatives of the pfaffic acid structural type were found. Five of the six pfaffosides are inhibitory to cultured tumor cell melanomas. The basic structural type of pfaffic acid is also inhibitory to cultured melanomas. Sitosterol, stigmasterol and allantoin was also present in the roots. Further studies have demonstrated the presence of germanium as one of the active constituents in suma.
Properties: chi tonic, nutrient, demulcent
Uses: It increases energy, strengthens the immune system, fortifies hormones (especially estrogen), reduces tumors and cancers, regulates blood sugar. It is considered a near panacea in Brazil, where it is called "Brazilian ginseng".

Dosage: The effective minimum dose for the treatment of cancer is at least 9 gms. daily.

SIBERIAN GINSENG   *Eleutherococcus senticosus;*
                                        Araliaceae

Energetics: acrid, sweet, bitter, warm
Meridians/Organs affected: liver, kidney
Part used: the bark of the root
Active constituents: essential oil, resin, starch, vitamin A
Properties: chi tonic, antirheumatic, antispasmodic
Uses: It is used to treat low vitality and lack of endurance. For athletes, 10-20 gms. is taken daily to increase stamina. It is antirheumatic and often is given to the aged in the form of a wine. It reduces swelling, treats difficult urination, edema, poor circulation, coldness, and damp swelling of the legs.
Dosage: 3-15 gms.

ADRENAL YANG TONICS
(Kidney Yang Tonics)

Herbs that strengthen the yang or root energy of the body are primarily sweet, but some have a pungent or salty taste. They all enter the kidney organ and channel primarily, and the liver and spleen secondarily. Their energy is usually warm. This means their properties are generally tonic, diuretic, astringent and aphrodisiac.

Symptoms of yang deficiency include the following: exhaustion, timidity, feeling like being alone and not talking, lack of will power, fear of cold, lower back and joint pains, impotence, frigidity, pallor, spermatorrhea, clear leucorrhea, enuresis, polyuria, wheezing, asthma and morning diarrhea.

While chi tonics address the aspects of digestion and vitality that especially relate to the energy derived from air, food and water (acquired chi), yang tonics are more fundamental and treat our source energy, sometimes called *congenital chi*. The yang of the kidney-adrenals is the fundamental yang of the entire body *(ming men)*, the fire of the gate of life. This is the original spark on which all life depends, the pilot light for our energy system.

Thus herbs in this category often have a direct regulating effect upon the endocrine system, and effect energy metabolism, sexual function, growth and the immune system. Some of the more powerful and direct yang tonics used by the Chinese are derived from animals. These sources include the antler velvet of young deer (thinly sliced and macerated in vodka or gin), the reproductive organs of animals, the human placenta, and male and female gecko lizards. This list recalls the times of the witches and warlocks who were burned at the stake in Europe and early America for using such strange substances. Traditional Chinese Medicine helps us to see that there may have been a rational basis for the therapeutic use of these things.

Some substances and herbs in this category, such as human placenta and saw palmetto berries, tonify both kidney yin and kidney yang. These are thus milder and safer to use, having a more complete tonic action. Commonly available kidney yang herbs include walnut and fenugreek.

Following the principle of yin and yang being mutually rooted, it is more effective to add some yin tonic to attract and develop the energy of yang. Hence these herbs are often combined, with either the yin or yang aspect predominating, according to which most needs to be tonified. Many yang tonic formulas, therefore, include herbs like prepared rehmannia or lycium berries for yin tonification. Usually it is more necessary to protect the yin while tonifying the yang, then it is to protect the yang while tonifying the yin, because the yin, being more delicate, can be more easily damaged.

These herbs also are used to strengthen the mind and develop will and stamina. They are helpful for individuals who lack decisiveness, focus and direction. Many of them, however particularly those derived from animal sources, can over-stimulate the reproductive system (the most powerful aphrodisiacs are found in this category), and irritate or dull the mind. Therefore, they are not recommended for those practicing yoga.

In Ayurveda, these herbs are considered to nourish and strengthen the deeper tissues of muscle, bone marrow, nerves and reproductive secretions. They increase pitta, the biological humor most closely corresponding to the yang. Those more nourishing in nature increase kapha (water), while those more warming or drying decrease it. Generally, because of their heavy nature, they all diminish vata (air). They should be used only in conditions where there are no excesses to be cleared. When used where conditions of excess are present, they can strongly aggravate any of the humors.

These herbs are contraindicated for deficient yin symptoms with emaciation, and wasting and inflammatory diseases. Signs of incorrect or excessive use include feeling hot, excessive sexual desire, anger, irritability and insomnia.

WALNUTS   *Juglans regia; Juglandaceae*

Energetics: sweet, warm
Meridians/Organs affected: lung, kidney
Part used: the seed. The outer hull and bark have other useful actions.
Active constituents: juglone, isojuglone, essential oil, inositol, phytin, phytosterols, oxidase, vitamins A, B, C and E, and ellagic, lauric, myristic, arachic, linoleic, linolenic, isolinolenic, and oleic acids. Juglone is believed to have an antifungal property. The hulls and leaves are highly astringent and contain tannin as well as juglandin, a bitter principle.
Properties: tonic, nutritive, demulcent; the outer shells and bark are alterative and antifungal; the bark is laxative
Uses: The seeds are a mild yang tonic good for wasting diseases, emaciation and underweight conditions, and weakness and dryness of the colon and lungs. The bark has mild astringent and laxative properties, the leaves and outer hulls are antiparasitical, antifungal and detoxifying.
Dosage: kernels 6-15 gms.; powdered hulls and leaves may be used internally (about one teaspoon per cup of boiling water), and externally as a liniment or lotion for skin diseases and parasites.

FENUGREEK SEEDS   *Trigonella foenum-graecum*
                                                    Leguminosae

Energetics: bitter, warm
Meridians/Organs affected: liver, kidney

Part used: seeds
Active constituents: 28% mucilage, fatty oil, saponins, choline, lecithin, phytosterols and an alkaloid, trigonelline
Properties: yang tonic, nutritive, carminative, stimulant, demulcent, alterative
Uses: The pulverized seeds may be taken as a tonic for osteomyelitis, tuberculosis and scrofula. They also are traditionally used to counteract catarrh and phlegm, prevent fever, treat stomach and digestive disorders, and regulate insulin in diabetes. They are helpful for wasting diseases, anemia, debility, neurasthenia and gout. The crushed seeds are applied externally as a cataplasm and poultice to sores, boils and abscesses. This is one of the oldest known medicinal herbs, used by Hippocrates, and widely esteemed by both East and West.
Dosage: 3-9 gms.

FALSE UNICORN ROOT
Chamaelirium luteum dioica (Helonias dioica); Liliaceae

Energetics: bitter, warm
Meridians/Organs affected: kidney, spleen
Part used: root
Active constituents: chamaelirin, fatty acid
Properties: tonic, diuretic, vermifuge, emetic in large doses
Uses: It is used for more feminine reproductive problems, including infertility, menstrual irregularities, amenorrhea, leucorrhea, prevention of miscarriages and morning sickness. The primary indication is a heavy dragging feeling in the lower abdomen. It is a good general tonic for genitourinary problems and liver and kidney diseases. It also is used to treat dyspepsia, loss of appetite, malabsorption, albuminuria, atony of the sexual organs, nocturnal emissions, aching pain in the lumbosacral region, and impotence. One other use for this remarkable herb is in the treatment of worms and parasites. For this purpose it is taken internally or applied externally as a lotion or paste.
Dosage: standard dosage or 3-9 gms.; tincture, 5-30 drops

DAMIANA (Turnera)

Turnera aphrodisiaca;
Turneraceae

Energetics: spicy, warm
Meridian/Organ affected: kidney
Part used: leaves
Active constituents: essential oil with cineol, cymol, pinene, arbutin, hydrocyanic glycoside, bitter principle, tannin, resin
Properties: yang tonic, aphrodisiac, diuretic, nervine, aperient
Uses: It treats frigidity in women and impotence in men. It also is used for chronic cystic catarrh and renal catarrh. It improves digestion, cures constipation and relieves respiratory disorders including irritable coughs.
Dosage: 3-6 gms.

YOHIMBE

Coryanthe yohimbe, Pausinystalia yohimbe;
Rubiaceae

Energetics: spicy, warm
Meridians/Organs affected: kidney, heart
Part used: bark
Active constituents: several isomeric alkaloids, the most important of which is yohimbine
Properties: stimulant, aphrodisiac, cardiac, local anesthetic
Uses: It treats impotence and frigidity, angina pectoris and painful menstruation. It is an antidiuretic, and either may lower or increase blood pressure in humans (needs more study).
Dosage: 3-6 gms.

MUIRA-PUAMA

Liriosma cupana; Oleacaceae

Energetics: spicy, warm
Meridian/Organ affected: kidney
Part used: balsam
Active constituents: the alkaloid muira-paumine
Properties: aphrodisiac, stimulant

Uses: It treats both frigidity and impotence, and probably tonifies kidney yang.
Dosage: root (according to Jeanne Rose[2]), 10-60 drops of the alcoholic liquid extract or one capsule daily; in formulas, 3-6 gms.

CELERY SEEDS   *Apium graveolens; Umbelliferae*

Energetics: spicy, warm
Meridians/Organs affected: kidney, spleen
Part used: seeds
Active constituents: essential oil, flavonic glycoside and a furanocoumarin (bergaptene)
Properties: stimulant, emmenagogue, antirheumatic, diuretic, carminative
Uses: It is used to treat chronic kidney and bladder problems of a cold nature, overweight, flatulence, dropsy, pulmonary catarrh, rheumatism, gout, arthritis, delayed menses, impotence and frigidity. Ajwan *(Carum copticum),* a similar Ayurvedic herb, is a powerful warming spice for cold debility conditions and is used in cooking. Celery stalk, however, is cooling and sedative.
Precautions: It is contraindicated for pregnant women, since it is strongly abortive.
Dosage: standard dose or 3-9 gms. in formulas

CUBEB   *Piper cubeba; Piperaceae*

Energetics: spicy, warm
Meridians/Organs affected: kidney, lungs
Part used: fruit
Active constituents: 10 to 185 volatile oil, amorphous cubebic acid, colorless crystaliine cubebin and resins
Properties: yang tonic, stimulant, diuretic, expectorant
Uses: Cubeb is used for joint pains, gleet (penile discharge), chronic urethritis, gonorrhea after the preliminary inflammatory stage, chronic cystitis, abscesses of the prostate gland and hemorrhoids. It treats most chronic urinary-genital disorders, especially of a cold nature; catarrh of the lungs and bronchitis; and weak digestion.
Dosage: standard dose or 3-9 gms. in formulas

SAW PALMETTO (Serona)   *Sabal serrulata;*
                                                  Palmaceae

Energetics: pungent, sweet, warm
Meridians/Organs affected: kidney, spleen, liver
Part used: the fruit
Active constituents: essential oil, fatty oil, with capric, caprylic and lauric acids, fatty acids, carotene, tannin, sitosterol invert sugar, estrogenic substance
Properties: yang and yin tonic, diuretic, expectorant, roborant, aphrodisiac
Uses: It is used for wasting diseases, impotence, frigidity, and prostate problems (combined with echinacea). It helps build muscles, is good for colds, asthma, bronchitis, and catarrh due to deficiency and coldness.
Dosage: 3-12 gms.

GARLIC   *Allium sativa; Liliaceae*

Energetics: spicy, hot
Meridians/Organs affected: lungs, kidney, spleen, stomach, colon
Part used: bulb
Active constituents: Allyl sulfide, allicin, alliin, Vitamins A and C, nicotinic acid
Properties: Garlic is a yang tonic and a stimulant, diuretic, alterative, digestant, carminative, expectorant and parasiticide.
Uses: It stimulates metabolism, and is used both for chronic and acute diseases; has both tonic and alterative properties; counteracts lower back and joint pains, arthritis and rheumatism. It also treats weak digestion, genito-urinary diseases, lung and bronchial infections and mucous conditions. In Ayurveda it is considered a rejuvenative for both kapha (water) and vata (air).

Garlic cloves may be taken internally both as a preventative and as a treatment for all intestinal worms. Blended with a little sesame or olive oil, it may be used externally. However, its strong odor may repel humans as well as parasites. A single dose is three to five cloves in infusion or taken raw. This is repeated three to six times a day until the problem is resolved. Garlic is good for amoebic dysentery. Enemas of garlic also are helpful. It is an effective antibiotic for staphylococcus, streptococcus and salmonella bacteria and is effective against bacteria that are resistant to standard antibiotic drugs. It is a good antifungal for the treatment of candida albicans yeast infections. For the treatment of pinworms, it should be made into a paste with olive oil or the bruised clove inserted directly into the rectum. For vaginitis and leucorrhea, one or two bruised cloves wrapped in muslin are inserted into the vagina. Since it is a local irritant, it should be combined with an oil when applied externally.

Precautions: Pregnant women should use in small amounts as garlic is a mild emmenagogue. The yogis used it as a medicine, but did not recommend it as a food or spice because of its irritating properties.

Dosage: as tonic 3-6 gms.

DODDER SEEDS

Cuscuta europaea or C. japonica; Convulvulaceae

Energetics: sweet, neutral
Meridians/Organs affected: kidney, liver
Part used: seeds
Active constituents: glucoside cuscutin
Properties: yang and yin tonic, demulcent, aperient, diuretic, ophthalmic, aphrodisiac
Uses: It is used for impotence, spermatorrhea, prostatitis and neurological weakness. It builds sperm, builds the blood, strengthens sinews and bones. It also treats enuresis and seminal emission; constipation, backache and cold knees; and rheumatoid arthritis. It improves vision. One of the safer and more affordable yang tonics, dodder, like mistletoe, is a common parasitic growth on plants.
Dosage: 6-15 gms.

PSORALEA SEEDS

Psoralea spp.; Leguminosae

Energetics: bitter, pungent, warm
Meridians/Organs affected: kidney, spleen, pericardium
Part used: the seeds
Active constituents: fatty oil, alkaloid and psoralein or poraline

Properties: yang tonic, diuretic, stimulant

Uses: It treats impotence, spermatorrhea, premature ejaculation and leucorrhea; and skin diseases including leukoderma, leprosy, alopecia (baldness), psoriasis and callosity. It is antifungal and for most skin diseases should be taken internally and externally. For the latter, the seeds are crushed and topically applied in a poultice. Bensky and Gamble,[2] report on Chinese pharmacological research into the treatment of alopecia using psoralea. An injection of psoralea extracts and exposure to ultraviolet light were used in 45 cases. Within six months hair was completely restored in 36% of the cases and there was a significant restoration in another 30%. There are North American varieties in addition to the Chinese variety. These include *P. esculenta,* known as Indian bread root, of which the tubers were eaten and described by Lewis and Clark as "a kind of ground potato". Most early North American records indicate consumption of the root and not the seeds.

In Ayurveda it is used as an anti-pitta herb, for skin diseases and hair loss.

Dosage: of the seeds 3-9 gms.

TEASEL ROOT   *Dipsacus sylvestris and spp.;*
Dipsacaceae

Energetics: bitter, warm
Meridians/Organs affected: liver, kidney
Part used: root
Active constituents: essential oil, alkaloid lamine
Properties: tonic, diuretic, sudorific, stomachic, ophthalmic
Uses: The root is used to strengthen the bones and tendons and liver, stimulate blood circulation, treat weakness of the limbs, for arthritis and rheumatic complaints, and to prevent miscarriage.
Dosage: 6-12 gms.

EPIMEDIUM   *Epimedium grandiflorum and spp.;*
Berberidaceae

Energetics: acrid, sweet, warm
Meridians/Organs affected: liver, kidney

Part used: the leaves
Active constituents: glycoside icariin or epimedin, benzene, sterols, tannin, palmitic acid, linolenic acid, oleic acid, vitamin E
Properties: yang tonic, aphrodisiac, antirheumatic
Uses: It is frequently used in traditional Chinese medicine. The herb is easily cultivated in many parts of North America as an perennial ornamental. It is indicated for impotence, frigidity, spermatorrhea, frequent urination, forgetfulness, withdrawal, feelings of coldness in the lower back with aching soreness of the back and knees, spasms and cramps in the hands and feet, numbness in the extremities, and dizziness and menstrual irregularity associated with hypertension. Pharmacological research in China has demonstrated the effectiveness of this herb in stimulating sexual activity and sperm production. It also stimulates the sensory nerves. While it has not been shown to have any estrogen properties, it does have a moderate androgen-like effect on the testes, prostate and levator ani. Low doses of epimedium appear to increase urinary output while larger doses decrease it.
Precautions: It is contraindicated when there is a tendency towards hypersexuality and wet dreams, and for individuals with severe emaciation, weakness and deficient yin. It can cause dizziness, vomiting, dry mouth, thirst, and nosebleed. It may be advisable not to take over prolonged periods.
Dosage: 3-12 gms.

COTTON ROOT   *Gossypium herbaceum; Malvaceae*

Energetics: sweet, sour, warm
Meridians/Organs affected: liver, kidney
Part used: root, seeds
Active constituents: resinous substance, phenolcarbonic acid, salicylic acid, betaine, sugar, essential oil
Properties: yang tonic, emmenagogue, abortifacient
Uses: It treats impotence and frigidity. The seeds have been used for malaria and to increase nursing mothers' milk. The oil derived from the seeds recently has been studied as a male contraceptive. It was observed by the Chinese that there was a noticable decrease in births in areas

where cottonseed oil was used in cooking.

The fresh root is most effective when prepared in an alcoholic tincture. According to Grieves,[3] it increases contractions of the uterus during labor and also is effective in terminating unwanted pregnancies, for which it was widely used by Southern slaves. It also checks excessive menstrual bleeding, especially when this might be caused by fibroids.

Precautions: Not recommended during pregnancy.

Dosage: boil 4 oz. of the inner bark of the root in a quart of water down to a pint. The dose is one half cup every thirty minutes; tincture, ½ to 1 teaspoon; in formulas, 3-6 gms.

ASHWAGANDHA   *Withania somnifera; Solanaceae*

Energetics: bitter, sweet, warm
Meridians/Organs affected: lungs, kidney
Part used: root
Active constituents: bitter alkaloid somniferin
Properties: yang tonic, aphrodisiac, sedative, astringent
Uses: It treats impotence, infertility, weakness of the back and knees, joint and nerve pain, arthritis, insomnia, neurasthenia, weakness of the mind, wasting diseases, convalescence, poor growth in children, and the diseases of aging. It is the primary strengthening tonic used in Ayurveda. Safe and effective, it does not have the irritant properties of other aphrodisiacs, nor can it be overstimulating, like many of the herbs in this category. In fact, it promotes sound sleep and supports yoga and meditation. It is not prohibitively expensive.

Dosage: 3 gms. of powder twice a day in boiled warm milk; in formulas, 3-12 gms.

DEER ANTLER   *Cornu cervi*

Although the antler most studied is that of the Chinese Sika red deer, other varieties of deer and elk antler are used.

Energetics: sweet, salty, warm
Meridians/Organs affected: liver, kidneys
Part used: antler of the young deer (usually sawed off in the spring, when it is four to six inches long)

Active constituents: pantocrinum has been derived from the Siberian Sika red deer antler. It also contains small amounts of estrone, calcium, magnesium and phosphorus

Properties: tonic, stimulant

Uses: This powerful yang tonic should be used with caution, especially if there is a tendency towards deficient yin. It treats all deficiencies of energy and blood with yang deficiency. It is good for general weakness, physical and mental retardation, children's diseases associated with retarded growth, skeletal deformities, and learning disabilities. It treats impotence, frigidity, infertility, hormonal deficiency in both men and women, premature ejaculation, frequent clear urination, aching soreness in the lower back and joints. It also is very good for women with cold deficient bleeding and leuchorrea. A Himalayan preparation is made by calcining the older deer antlers at a high temperature in a kiln until it is reduced to a white ash. This is then ground to a fine powder, mixed with a small amount of whey (derived from the liquid residue of yogurt), and dried. Since deer shed their antlers naturally, yogis and ascetics are willing to use this preparation, called Sring Bhasma. It is taken during the winter to stimulate inner warmth and metabolism.

Dosage: about one quarter to one half teaspoon two or three times daily. Of the young deer horn, ½ to 1 gm. of the powder alone or in rice wine. A gelatin prepared from the old deer horn, called *lu jiao jiao*, is a less expensive but still effective medicine, dose 6-15 gms.

GECKO LIZARD
Gekko gekko or Phrynosoma cornuta;
Gekkonidae

Energetics: salty, neutral, mildly toxic

Meridians/Organs affected: lung, kidney

Parts used: both the male and female lizards

Properties: yang and yin tonic, stimulant

Uses: It is used to treat impotence, frigidity, frequent clear urination, kidney and lung deficiency with symptoms of asthma, emphysema, wheezing, consumptive cough with intermittent spitting up of blood, and morning diarrhea.

Dosage: 3-6 gms. in powder or pills. Removing the head and the feet (the toxic principle) 9-15 gms. can be boiled in decoction. Again, removing those parts, macerate both dried animals in a quart of rice wine and take 5-30 drops three or four times daily.

TONIFYING/NURTURING HERBS
(Blood Tonics)

The herbs in this category specifically treat deficient blood patterns and anemia. Most enter into the meridians of the heart, the liver and the spleen. Blood deficiency can arise from bleeding, over-exertion, yin deficiency or spleen chi weakness (poor digestion).

A blood deficiency condition manifests in pallor of the complexion and lips, dizziness, weakened vision, lethargy, palpitations, skin dryness, poor memory, ringing in the ears, delayed and scanty menses, pale tongue and a weak, fine, thready pulse.

In traditional Chinese medicine, both the heart and the liver directly affect blood. The heart directs or governs the blood while the liver stores it. This means that herbs that treat the heart tend to promote blood circulation, while many hemostatic, astringent herbs enter the liver organ and meridian. That blood renews itself by being stored in the liver in greater volume at night during sleep is an important concept. The spleen maintains the blood in the vessels. It "controls" the blood and, through digestion, also helps build it.

Most of these herbs work indirectly, building the blood by improving the general health of the whole body. They accomplish this through their nutritional capacity and their ability to promote improved blood circulation. Because of the monthly loss of blood through the menses, women usually have a greater need to tonify blood, while men usually require more chi tonification. This explains why dong quai is usually prescribed as a tonic for women, while ginseng is prescribed for men (although the reverse, of course, may be done in case of opposite deficiencies).

According to Ayurvedic medicine, these herbs would increase kapha (body fluids) and reduce pitta (fire) and vata (air). As blood is intimately related to pitta, tonifying herbs often are specific for pitta disorders. They strengthen the tissues (*dhatus*) not only of blood, but also plasma, muscle and reproductive secretions (semen).

Both blood and yin tonic herbs tend to nourish feelings of tolerance and love. Spiritually, they foster the energy of patience and devotion traditionally characterized as maternal.

YELLOW DOCK (see herbs to detoxify blood, pg. 194)

DONG QUAI   *Angelica sinensis and A. polymorpha;*
                                     Umbelliferae

There are many varieties of wild angelicas growing in the mountains throughout North America. One of these, *A. brewerii,* found in the
California Sierras, seemed a promising substitute for the Chinese dong
quai and the author has used it in his clinic with comparable results.
The common garden angelica *(A. archangelica)* has the emmenagogic
blood-moving properties of dong quai, but lacks the degree of sweetness necessary for tonics.

Energetics: sweet, acrid, bitter, warm
Meridians/Organs affected: heart, liver, spleen
Part used: the root
Active constituents: 40% sucrose, 0.2-0.3% essential oil made up of
carvacrol, safrol, isosafrol, alcohols, sesquiterpenes, cadinene, n-
dodecanol, n-tetradecanol, n-butylphalid; also a non-blycosidal, non-
alkaloid, and a water soluble crystalline material with B 12 and
carotene
Properties: blood tonic, emmenagogue, sedative, analgesic, laxative
Uses: It is used for all gynecological complaints; it regulates menstruation and treats dysmenorrhea and amenorrhea. It tonifies the blood and
is good for tinnitus caused by blood weakness, blurred vision and palpitations. It also promotes blood circulation and thus relieves the pain of
injuries and pains caused by stagnant blood. Finally, it is used for dryness of the bowels causing constipation.
Precautions: Avoid use during the early stages of pregnancy and if
there is bloating, abdominal congestion and conditions of deficient yin
with heat symptoms caused by wasting.
Dosage: 3-15 gms.

PEONY ROOT   *Paeonia spp.; Rununculaceae*

Energetics: bitter, sour, cold
Meridians/Organs affected: liver, spleen, lung
Part used: root
Active constituents: 5% asparagin and benzoic acid also paeoniflorin, paeonol, paeonin, triterpenoids, sistosterol
Properties: blood and yin tonic, emmenagogue, antispasmodic, astringent The cultivated peony is used more as a blood tonic while the wild "red peony" is used more as an emmenagogue.
Uses: It tonifies the blood, treats menstrual cramps and irregularities, amenorrhea, both functional and emotional nervous conditions, including chorea, epilepsy, spasms and other neurological affections. In large doses it is said to be emetic and cathartic, but the author's observations do not bear this out. The Chinese species, which corresponds to the ornamental garden variety, is widely used as an antispasmodic; and catalyst to relax tension in order to enhance the activity of the primary herbs in a formula. Peony is used for this purpose by the Chinese much as Thompsonian herbalists use lobelia. However peony, being a root, has more tonic properties.
Dosage: the fresh root is tinctured in alcohol and given in doses of 1-30 drops; the dried root is given in 6-15 gms. in decoction

REHMANNIA   *Rehmannia glutinosa;*
(Chinese foxglove)   *Scrophulariae*

Energetics: sweet, slightly warm
Meridians/Organs affected: liver, kidney, heart
Part used: the prepared root
Active constituents: glycosides, saponins, arginine, b-sitosterol, mannitol stigmasterol, campesterol rehmannin, catalpol, glucose, tannin, resins, coloring matter and a substance similar to myrtillin
Properties: yin and blood tonic, hemostatic, demulcent, laxative, alterative
Uses: It treats anemia, dizziness, pallor, palpitations, insomnia, irregular menstruation, uterine flooding and bleeding after childbirth

It is the principal herb for nourishing kidney yin. It treats conditions of yin deficiency including night sweats, thirst, wasting and nocturnal emissions. It also is used for kidney deficiency back pains, and to promote the healing of bones and flesh.

As an alterative, it may be used fresh or dried to clear deficient yin heat. This would include such inflammatory conditions as tuberculosis and other strumous or wasting diseases. The tonic is prepared by soaking it in rice wine with spices such as cardamon to increase its warming properties. It may be combined with gelatin to use in arresting excessive uterine bleeding.

Rehmannia is widely used in traditional Chinese medicine. It is cultivated in many areas of North America as a perennial garden ornamental.

Precautions: Individuals with weak digestion, tendency towards gas and abdominal bloating should use it with caution, as it is greasy and hard to digest.

Dosage: 9-30 gms. in decoctions. It is highly water soluble and does not tincture well.

LYCIUM BERRIES   *Lycium chinensis and spp.;*
(Wolfberry, Matrimony vine)   *Solanaceae*

Energetics: sweet, neutral
Meridians/Organs affected: kidney, liver
Part used: berries
Active constituents: carotene, vitamins A and C, thiamene, riboflavin, B- sitosterol, linoleic acid
Properties: blood and yin tonic, hemostatic, nutritive, antipyretic
Uses: It nourishes the blood and yin, helps reproductive secretions, strengthens and brightens the eyes, treats night blindness, dizziness and blurred vision. It also is used for yin deficient, consumptive or strumous diseases with thirst (such as tuberculosis). It tonifies liver and kidney yin; treats sore back, knees and legs; and impotence and nocturnal emission.

The North American varieties appear to have identical properties.
Precautions: Avoid in excess inflammatory conditions or conditions with weak digestion and tendency towards bloating.
Dosage: 6-15 gms.

AMLA   *Emblica officinalis; Combretaceae*

Energetics: sour, sweet, cool
Meridians/Organs affected: heart, liver, kidneys
Part used: fruit
Active constituents: vitamin C (one egg-sized fruit contains as much as eight lemons), tannin, gallic acid, ellagic acid
Properties: blood and yin tonic, nutritive, laxative, rejuvenative
Uses: This is one of the most effective tonics used in Ayurvedic medicine (see Chyavanprash in planetary formulas section, pg. 133). It is helpful for anemia, debility, and wasting diseases; and in convalescence or whenever a good tonic is indicated. A unique quality of the fruit is that the unusually high vitamin C content seems impervious to prolonged storage or cooking. The dry fruit is available at many Indian markets.
Dosage: 6-15 gms. in formulas

MULBERRY FRUIT   *Morus alba (M. microphylla*
which grows in Texas); Moraceae

Energetics: sweet, cool
Meridians/Organs affected: liver, kidney
Part used: fruit
Active constituents: carotene, vitamins A and C, thamene, riboflavin, tannin, linoleic and stearic acids
Properties: blood and yin tonic, nutritive
Uses: It is used for anemia, consumptive diseases with thirst, premature graying of the hair, dizziness and insomnia. It is very good for constipation in the aged caused by dryness from deficient blood.
Precautions: It is contraindicated for individuals with a tendency towards diarrhea and weak digestion.
Dosage: 9-15 gms.

BLACKBERRY and RASPBERRY   *Rubus spp.; Rosaceae*
(also wild Western Thimbleberries)

Energetics: sweet, neutral
Meridians/Organs affected: liver, kidney
Part used: fruit

Active constituents: Raspberry citrus, malic, and salicylic acids; sugars, fragarin, vitamin C and niacin. **Blackberry** Isocitric, and malic acids; sugars, pectin, monoglycoside of cyanidin and vitamin A and C.
Properties: blood and yin tonic, nutritive, refrigerant (the leaves and roots are astringent)
Uses: The fruit and juice are taken for anemia. It also sweetens and cools the blood and regulates menses. The leaves may be used as an astringent and uterine tonic. It also treats diarrhea and dysentery, for which the root bark is stronger.
Dosage: 9-15 gms. of the berries

HUCKLEBERRY (Bilberry)   *Vaccinium spp.;*
Ericaceae

Energetics: sweet, sour, cool
Meridians/Organs affected: liver, kidneys
Parts used: the berries and leaves
Active constituents: vitamin C, sugar; quinnic acid is found in the leaves with a little tannin
Properties: blood and yin tonic, nutritive, diuretic, mild astringent
Uses: The fruit is used for anemia, consumptive wasting and thirst, and also urinary problems such as cystitis and nephritis. The leaves are highly regarded as a remedy for diabetes, lowering occasionally high blood sugar. The leaves also are used, almost identically to uva ursi or pipsissewa, as an astringent and diuretic. The berries of uva ursi and its near relative manzanita are similar hemotonic nutrients. The roots are useful for dropsy and urinary stones.
Dosage: 9-15 gms. of the berries; of the leaves 3-9 gms.

BLACK CURRANT   *Ribes rubrum; Saxifragaceae*

Energetics: sweet, sour, cool
Meridians/Organs affected: liver, kidney

Part used: berries
Active constituents: vitamin C, tanni, traces of essential oil, enzyme emulsion
Properties: blood and yin tonic, nutritive, demulcent
Uses: It treats anemia, wasting and inflammatory diseases, excessive thirst, and sore throat with dry cough
Dosage: 9-15 gms.

GRAPES (dark)   *Vitex vinifera; Vitaceae*

Energetics: sweet, sour, neutral
Meridians/Organs affected: liver, kidney
Parts used: the fruit, leaves
Active constituents: vitamins A, B, C, dextrose, fructose, pectin, tartaric and malic acids, mineral salts, tannin, flavone, glycosides and pigment
Properties: blood and yin, nutritive, diuretic
Uses: It treats blood and energy deficiency, night sweats, thirst, palpitations, rheumatic and joint pains, difficult urination, edema, dry cough
Dosage: 9-30 gms. or drink the fresh juice

LONGAN BERRIES   *Nephelium longana; Sapindaceae*

Energetics: sweet, warm
Meridians/Organs affected: spleen, heart
Part used: berries
Active constituents: 27% glucose, sucrose, vitamins A and B, tartaric acid
Properties: blood and chi tonic, nutritive, mild sedative
Uses: It treats anemia, restlessness and anxiety; reduces the cravings for sweets especially when cooked with millet; and also is used for insomnia, heart palpitations, forgetfulness and dizziness. Often is is used in combination with other herbs to nourish the heart blood and strengthen the heart muscle. Longan berries are available in most Chinese herb or grocery stores.
Dosage: 6-15 gms.

GELATIN   Animal skin gelatin (the best kind is made from black donkey skin)

Energetics: sweet, neutral
Meridians/Organs affected: lung, liver, kidney
Active constituents: gelatin, chondrin, collagen
Properties: blood and yin tonic, nutritive, hemostatic, demulcent
Uses: It is used for anemia, bleeding, dryness, dizziness, pallor, palpitations, and consumptive bleeding of the lungs. It is a specific for menorrhagia or excess menstrual bleeding and is the best herb for deficiency bleeding. It is used in a special tonic Chinese patent medicine called Don Quai Gin, available in most Chinese herb stores. It may be combined with other blood tonic herbs, such as dong quai, to enhance its tonic properties. For those with a weak stomach it may be difficult to digest.
Dosage: 6-15 gms. It is separately dissolved in warm water and the strained decoction of the other herbs is then added to it.

BLACKSTRAP MOLASSES

Energetics: sweet, warm
Meridians/Organs affected: liver, spleen, kidney
Active constituents: a variety of sugars, calcium, iron, potassium, B vitamins and trace minerals such as zinc, copper and chromium
Properties: blood tonic, digestive
Uses: it is used to treat blood weakness, wasting and degenerative diseases. Use it as a base for syrup of yellow dock. Make a decoction of on ounce of yellow dock root. Simmer in a pint of water for twenty minutes, strain and discard liquid. Cook the herbs again in one cup of water until it reduces to ½ cup. Add one ounce of blackstrap molasses. Keep refrigerated.
Dosage: take two or three tablespoons two or three times a day

IRON   *Ferrum*

Energetics: pleasant and acrid, cool
Meridian/Organ affected: liver
Properties: blood tonic, antispasmodic

Uses: It relieves convulsions, calms the liver, relieves anger, mania and fright, treats epilepsy and convulsive spasms in infants.

Ayurveda uses incinerated iron similarly in blood-building preparations with other herbs. This specially prepared iron is safe for internal usage.

Dosage: Boil 15-30 gms. of iron filings in decoction. Strain carefully and take only the water.

YIN TONICS
(Herbs that Tonify Vital Fluids)

Yin refers to the vital essence and all the fluid aspects of the body: blood, lymph, muscles, connective tissues, reproductive secretions, lubricating secretions of the mucous membranes, skin and joints, and hormonal secretions.

A deficiency of yin gives rise to a deficiency in bodily essence and any of the above bodily fluids. It also may create an apparent yang excess because yin and yang are rooted in each other. These symptoms of yang excess usually would manifest as a wasting inflammatory condition. Imagine an electrical wire as the solid, yin-like substance that must be sufficiently dense and well-insulated to serve as a conduit for the amount of yang-electricity that it must accommodate. If the wire is not strong enough for the amount of voltage it must carry, it will burn and short out.

Thus while yang is tonified or strengthened, yin is nourished with sweetish, solid, moist and nutritive types of herbs and foods. We distinguish here between *empty yin,* which is moist like an orange and sweet like sugar but lacks in rich nutrients, such as proteins or minerals; and *full yin,* which includes such yin tonic foods as dairy products, ghee and seaweed, or meats such as oyster or pork.

The false yang or weak heat found in yin-deficient conditions requires a building of the bodily essence, not the purging or alterative therapy used for strong or excess heat. Here bodily fire rises in proportion to deficient bodily water. It is not a true excess of fire. Hence this category is related to that of heat-clearing herbs, described under the category of *clear heat and cool blood,* for their demulcent febrifuges, which not only reduce fire but build body fluids. Some of these herbs may be needed to clear the deficient heat and are used with other herbs for nourishing the yin essence.

Consumptive diseases are essentially yin deficient. The Eclectic herbalists called them "strumous" conditions. What in the West is called tuberculosis the Chinese would call a lack of lung yin. This also refers to the symptoms of a dry cough, loss of voice, thirst, dry throat and dry skin.

Lack of stomach yin is another yin deficient syndrome and refers to a lack of stomach fluids. The signs of heat that are its symptoms include inflamed gums and mouth, lack of appetite, irritability, thirst, dry mouth and constipation. These symptoms may occur as a result of prolonged fever.

Deficient liver yin exhibits symptoms of dry, dull eyes and poor vision, night blindness, dizziness, tinnitus and dry brittle nails. The individual may also complain of feeling unusually warm. This condition requires herbs that nourish liver blood and yin. An extreme manifestation of liver yin deficiency may produce hypertension called *ascendent liver yang*. This condition produces symptoms of unusual irritability, anger, vertigo, tinnitus, dry mouth and throat, insomnia, crimson tongue and a rapid, thin pulse.

Deficient kidney yin[4] is a root cause of most chronic diseases and diseases related to aging. As one ages, the yin essence dries up and produces dryness, graying of the hair, and wrinkled skin, for example. Symptoms include dizziness, tinnitus, weakness of the lower back, knees and joints, a feeling of warmth in the chest, palms and soles of the feet that increases in the afternoon, lack of sexual libido, scanty, dark urine, dry, red tongue and a rapid, thready pulse.

In any of these cases, not all the symptoms need be present; but having several in any category gives the basis for a diagnosis. There also may be additional symptoms, indicating still other imbalances. One can be deficient in both yin and yang and in yin and chi, and so on.

In the West there has grown a great interest in developing the yang, the aggressive potential. This is reflected in the kinds of foods, like red meat, that are part of the standard Western diet; in the kind of aerobic exercise and body-building regimens we favor; and it is indicated by our highly stressed, competitive lifestyle. This contrasts with the traditional and oriental modes of living that emphasized yin vegetable types of foods and such passive exercises as yoga or tai chi. An understanding of the value of preserving and nourishing the yin essence is the key to happiness and longevity.

Herbs in this category tend to foster compassion, tolerance, patience and devotion, much as do those in the blood tonic category.

Ayurvedic medicine classifies these tonic herbs as water-predominant or pro-kapha. They strengthen the tissues of plasma, blood, fat, bone and reproductive secretions. They reduce pitta and vata.

Contraindications for yin tonics are conditions of excess fluid, excess mucus and cold, damp stagnation.

ASPARAGUS ROOT   *Asparagus officinalis; Liliaceae*

Energetics: sweet, bitter, cold
Meridians/Organs affected: lung, kidney
Part used: the tuberous root
Active constituents: asparagin, sucrose, starch, and mucilage
Properties: yin tonic, nutritive, diuretic, expectorant, demulcent
Uses: It treats dryness of the lungs and throat, consumptive diseases, tuberculosis and blood-tinged sputum. It also counteracts thirst and treats kidney yin deficient lower back pains. The Chinese variety is *Asparagus lucidus.* Our asparagus root appears to have similar properties. A variety used in Ayurveda, which resembles the Chinese asparagus, is called shatavari (*Asparagus racemosus*). It is the major herb used in that tradition for gynecological purposes and to strengthen female hormones. It is considered to promote fertility, increase breast milk, nourish the female reproductive system and relieve menstrual pain. It is also regarded as an important herb for pitta (fire) and is considered rejuvenative for pitta-types.

Asparagus root is said to increase love, devotion, and compassion. The most adept Chinese herbal pharmacists will taste a new shipment of asparagus root, testing it for sweetness. They might then reserve the sweetest roots for themselves, since these are believed to foster the deepest feelings of spiritual compassion.

The upper stalks (eaten as a food) and the seeds have a diuretic action, thus eliminating excess yin. The roots, on the other hand, are deeply nourishing to the yin quality.

There are a number of other asparagus species that have similar tonic properties. Further study is needed to differentiate their therapeutic applications.

Precautions: It is contraindicated for individuals with a cold damp deficient diarrhea.

Dosage: 6-15 gms.

TIGER LILY   *Lilium spp.; Liliaceae*

Energetics: sweet, bland, cool
Meridians/Organs affected: heart, lung
Part used: bulb
Active constituents: various alkaloids, protein, starch, colchicine
Properties: yin tonic, nutritive, demulcent, expectorant, mild sedative
Uses: It treats dry and inflamed lung and throat conditions, low grade fever, insomnia and irritable restlessness after a prolonged acute febrile disease and wasting and consumptive diseases.

Most members of the lily genus have edible bulbs[5] which may be eaten as a survival food either raw or cooked. Lilies are cultivated throughout Asia for their food value, and since ancient times they were believed to foster purity and virtue. The rarity of the beautiful wild varieties tell us to use only the cultivated varieties for food and medicine. Bulbs of the North American tiger lily and the "sego" or "mariposa" lily were used for food by the early Mormon settlers. We would do well to cultivate these and other precious native plants for use both as food and medicine.

Dosage: 6-15 gms.

SOLOMON'S SEAL   *Polygonatum officinale; Liliaceae*

Energetics: sweet, cool
Meridians/Organs affected: lungs, stomach
Part used: root
Active constituents: convallarin, asparagin, gum, sugar, starch, pectin

Properties: yin and chi tonic, nutritive, expectorant, mild diaphoretic
Uses: It is used to treat for chronic wasting and consumptive diseases, tuberculosis, diabetes and dry cough. In Western herbalism it is an important herb for promoting the healing of broken bones. In Ayurveda it is regarded as a kidney tonic and thought to build reproductive secretions. In modern China it is an important herb in treating cardiac diseases and is thought to be a strong heart tonic.

A number of varieties of this plant are in use. Another Chinese variety is used as a chi tonic. False solomon's seal *(Smilacina spp.)* is one of several related North American plants. They may be used similarly to the Chinese.
Dosage: 6-15 gms.

MARSHMALLOW ROOT   *Althea officinalis; Malvaceae*

Energetics: sweet, bitter, cool
Meridians/Organs affected: lungs, stomach, kidneys
Part used: root
Active constituents: starch, mucilage, pectin, oil, sugar, asparagin, phosphate of lime, glutinous matter, cellulose
Properties: yin tonic, nutritive, alterative, diuretic, demulcent, emollient, vulnerary, laxative
Uses: It is used to treat wasting and thirsting diseases, tuberculosis, diabetes, cough, dryness and inflammation of the lungs, gangrene, septicemia, ulcers, pain of kidney stones, difficult or painful urination, blood in the urine, stool or nose, and vomiting or spitting of blood.
Dosage: 6-15 gms.

ICELAND MOSS   *Cetraria islandica; Parmeliaceae*

Energetics: sweet, bland, cool
Meridians/Organs affected: lungs, stomach
Part used: the whole plant
Active constituents: mucins (mainly lichenin), bitter fumaric acids, some iodine
Properties: yin tonic, nutritive, demulcent

Uses: It treats irritated throat and mucous membranes, dry cough, consumptive and wasting diseases, chronic lung weakness, catarrh, digestive weakness and dysentery.
Dosage: 6-15 gms. in decoction

IRISH MOSS   *Chondrus crispus; Gigartinaceae*

Energetics: sweet, salty, cool
Meridians/Organs affected: lung, stomach
Part used: the whole plant
Active constituents: proteins, mucins, amino acids, iodine, bromine and manganese salts
Properties: yin tonic, alterative, laxative, demulcent, emollient
Uses: Irish moss is used to treat chronic lung problems with dryness and irritated membranes and wasting diseases. It often is combined with Iceland moss, comfrey root and honey to form a mucilage for treating inflamed lungs, sore throat and wasting diseases. It also is good for dysentery and as a digestive aid, and has a mild laxative property.
Dosage: 3-9 gms.

SLIPPERY ELM   *Ulmus fulva; Ulmaceae*

Energetics: sweet, neutral
Meridians/Organs affected: lung, stomach
Part used: inner bark
Active constituents: mucilages, tannins
Properties: yin tonic, nutritive, demulcent, expectorant, emollient, astringent, vulnerary
Uses: It is used to treat sore throat, coughs, bleeding from the lungs and other lung problems, dryness of the throat, wasting diseases, digestive problems, nausea. This is one of the most mucilaginous herbs and a gruel may be made by slowly mixing cool water into the powdered herb until a thick porridge consistency is achieved. This may be flavored with a little honey or a dash of cinnamon and is a good food to give, even to infants when there is difficulty in keeping food down. This gruel may be given for any wasting diseases and its tonic properties can be supplemented by preparing it with a tea of ginseng instead

of water. Slippery elm also is good for colitis and ulcers. It is a strengthening herb that may be eaten freely. It is one of the most versatile herbs and can be used alone or with other appropriate powdered herbs as a heating poultice for injuries, burns and all inflamed surfaces.

For gangrenous wounds, suppurating sores and bed sores, combine it with equal parts of echinacea and comfrey root powders. To stimulate suppuration, add brewer's yeast. For rheumatic, gouty and arthritic aches, mix with equal parts of wheat bran and moisten with warm apple cider vinegar.

A slippery elm-marshmallow ointment is made with 3 oz. marshmallow or malva leaves, 2 oz. comfrey leaves, 2 oz. echinacea, 2 oz. golden seal powder, 3 oz. slippery elm bark powder, 6 ounces of beeswax, 1 quart of ghee, olive or sesame oils, 1 oz. tincture of benzoin.[6] Boil the herbs in 2 quarts of water for 15 minutes. Press-strain and reduce the resulting tea down to a pint. Melt the beeswax and oil slowly so as not to burn them, and add the tea. Continue to heat slowly until all of the water has evaporated. Bottle in a wide-mouthed jar.

It is often better to use the cut and sifted bark, rather than the powder which will be too mucilaginous to make slippery elm tea.

A native California tree in the *Tiliaceae* family, *Fremontia californica* is nearly identical in properties and use with the East coast North American slippery elm. It grows abundantly in the Southern Sierra Nevada region and has begun to be cultivated as an ornamental tree.
Dosage: 9-30 gms.

COMFREY ROOT

Symphytum officinale;
Boraginaceae

Energetics: bitter, sweet, cool
Meridians/Organs affected: lungs, stomach, kidneys
Part used: the root
Active constituents: allantoin, mucilage, tannins, starch, inulin and traces of oil
Properties: yin tonic, demulcent, expectorant, vulnerary, astringent

Uses: It is used to treat chronic lung diseases with dry cough and inflamation, sore throat, pulmonary catarrh, stomach ulcers, and wasting diseases. It is excellent both internally and externally for promoting the healing of sores, bones, muscles and other tissues, and is as powerful as some of the best oriental tonic herbs. Recent controversy suggests that prolonged internal use of comfrey root for more than two or three months at a time may cause liver impairment in some individuals. Until this is resolved, it may be advisable to refrain from using it internally for no more than two weeks at a time and definitely not during pregnancy or small infants and children.

Hound's tongue *(Cynoglossum officinale),* a related species used for diarrhea, is less tonic and more astringent, owing to its higher tannin content.

Dosage: 6-15 gms.

PRIVET   *Ligustrum lucidum; Oleaceae*

Energetics: bitter, sweet, neutral
Meridians/Organs affected: liver, kidney
Part used: berries
Active constituents: oleanolic, palmitic, linoleic and ursolic acids, mannitol and glucose
Properties: yin tonic, alterative
Uses: It is used to nourish the liver and kidneys, for yin deficiency, consumptive and wasting diseases, premature gray hair, dizziness, blurry vision, lower back pain, knee and joint pains, and tinnitus.
Dosage: 6-15 gms.

BLACK SESAME SEEDS   *Sesamum indicum;*
Pedaliaceae

Energetics: sweet, neutral
Meridians/Organs affected: liver, kidney
Part used: the seeds
Active constituents: over 50% fatty oil, including olein, linolein, palmitin, stearin and myristin. It also contains lecithin, choline, 1% oxalate acid, chorogenic acid, vitamins E, A and B and appreciable amounts of calcium
Properties: yin tonic, nutritive, demulcent
Uses: It nourishes the liver and kidneys, lubricates dry intestines, darkens prematurely graying hair. It treats backache, tinnitus, blurry vision and dizziness, constipation and dry cough, blood in the urine, weak

knees and joint stiffness. Because of its easily assimilable calcium content, it nourishes the blood, calms nervous spasms, and alleviates headaches, dizziness and numbness caused by deficient blood or yin. It is a good general tonic and particularly suitable for the aged.

The seeds are thoroughly ground into a powder and mixed into a paste with honey (the mixture is eaten as a candy called *halva* in the Middle East) and two teaspoons taken daily. For dry cough, asthmatic and lung conditions, combine the powdered seeds with a pinch of black pepper, ginger juice and honey. One tablespoon is taken three times daily.
Dosage: 9-30 gms.

ECLIPTA   *Eclipta alba, E. prostrata; Compositae*

Energetics: sweet, sour, cool
Meridians/Organs affected: liver, kidneys
Part used: the whole plant
Active constituents: saponins, nicotine, tannin, vitamin A, ecliptine
Properties: yin tonic, alterative, astringent, hemostatic
Uses: It nourishes the kidneys and liver, stops bleeding from any cause, and treats tinnitus, premature graying of the hair, and neurotic symptoms. This herb, popularly called "false daisy", is found in many parts of the world, including the Asian and North American continents where it is used as a potherb. In India it is a famous herb for the hair and used in many hair oils.
Dosage: 6-15 gms.

PYROLA   *Pyrola rotundifolia* and *spp.; Pyrolaceae*

Energetics: sweet, bitter, slightly warm
Meridians/Organs affected: liver, kidney
Part used: whole plant
Active constituents: arbutin, tannin, renifolin, essential oil, homoarbutin, isohomoarbutin and saccharose
Properties: yin tonic, antirheumatic, vulnerary, astringent
Uses: It tonifies the essence, strengthens the bones and ligaments, relieves back, knee and joint pains, helps blood circulation, regulates

menses, and treats uterine bleeding and leucorrhea. For topically use, the fresh plant is crushed and applied as a poultice or ointment to promote healing.
Dosage: 9-30 gms.

OPHIOPOGON   *Ophiopogon japonicus and spp.;*
                                                      Liliaceae

Energetics: sweet, slightly bitter, slightly cold
Meridians/Organs affected: lung, stomach, heart
Part used: bulbs
Active constituents: mucilage, ophiopogonin, b-sitosterol, stigmasterol and ruscogenin
Properties: yin tonic, nutritive, demulcent, expectorant, antipyretic
Uses: It is used to moisten lung dryness, for dry cough and tuberculosis, to nourish body fluids, satisfy thirst, harmonize the stomach, counteract nausea and vomiting, lubricate the intestines and to treat dry constipation. This is another herb traditionally used in Chinese medicine that is grown as a common perennial in the warmer areas of North America, where it is known as "Japanese lily turf".
Dosage: 6-15 gms.

TURTLE SHELL   *Plastrum testudinis*

Energetics: salty, sweet, neutral
Meridians/Organs affected: kidney, heart, spleen, liver
Part used: The belly of the hard-shelled or the back of the soft-shelled turtles is used.
Active constituents: calcium
Properties: yin tonic, demulcent, sedative, astringent
Uses: It is used to treat lack of kidney yin, tinnitus, dizziness, blurry vision, headaches and numbness, anemia, dry constipation, deep fever with consumptive wasting, nocturnal emissions, menorrhagia, leucorrhea, aching soreness of the back and legs, and delayed formation of the

fontanelle in children. **Precautions:** Avoid or use with caution during pregnancy.
Dosage: 9-30 gms. of the crushed shell boiled alone in decoction for at least thirty minutes before other herbs are added

DEVIL'S CLUB   *Oplopanax horridum*

Energetics: acrid, bitter, cool
Meridians/Organs affected: spleen, lungs
Part used: root bark
Active constituents: not found but probably saponins and substances with insulin-like action
Properties: tonic, alterative, adaptogen, hypoglycemic agent, anti-arthritic
Uses: While devil's club is not an easy plant to harvest, it is perhaps one of our most valuable botanicals native to the Pacific Northwest. It was widely used by the Native Americans for a variety of both chronic and acute complaints as well as its use by them as a protective charm. It was widely used for arthritis, rheumatism, stomach pains, constipation, and especially for the prevention and treatment of diabetes. A story reported by Weston A. Price in *Nutrition and Physical Degeneration* is of an Indian who was brought into a hospital in Prince Rupert, British Columbia for an operation. He showed signs of diabetes and had evidently kept himself in good health for several years by taking a regular decoction of devil's club. He said it was in common usage among the Indians in the region. Further experiments, reported by Vogel, were done on rabbits and demonstrated that an extract of the herb would substantially reduce blood sugar without any toxic side effects.

Judging from its widespread use as a tonic alterative by the Native Americans in Moerman, devil's club would serve ideally both as a yin tonic and an alterative in the category of cooling blood.
Dosage: 3-9 gms. in decoction

Other important substances that may be used as yin tonics include cod liver oil and black beans.

---

[1] Editor's note: American ginseng may be cooler than the Korean, more calming and more of a yin tonic but this does not mean it is cool in nature or that it is classified as primarily a yin tonic. Licorice, another chi tonic, is cooler, more calming and more moistening than ginseng but not, therefore, regarded as a yin tonic. American ginseng certainly appears to be more energizing than such recognized chi tonics as licorice, jujube or even codonopsis, the main ginseng substitute. Furthermore, yin tonics are inexpensive and readily available, so why would such high prices be paid for an herb whose qualities are so easily found close at hand?

Some people have reported chi stagnation and heat symptoms from excess use of American ginseng, symptoms similar to those resulting from excess use of the Chinese or Korean. There are variations in American ginseng as there are in the Chinese. The more rugged, wild and northern roots may be more chi-tonifying than the more succulent, cultivated and southern roots.

The Chinese have a point but they have perhaps taken it too far. It is my view that American ginseng is an effective chi tonic. It may be used like the Chinese in all but conditions of collapse of the chi. It is stronger than codonopsis and the other ginseng substitutes. This is how I use it in my practice and the results appear to bear it out. American ginseng is slightly milder and safer for long term use than the Chinese. But this does not mean that we have to dismiss it as a chi tonic and let our valuable native plant be exported away, as we have been doing for centuries.

[2] See bibliography

[3] See bibliography

[4] This type of deficiency is closely related to liver yin deficiency and the same herbs are used to treat both conditions.

[5] The exception is the so-called "calla" lily which is not a true lily. Its bulb is acrid and will cause blisters on direct contact.

[6] Tincture of benzoine, available in most pharmacies, is added optionally as a preservative.

ASTRINGENTS

Astringents are herbs that contract, dry and tighten tissues. As they do so they help to stop excessive discharges. Therefore they are used to treat diarrhea, excessive sweating, excessive urination, mucous discharges and bleeding. They also treat prolapsis of the uterus and rectum. In Chinese medicine these conditions are considered to result from a progressive weakness or flaccidity. Hence they often use astringents to supplement tonics (see the Chinese classification following the section on tonics).

Such problems often arise from weakening of the nervous system which may be caused by surgical operations or the excessive use of purgatives or eliminating-type foods, including too much liquid or raw food. The Chinese classify hemostatics (stopping-bleeding herbs) separately from astringents. Astringents, however, always tend to have a hemostatic action. Their active constituent is tannin, which is a coagulant.

Astringents also may be used to supplement various clearing or detoxifying therapies. Many have heat-clearing, alterative, expectorant or diuretic properties. They are particularly good for treating ulcerations of the skin or the mucous membranes. For best results they should be applied locally, for example, as gargles for sore throat, in treating spongy gums, or as a dentifrice.

Externally, astringents function as vulneraries to promote the healing of tissues, whether from wounds or sores, and for this purpose are nature's first-aid medicine. Applied in a bath, they help to toughen the hands and feet. They are used to tan leather. Astringency is perhaps the most common therapeutic property in nature. In early herbalism many astringent herbs were considered heal-all remedies. Before the advent of first-aid chemical medicines, such herbs were the only means to stop an acute loss of vital fluids and to promote the healing in injuries. Their use for this purpose is still worthy of consideration.

In Ayurveda, astringents are considered to be drying and to increase vata (air), which means that they can have a depleting effect upon the nervous system. They decrease kapha (water) by means of their diuretic and expectorant action. Their anti-inflammatory properties can decrease pitta (fire). According to Ayurveda, excessive discharges can arise from either pitta or kapha.

A precautionary note about tannins: although the liver tends not to absorb them, even a gram of tannic acid can cause serious side effects. These include abdominal pains, constipation, diarrhea, thirst, polyuria, and liver, heart or kidney failure. Herbalists tend to avoid an excessive use of herbs high in tannins, preferring deeper therapeutic strategies. Astringents are more often used secondarily to treat acute symptoms, while other therapies are used primarily, to treat the cause.

Astringents may be contraindicated in treating excessive discharges. For example, diarrhea from toxins or poisoning should not be suppressed, but promoted as part of the cleansing process. Sweating from excessive fever also should not be suppressed by astringents. The fever should be directly reduced with heat-clearing herbs. Astringents, by acting on symptoms, have more potential for mistaken application than other herbal therapies. They should not be used before the total condition of the patient is understood. This is particularly true of those herbs that contain high amounts of tannin and have a very strong action.

Some astringents—such as raspberry and blackberry leaves, huckleberry, nettles, amaranth, rose hips, cranesbill and eyebright—are widely used because of their mildness and broad regulating action. Others, like alum, oak bark and oak galls, are stronger and are used internally for acute problems or externally in salves and ointments. As a general rule, however, the diverse biochemical constituents of most plants tend to provide counteracting elements that prevent harm.

Contraindications for the internal use of astringents usually are conditions of dryness, contraction or severe nerve (vata) disorders. In these cases they should be combined with other herbs (such as demulcents like licorice or marshmallow) to protect the vital fluids.

NETTLES   *Urtica urens; Urticaceae*

Energetics: bland, slightly bitter, cool
Meridians/Organs affected: small intestines, bladder, lungs
Part used: leaves
Active constituents: The stinging element is formic acid, which is dissipated by cooking or drying. It also contains, silicon, potassium, tannin, glucoquinines, chlorophyll and vitamins A and C
Properties: astringent, hemostatic, diuretic, galactagogue, expectorant, tonic, nutritive
Uses: The young nettle leaves may be steamed as a potherb. The tea is taken cool as a diuretic for such urinary problems as strangury (stopped urine), gravel, and inflammatory conditions, including nephritis and cystitis. The warm tea is used for asthma, mucous conditions of the lungs, diarrhea, dysentery, hemorrhoids, various hemorrhages, scorbutic affections and summer dysentery (especially for children). It is very helpful in treating mucus in the colon in adults.

The German herbalist, Maria Treben, recommends daily use of nettle tea, taking a cup two or three times a day as a tonic. It is effective against low energy and fatigue, probably because it counteracts flaccidity, removes dampness and brightens the chi. It is said to be effective against eczematous affections of the upper quadrant of the body including the face, neck and ears.

For arthritic and rheumatic problems nettles are used both internally and externally. Externally, fresh nettles brushed over painful areas are an effective rubefacient to reduce local pains. The juice of nettles rubbed on a wart for 10 to 12 days is a reliable remedy to eliminate them.

A tincture made of the seeds is recommended for goiter and low thyroid. In raising thyroid function, it effectively reduces the associated obesity.

Dosage: 9-30 gms.

CRANESBILL   *Geranium maculatum; Geraniaceae*

Energetics: astringent, bitter, neutral
Meridians/Organs affected: stomach, intestines, liver, heart
Part used: root
Active constituents: tannic and gallic acid, starch, sugar, pectin, gum
Properties: astringent, hemostatic, styptic
Uses: It is used to treat diarrhea, dysentery, internal bleeding, hemorrhages, indolent ulcers, mouth sores, ophthalmia, leucorrhea, gleet, hematuria, menorrhagia, diabetes, and all excessive chronic mucous discharges. The powder of cranesbill is directly applied for external bleeding. For dysentery it is boiled with milk to which a little cinnamon has been added and the milk cooked down to half its liquid volume. For hemorrhoids, combine finely powdered cranesbill with powdered yarrow. These are made into an ointment or bolus by then adding melted coconut butter until a doughy consistency is achieved. Roll this mixture into anal suppositories of about the thickness of the middle finger. Insert inch-long pieces into the rectum each evening before retiring.

As a vaginal suppository for vaginal discharge, leucorrhea of various types and to treat vaginal flaccidity, combine cranesbill powder with powders of white oak bark, echinacea, golden seal and raspberry leaf and add coconut butter. Insert three one-inch segments each evening. Seal with a napkin to prevent leakage.

Cranesbill is one of the safest and most effective astringent herbs for gastrointestinal problems.

Dosage: root powder 20-30 grains; dried and cut root, standard decoction or 3-9 gms.; tincture 10-30 drops

ALUM ROOT   *Heuchera americana; Saxifragaceae*

Energetics: bitter, astringent, neutral
Meridians/Organs affected: stomach, intestines
Part used: root

Active constituents: 9 to 20% tannins and various unidentified substances
Properties: astringent, styptic
Uses: A teaspoon of the chopped root boiled in water for 20 minutes is used for gastroenteritis, stomach flu, diarrhea and dry bilious vomiting. It will stimulate the healing of the esophagus and treat stomach ulcers but not duodenal ulcers, since tannins tend to dissipate before reaching the colon. For dysentery, a cup may be taken every two hours until the symptoms have abated. It is a good douche for leucorrhea and vaginitis. It is an excellent gargle for sore throat. The Native Americans of Nevada and Utah use it both internally and externally as a healing astringent for injuries, sores and wounds.
Precautions: Excessive use can cause gastric irritation and kidney and liver failure.
Dosage: No more than 5-10 gms. of the powdered root should be taken at a time.

WITCH HAZEL

Hamemelis virginiana;
Hamamelidaceae

Energetics: bitter, astringent, neutral
Meridians/Organs affected: heart, stomach and intestines
Parts used: leaf and bark
Active constituents: tannin, traces of essential oil, flavonoids, choline and a saponin. The bark contains less tannin.
Properties: astringent, hemostatic, anti-inflammatory
Uses: It is used for diarrhea, dysentery, hemorrhages, excessive mucous discharges, leucorrhea, gleet, prolapsed condition of the internal organs, varicose veins, menorrhagia, and as a tonic after abortions. For severe menorrhagia, a teaspoonful of the alcoholic tincture is added to a cup of boiling water and taken every hour or two, tapering off gradually as the condition subsides. A tea made from the bark or leaf is used as a gargle for tonsillitis and sore throat.

It usually is used externally as an ointment, poultice, liniment and wash. It is made into an ointment and suppository for treating fissured anus and hemorrhoids. The alcoholic tincture is applied to relieve sprains, contusions, wounds and swellings. Diluted with water or mixed with honey, the powder may be topically applied as a dressing for burns, scalds, abrasions, and crushed toes and fingers. It is an effective wash for burning skin, inflamed breasts, varicose veins and various rashes. It is often used as an after-shave lotion. Witch hazel is one of the most valuable and versatile astringents.

Dosage: decoction, one tablespoon to a cup of boiling water simmered 15-20 minutes. Two to four fluid ounces are taken three or four times daily. Of the tincture take 1-30 drops. In formulas use 3-9 gms.

OAK   *Quercus alba and spp.; Fagaceae*

Energetics: astringent, bitter, neutral
Meridians/Organs affected: spleen, stomach, intestines
Parts used: bark, gall, acorn
Active constituents: about 15 to 20% tannins
Properties: The bark and gall are astringent, styptic, hemostatic, and antiseptic. (The acorns also are astringent; but when shelled, ground into a meal and soaked in running water for a few hours, the tannic acid is leached out. They then may be used as a nutritive tonic for wasting diseases.)
Uses: It treats dysentery, diarrhea, hemorrhages, leucorrhea, prolapsed uterus or anus, indolent ulcers, relaxed uvula and chronic cough. It is used topically for sores, ringworm, poisonous swellings and deep skin ulcerations; internally for poisoning by strychnine, veratrine and other vegetable alkaloids. For diarrhea, boil a tablespoon or two in milk. It may be used similarly to witch hazel bark as a gargle for sore throats and as a wash for burns, both to promote healing and as an antiseptic to prevent infection. The tannins seem to bind with the proteins and amino acids of the weeping tissue to protect them from pathogenic invasion. A poultice of powdered oak bark and wheat flour combined with a little boiled water draws out slivers and other foreign substances. The quercin in oak makes it adjunctive to bioflavenoid (vitamin P), which helps strengthen the capillaries. A wash of oak, or oak combined with witch hazel bark, is an excellent night-time compress for

varicose veins and broken capillaries under the skin. It also is made into a suppository for hemorrhoids.

The galls have the same properties as the bark.

Dosage: 1 teaspoon simmered in a cup of boiling water. One cup is taken three times daily. As an external wash, enema or douche, steep one or two tablespoons in a quart of water for 30 minutes, strain and apply often. Standard dose in formulas or 3-9 gms.

HORSE CHESTNUT
Aesculus hippocastanum;
Hippocasanaceae, Sapindaceae

Energetics: bitter, astringent, neutral, toxic
Meridians/Organs affected: spleen, lungs
Parts used: seed and bark
Active constituents: the seeds contain various saponins incuding aescine, tannins, flavones, purines, starch, sugar, albumin and a fatty oil. The bark contains coumarins, glycoside, resin and pigment

Because of the high tannin content in horse chestnuts, they must be shelled, crushed and leached overnight in cold water before they can be used. They are then strained and boiled for half an hour. The meal from the nuts is dried and used as medicine for humans or fodder for animals.

Properties: astringent, narcotic, nutritive, febrifuge, expectorant
Uses: The bark and the fruit are used similarly to both witch hazel and oak, but horse chestnut tends more to increase the blood circulation. For this reason, a poultice of the crushed and powdered bark or fruits is useful for the treatment of varicose veins, hemorrhoids and other rectal problems. It also is directly applied for the treatment of leg ulcers, rheumatism, neuralgia and burns. A fluid extract from the fruit protects against sunburn.

Since it is astringent, blood-moving and febrifuge, the fruit is used as a treatment for gastritis, enteritis, bronchitis, phlegm in the lungs, and swollen prostate.

Precautions: The green outer casing of the fruit is poisonous and narcotic but the toxic principles appear to be neutralized by preroasting.

Toxic symptoms include gastroenteritis, enlarged pupils, drowsiness, and flushing of the skin.

A related species, California buckeye (*Aesculus californica*), was reported to cause abortions in cattle. Although considered poisonous unless fully ripened and properly leached, it was used by the local Native Americans as a remedy for rheumatic aches and toothache. **Dosage:** The bark is boiled using one ounce to a pint of water. Not more than a tablespoonful is given three or four times daily. The fruit is usually made into a liquid extract or tincture of which 5-20 drops are given 3 or 4 times daily.

BLACKBERRY   *Rubus villosus; Rosaceae*

Energetics: bitter, astringent, neutral
Meridians/Organs affected: stomach, intestines
Parts used: leaves, root bark (for fruit, see section on blood tonics, pg.315)
Active constituents: the leaves and root bark are high in tannins
Properties: astringent, hemostatic
Uses: The leaves and roots are used to treat dysentery and diarrhea, the root being the stronger remedy. They also inhibit excessive menstrual bleeding.
Dosage: leaves, standard infusion; root, the standard decoction, 3-9 gms.

HUCKLEBERRY   *Vaccinum myrtillus; Ericaceae*

Energetics: astringent, bitter, cool
Meridians/Organs affected: spleen, bladder, colon
Part used: leaves (for fruit, see section on blood tonics, pg.316)
Active constituents: the leaves contain a glucoquinine which lowers blood sugar
Properties: the leaves are astringent, antidiabetic, and diuretic
Uses: The leaves are used specifically to control blood sugar in diabetes. As a diuretic, the leaves are used similarly to uva ursi. They also are effective for diarrhea.
Dosage: standard decoction or 3-9 gms.

AMARANTH
Amaranthus hypochondriacus and spp.;
Amaranthaceae

Energetics: sweet, neutral energy
Meridians/Organs affected: spleen, kidney
Part used: upper aerial portion
Active constituents: not identified but probably a small amount of tannin
Properties: astringent, hemostatic, nutritive, alterative
Uses: None of the many species is poisonous and many are used as potherbs. An infusion or decoction made from the leaves is used as a mild astringent. *A. caudatus* is a hardy annual which is effective in treating spitting up of blood, hemorrhages and menorrhagia. Its folk name "love lies bleeding" refers to its use in treating excessive menstruation.

The leaves of some species are known as "pigweed" and are very potent nutritionally, being high in vitamins A and C. They are sold in marketplaces throughout the world and in India are highly recommended as a potherb for convalescents. The seeds of another species were used as a staple by the Aztecs of Mexico.
Dosage: 6-30 gms.

LOOSESTRIFE
Lythrum sallicaria; Lythraceae

Energetics: sweet, astringent, cool
Meridians/Organs affected: spleen, liver
Part used: aerial portions
Active constituents: a glycoside, polyphenolic tannins, pectin and essential oil
Properties: astringent, demulcent, alterative
Uses: It treats diarrhea and dysentery. Externally it is used as an eyewash for ophthalmia, sore eyes, sores and ulcers and various skin diseases. It is effective as a local wash or douche for leucorrhea. Because of its paradoxical astringent and mucilaginous properties, loosestrife is an importent herb.
Dosage: standard infusion or 3-9 gms. For acute conditions, one to three ounces may be taken three or more times a day until relief is achieved; of the powder, 30-60 grains is taken every three or four hours.

SUMAC   *Rhus glabra; Anacardiaceae*

Energetics: cold, sour, astringent
Meridians/Organs affected: kidney, bladder, liver
Parts used: root bark, berries
Active constituents: malic and acid calcium malate with tannic and gallic acids, fixed and a small amount volatile oils
Properties: The bark is astringent, antiseptic and alterative; the berries are refrigerant and diuretic
Uses: The root bark is useful in the treatment of gonorrhea, gleet, leucorrhea, diarrhea, dysentery, restless fever, scrofula, and profuse perspiration from debility. Combined with the barks of white pine and slippery elm and applied externally, it is effective in the treatment of syphilitic ulcerations. This mixture is good for old sores or ulcers. As a douche, it is used for leucorrhea, prolapsed uterus and hemorrhoids. As a mouthwash, it is used for sore and bleeding gums. The berries are given in infusion for diabetes, strangury, bowel complaints and febrile diseases and also make a pleasant acid drink. They also are effective as a wash for ringworm, tetters and offensive ulcers. In hot weather the bark can be punctured; the juice that then flows out is used for venereal disease and several chronic urinary affections. Sumac galls are astringents in common use in Ayurvedic and Chinese medicine.
Precautions: Care should be taken to identify the plant correctly, as other varieties of rhus can be very toxic (poison oak and poison ivy). Free use of the bark will produce catharsis.
Dosage: bark or the berries, from one to four fluid ounces of the decoction or 3-9 gms. in formulas

WHITE POND LILY   *Nymphea odorata; Nymphaceae*

Energetics: bitter, astringent, cool
Meridians/Organs affected: kidneys, spleen
Part used: rhizome
Active constituents: several alkaloids including nupharine, a glycoside, nymphaline and tannin
Properties: astringent, demulcent, alterative, anodyne

Uses: It treats dysentery, diarrhea, gonorrhea, leucorrhea and scrofula. Combined with wild cherry bark, it is effective for bronchial affections. Externally, the the leaves and roots are used as a poultice for boils, tumors, ulcers and inflamed skin. The infusion is an effective gargle for mouth sores, ulcers and sore throat. This herb has been known to be effective for uterine cancer, for which it is taken freely internally and injected as a douche.
Dosage: 3-12 gms.

YELLOW WATER LILY
Nelumbium luteum,
Nuphar lutea; Nymphaceae

Energetics: bitter, neutral
Meridians/Organs affected: liver, spleen, stomach
Parts used: leaf and rhizome
Active constituents: sesquiterpenoid alkaloids (nupharine, thio-binuphaidine and desoxynupharidine)
Properties: astringent, alterative, antispasmodic
Uses: It is used to treat diarrhea, dysentery, vaginal discharges, gleet and bleeding.
Dosage: 3-9 gms.

BISTORT
Polygonum bistorta; Polygonaceae

Energetics: astringent, bitter, cool
Meridians/Organs affected: liver, intestines
Part used: root
Active constituents: up to 20% tannins
Properties: astringent, hemostatic
Uses: Like white oak bark, it is used as a strong astringent and hemostatic.
Dosage: 3-9 gms.

JAMBUL
Syzygium cumini, Eugenia jambolanum
Myrtaceae

Energetics: bitter, aromatic, neutral
Meridians/Organs affected: spleen, stomach
Parts used: fruit, seeds
Active constituents: essential oil, fat, resin, gallic and tannic acids, albumen and ellagic acid
Properties: astringent, carminative, antidiabetic
Uses: It is used for diarrhea and colic, and regulates blood sugar in diabetes.
Dosage: 0.3-2 gms. of dried fruit three times daily

CEANOTHUS (Red root)
Ceanothus americanus;
Rhamnaceae

Energetics: bitter, astringent, cool
Meridians/Organs affected: spleen, lungs, liver
Part used: root
Active constituents: ceanothic (emmolic), succinic, oxalic, malonic, malic, orthophosphic, and pyrophosphoric acids; tannin
Properties: astringent, expectorant, sedative, antispasmodic, antisyphilitic
Uses: It is used for enlarged spleen, lymphatic congestion, despondency and melancholy.
Dosage: 3-9 gms.

EPHEDRA ROOT
Ephedra, spp.; Ephedraceae

Energetics: sweet, neutral
Meridians/Organs affected: lung, heart
Part used: root
Active constituents: alkaloid ephedrine, pseudo-ephedrine, tannins, saponin, flavone, essential oil
Properties: astringent
Uses: It is used to treat diarrhea, sweating from deficiency, night sweats, and postpartum sweating.
Dosage: 6-15 gms.

ROSE HIPS
Rosa spp.; Rosaceae

Energetics: sour, neutral
Meridians/Organs affected: kidney, bladder, colon
Part used: fruit
Active constituents: saponins, citric and malic acids, fructose, sucrose, flavonoids, vitamin C, tannin
Properties: astringent, antidiuretic, tonic
Uses: It is used for diarrhea, enuresis, frequent urination, spermatorrhea and leucorrhea (all complaints of deficient kidney chi).
Dosage: 3-12 gms.

LOTUS SEED
Nelumbo nucifera; Nymphceae

Energetics: sweet, astringent, neutral
Meridians/Organs affected: heart, spleen, kidney
Part used: seed
Active constituents: raffinose, calcium, phosphorus, iron
Properties: astringent, tonic, sedative
Uses: It clears heat and strengthens heart and kidneys. It also treats irritability, restlessness, insomnia, palpitations, dry mouth, dark urine, wet dreams, and stops diarrhea in chronic conditions.
Dosage: 6-15 gms.

EYEBRIGHT
Euphrasia officinalis; Scrophulariaceae

Energetics: bitter, mildly astringent, cool
Meridians/Organs affected: liver, lung
Part used: aerial portions
Active constituents: tannins, substances similar to aucubine and essential oil
Properties: astringent, anti-inflammatory, expectorant
Uses: It treats conjunctivitis, superficial eye problems, watery catarrh of nose, sinus and middle ear problems.
Dosage: 2-5 gms.

POMEGRANATE
Punica granatum; Punicaceae

Energetics: bitter, sweet, astringent, neutral
Meridians/Organs affected: stomach, colon
Part used: husk of fruit
Active constituents: tannin, inulin, mannitol, malic acid, calcium oxalate, pelletierine, isoquercitrin
Properties: astringent, anthelmintic
Uses: It treats hiccoughs, diarrhea, dysentery and tapeworm. In a douche it treats leucorrhea; in a gargle, throat irritation and mouth sores. The fruit is considered a blood tonic in Ayurvedic medicine.
Dosage: 3-9 gms.

LADY'S MANTLE
Alchemilla vulgaris; Rosaceae

Energetics: bitter, astringent, neutral
Meridians/Organs affected: spleen, kidneys
Part used: aerial portions
Active constituents: tannin, tannin glycoside, traces of salicylic acid and unidentified substances
Properties: astringent, febrifuge
Uses: It treats loss of appetite, rheumatism, stomach ailments, diarrhea, enteritis and menstrual problems (especially leucorrhea and excessive menstrual bleeding). It makes a good douche for leucorrhea and is used as a wash or poultice for wounds.
Dosage: tincture, 10-30 drops; standard infusion or 3-9 gms.

YERBA MANSA
Anemopsis californica; Saururaceae

Energetics: bitter, astringent, warm
Meridians/Organs affected: lungs, spleen
Parts used: root, leaf
Active constituents: not available
Properties: astringent, carminative, antiemetic
Uses: It is used for diarrhea, dysentery, malarial fevers, pulmonary affec-

tions, gonorrhea, catarrhal conditions, indigestion, cough, and digestive weakness. Externally it may be used as a tincture or ointment for infections, especially fungal infections.

Dosage: fluid extract, 10-60 drops every three or four hours; standard infusion or 3-9 gms.

GINKGO NUT   *Ginkgo biloba; Coniferales*

Energetics: bitter, astringent, neutral, mildly toxic
Meridians/Organs affected: lung, kidney
Part used: seed
Active constituents: volatile oil, tannin, resin
Properties: astringent, expectorant, sedative, antitussive
Uses: It expels mucus from the bronchioles and lungs, stops wheezing, inhibits cough, stops leucorrhea, regulates urination, stops spermatorrhea. The ripe fruit, having been macerated in sesame oil for one hundred days, has been successfully used in China for the treatment of tuberculosis. The 24 to 1 extract of the leaf is now a popular herbal product for a wide variety of vascular problems, especially increasing vascular circulation to the brain for the treatment of dementia and possibly Alzheimer's disease.
Precautions: Since it is slightly toxic, it should not be taken in large doses over a long period of time. The shells are an antidote to the nuts and may be taken with them to help alleviate side-effects. Toxic symptoms include headache, fever, tremors, irritability and dyspnea. Licorice also may be used antidotally with this herb.
Dosage: 3-9 gms. (less if fresh)

WHEAT CHAFF   *Triticum vulgare; Graminae*

Energetics: sweet, slightly cold
Meridian/Organ affected: heart
Part used: chaff
Active constituents: not available
Properties: astringent, sedative, tonic
Uses: It treats night sweats and insomnia. The seed has similar but milder properties.
Dosage: 15-30 gms.

GLUTINOUS RICE ROOTS

Oryza sativa;
Graminae

Energetics: sweet neutral
Meridians/Organs affected: liver, lung, kidney
Part used: root
Active constituents: 90% starch, vitamins A, B, C, D and E
Properties: astringent, tonic
Uses: It is used for spontaneous sweating, night sweats, and yin fevers
Dosage: 15-30 gms.

NUTMEG

Myristica fragrans; Myristaceae

Energetics: spicy, warm, slightly toxic
Meridians/Organs affected: spleen, stomach, colon
Part used: seed
Active constituents: volatile oil consisting of d-camphene, a-pinene, myristicin
Properties: astringent, stomachic, carminative
Uses: It is used to treat diarrhea, indigestion, loss of appetite, colic, flatulence and insomnia.
Precautions: More than 7.5 gms. can be toxic.
Dosage: ½-6 gms. in infusion

SCHIZANDRA

Schizandra sinensis; Magnoliaceae

Energetics: sweet, sour, warm
Meridians/Organs affected: kidney, lung, heart
Part used: fruit
Active constituents: sesquicarene, schizandrin, schizoandrol, citral, stigmasterol, vitamin C, vitamin E
Properties: astringent, tonic, sedative
Uses: It is used for wasting and thirsting diseases, tuberculosis, diabetes, asthma, diarrhea, nocturnal emmission, involuntary sweating, insomnia, and low energy. This Chinese herb is now used in the West as an adaptogenic tonic, although in China its chief use is as a tonic astringent. It makes a good tincture or herbal wine.
Dosage: standard decoction or 3-9 gms.

SEDATIVES AND NERVINES

Chinese medicine discriminates between two classes of sedatives. The first are stronger sedatives or tranquilizers. These are exclusively minerals, which can more effectively weigh down and calm the mind than herbs. This group is classified as "strong sedatives". The second category consists of mild sedative herbs that usually possess tonification properties. They calm and nourish the heart and are better suited for weaker types and less acute conditions. They are classified here as "calmatives".

To these traditional Chinese classifications two additional categories are added here. Most of the typical Western nervines like valerian and skullcap, which fall between the two categories above, are classified here as "nervines". Another special category added here is "herbs to regulate the heart".

Western herbal medicine tends to put nervine and antispasmodic herbs in a single category, since what calms the nerves usually relieves muscle spasms. Following the stricter differentiation of the Chinese categories, many other nervine herbs will be found under the antispasmodic category.

In Ayurvedic terms these are mainly herbs that treat vata (nervous system disorders). Many also reduce pitta, as excess fire also deranges the nervous system. Most increase kapha (water), which usually induces lethargy and hypoactivity.

STRONG SEDATIVES

This category consists entirely of minerals or shells. It is a category that is unique to Chinese herbal medicine. These substances calm the spirit, relieve palpitations, treat insomnia, anxiety, nervousness, irritability, fright and hysteria. They anchor the chi of the lungs and stomach and treat vomiting, coughing, belching, hiccoughs and wheezing.

The side-effects of the stronger of these substances are numerous. Many, like cinnabar, are toxic and can accumulate in the tissues. Because of their inorganic nature they can damage the stomach, causing indigestion and loss of appetite. (It should be noted that some of the same side-effects, to a lesser degree, can occur through taking too large quantities of mineral supplements, which are similarly heavy and hard to digest). Hence they are used largely for acute conditions and should be used with caution.

Except when otherwise mentioned, the method of preparation is to boil the stone or mineral in water, usually for 20 to 30 minutes before adding herbs. Only the resulting tea is taken. The minerals are not to be taken internally. The doses indicated refer to how much of the mineral is used in the decoction, not how much is taken internally. They are sometimes high because Chinese medicine considers that heavy substances should be used in larger weights in formulas.

The Chinese appear not to have developed the process of "humanization" of minerals, as in Ayurveda. In Ayurveda minerals are purified in various ways, mainly through repeated incinerations. The resultant oxide of the mineral is then rendered safe and non-toxic to take internally in small amounts. Such preparations, called *rasas* and *bhasmas,* can have a very strong action on the brain and serve to carry the effects of herbs deep into the nervous tissues. They are at the foundation of the most important compounds used in Ayurveda.

Ayurvedic humoral theory would consider the herbs in this category as reducing vata (air), but only in acute conditions. They also reduce pitta (fire) but usually increase kapha (water), and so have a dulling effect upon the mind. Wrongly prescribed, they can aggravate all the humors.

These herbs are contraindicated except for acute nervous disorders. Oyster shell and dragon bone, however, are safer and possess mild tonic properties.

OYSTER SHELL   *Ostrea gigas*

Energetics: salty, astringent, cool
Meridians/Organs affected: heart, liver, kidney
Part used: shell
Active constituents: calcium carbonate, calcium phosphate, calcium sulphate, magnesium, aluminum, ferric oxide
Properties: sedative, anti-inflammatory, demulcent, astringent, tonic
Uses: It is a sedative for insomnia, cramps, nervousness and hyperchlorhydria. It also is used as an astringent for spontaneous sweating, night sweating, spermatorrhea, leucorrhea, uterine bleeding caused by kidney deficiency and nocturnal emissions. It is beneficial for goiter, hard swollen thyroid, and other hardened lumps (it probably contains some iodine). It is antacid, and therefore relieves stomach acidity. Oyster shell is the safest substance to use in this category.
Dosage: 15-30 gms.

DRAGON BONE   *Os draconis*
Energetics: sweet, astringent, neutral
Meridians/Organs affected: heart, liver, kidney, large intestine
Part used: the ossified bones of prehistoric mammals
Active constituents: calcium carbonate, calcium phosphate, iron, potassium, sulphates
Properties: sedative, astringent, tonic
Uses: It is used to treat restlessness, insomnia, irritability, dizziness, blurred vision, short temper, night sweats, nocturnal emissions, leucorrhea, uterine bleeding, and spermatorrhea. The powder is topically applied to promote the healing of sores and ulcers.

Dragon bone and oyster shell often are combined. Dragon bone is considered to be a little stronger. "Dragon teeth", the fossilized teeth, are astringent and cool. While they basically have the same properties as dragon bone, they are more effective in treating anxiety, insomnia and frequent dreams.

This natural resource is collected from Dragon Bone Mountain outside of Peking. A similar deposit has been discovered in central Florida.
Dosage: 15-30 gms.

PEARL   *Pteria margaritifera*

Energetics: sweet, salty, cold
Meridians/Organs affected: heart, liver
Part used: the granulated pearl
Active constituents: calcium carbonate, magnesium carbonate, calcium phosphate, ferric oxide, silica
Properties: sedative, anti-inflammatory, demulcent
Uses: It is used to treat extreme rising heat symptoms, childhood convulsions, seizures, hypertension, and excessive anger with blurred vision. It is made into a salve and topically applied to clear heat rash, pimples, blemishes caused by heat, and ulcers and sores that are difficult to heal. It is an important ingredient in many oriental beauty creams, as it is thought to make the skin smoother, softer, clearer and less wrinkled. Internally it is taken as a finely granulated powder.
Dosage: 300 mgs.-1 gm.

MAGNETITE (Lodestone)

Energetics: acrid, cold
Meridians/Organs affected: kidney, liver
Part used: the finely ground mineral
Active constituents: tri-iron tetroxide, ferric oxide, ferrous oxide, magnesium oxide, aluminum oxide
Properties: sedative, blood tonic
Uses: it treats tachycardia, nervousness and asthma. Magnetite is used for restlessness, palpitations, insomnia, and fear-induced tremors and convulsions in children. Since it also has tonic properties, it is very effective for individuals with deficient yin and rising yang. It quiets the liver, and is used for the treatment of dizziness, vertigo, epilepsy, tinnitus and blurry vision. It is good for anemia and kidney-adrenal deficient asthma.

Preparation: it is heated in a skillet or clay pot, dipped in vinegar and then finely pulverized. As with most of the other hard substances in this category, it is usually cooked for about a half hour before adding herbs to the decoction.
Dosage: 9-30 gms.

FLUORITE   *Floritum*

Energetics: sweet, warm
Meridians/Organs affected: heart, liver
Active constituents: calcium fluoride, diferric trioxide
Properties: sedative, astringent
Uses: It sedates the mind, relieves states of extreme fearfulness, mental instability, insomnia, anxiety, palpitations, and convulsions caused by deficient blood and extreme hypertension. It is warming to the lungs and helps move the chi downwards in treating asthma, cough and wheezing in individuals with kidney-adrenal deficiency. It also treats excessive menstruation caused by coldness and deficiency, aiding pelvic circulation. It also is regulatory for women who exhibit cold deficient type uterine bleeding and infertility.
Dosage: 6-15 gms.

AMBER   *Succinum*

Energetics: sweet, neutral
Meridians/Organs affected: heart, liver, small intestine, bladder
Part used: the crushed stone
Active constituents: succoxyabietic acid, succinosilvic acid, succinoabieti nolic acid, succinoresinol, succinoabietol, succinic acid, succinit, resin, benzene
Properties: sedative, emmenagogue, diuretic, lithotriptic
Uses: It treats insomnia, anxiety, frequent dreams, forgetfulness, palpitations, seizures from a disturbed spirit, childhood convulsions and epilepsy. It also promotes urination and treats acute urinary tract infections and urinary tract stones. It aids blood circulation and promotes menstruation, relieving menstrual cramps, stopped menses, and abdominal tumors. It is good for a disturbed heart and spirit and for individuals with coronary heart disease.

Precautions: It is contraindicated for individuals with blood stagnation symptoms with acute internal fire or inflammations.
Dosage: Use only as a powder or pill, up to 3 gms. maximum taken internally, not in decoction

HEMATITE   *Haemititum*

Energetics: bitter, cold
Meridians/Organs affected: heart, liver
Active constituents: red colored iron ore composed of ferric oxide
Properties: sedative, antiemetic, hemostatic
Uses: It lowers the energy, treating symptoms such as belching, coughing, hiccoughs, vomiting and acute asthma. It also quiets the liver and relieves acute hypertension with symptoms of dizziness, vertigo, pressure around the eyes and tinnitus. It is a hemostatic, inhibiting bleeding of both hot and cold types (depending upon the herbs used in decoction). It also is used to treat vomiting blood and nosebleeds.
Dosage: 10-30 gms.

CINNABAR   *Cinnabaris*

Energetics: sweet, cool, toxic
Meridian/Organ affected: heart
Active constituents: red mercuric sulfide HGS
Properties: sedative, antispasmodic, alterative, antipyretic
Uses: It is used for extreme insomnia, palpitations, epilepsy, and infantile convulsions caused by high fever. Its alterative properties make it useful for detoxifying poisons in the blood, preventing putrefaction, and treating boils, carbuncles and furuncles. It helps expel mucus from the lungs and clears heat associated with dizziness and general nervousness. Externally it can be applied as a powder or salve as an antibiotic and antiparasitical.
Precautions: Long term use causes mercury poisoning.
Dosage: 250 mg.-1 gm.

NERVINES
(Mild Stabilizing and Sedative Herbs)

These herbs are used for conditions of nervousness, anxiety, insomnia, emotional instability, pain, cramps, spasms, tremors and epilepsy. Many are helpful for relieving stress and muscle tension. They include the well-known Western nervines not used in classical Chinese herbalism. These are safer than the previous category of strong sedatives and should be tried before resorting to them.

In terms of Ayurveda, these herbs reduce vata (air) for the short term, but those which are cooling can increase it over the long term. Most of them reduce pitta (fire). Pitta engenders turbulent emotions, while vata causes nervousness. Most nervines also reduce kapha (water), as many are light and drying. Many of these herbs will keep kapha types awake and aware, as herbs affect the different humors in different ways.

Contraindications are mainly for deficient nervous conditions and neurasthenia; most of these herbs are not nutritive enough for these conditions. Many of these herbs work well in tincture form, which directs their effects more specifically to the brain.

VALERIAN *Valeriana officinalis; Valerianaceae*

Energetics: spicy, bitter, warm
Meridians/Organs affected: liver, heart
Part used: roots
Active constituents: essential oil, valepotriates, which are special valerian compounds and alkaloids
Properties: nervine, antispasmodic, carminative, stimulant, anodyne
Uses: Valerian is calming and sedating. It relieves pain, cramps, and spasms, and is a brain stimulant. This herb can have opposite effects on individuals who have a heated condition, since it is heating as well as sedative. This is a clear example of the necessity of prescribing herbs energetically rather than purely symptomatically. The therapeutic indications as well as the constitutional energetic balance must be taken into account. Valerian is best for individuals with a cold, nervous condition.
Dosage: standard infusion or 3-9 gms.; tincture, 10-30 drops

LADY'S SLIPPER   *Cypridium pubescens; Orchidaceae*

Energetics: acrid, sweet, neutral
Meridians/Organs affected: liver, heart
Part used: root
Active constituents: volatile oil, volatile acid, tannic and gallic acids, resins and inorganic salts
Properties: nervine, sedative, antispasmodic
Uses: It treats anxiety, hysteria, neurosis, insomnia, restlessness, tremors, epilepsy, and palpitations, especially in debilitated conditions. It clears depression and induces a calm and cheerful state of mind conducive to restful sleep. As an endangered species it should be used with discretion. Several related orchids of the Rocky Mountain West, called coral root *(Corallorhiza spp.),* may be used in the same way.
Dosage: standard decoction or 3-9 gms.; tincture 10-30 drops. Since it is like a "nerve food" as with so many of the other nervines, it should be taken 3 to 4 times daily for maximum effectiveness

SCULLCAP   *Scutellaria lateriflora; Labiatae*

Energetics: bitter, cool
Meridians/Organs affected: heart, liver
Part used: aerial portions
Active constituents: volatile oil, scutellarin, a bitter glycoside, tannin, fat, a bitter principle, sugar
Properties: nervine, sedative, antispasmodic
Uses: It relaxes nervous tension, induces calm and counteracts sleeplessness. It eases premenstrual tension, strengthens the brain, is useful in the treatment of chorea, epilepsy and seizures generally. It usually is combined with valerian, lady's slipper and other nervines for a broader action.

This is one of the best herbs to use to break addictions and to ease the problems associated with drug and alcohol withdrawal. For such a condition, a quarter to half a cupful of the tea should be taken every hour or two, tapering off as the symptoms subside. It also is a good brain tonic for promoting meditation.

Precautions: It should be noted that most of what is sold as skullcap in this country is germander *(Teucrium)*. Ask for the geniune herb.
Dosage: standard infusion or 3-9 gms.; tincture, 10-30 drops

HOPS   *Humulus lupulus; Moraceae*

Energetics: bitter, cool
Meridians/Organs affected: heart, liver
Part used: strobiles (female flowers, leafy cone-like catkins)
Active constituents: lupuline, humulone, lupulone, resin with picric acids, essential oil, tannins, estrogenic substances, choline and asparagine
Properties: nervine, sedative, hypnotic, bitter tonic, antiseptic
Uses: It is used to treat insomnia, nervous tension, anxiety, restlessness, headache, indigestion, and mucous colitis. It is much used as an aromatic bitter in alcoholic beverages such as beer.
Dosage: standard infusion or 3-9 gms.; tincture, 10-30 drops. It is a delicate herb and should be used fresh or freshly tinctured

PASSION FLOWER   *Passiflora incarnata;*
Passifloraceae

Energetics: bitter, cool
Meridians/Organs affected: heart,liver
Part used: aerial portions
Active constituents: alkaloids including passiflorine, harmine and harmol and flavonic derivatives
Properties: nervine, sedative, hypnotic, antispasmodic, anodyne
Uses: It treats sleeplessness, chronic insomnia, Parkinson's disease, seizures, epilepsy, hysteria, neuralgia, shingles, anxiety, and nervous tension. The fruit is rich in flavonoids and is diuretic and a nutritive tonic.
Dosage: standard infusion or 3-9 gms.; tincture, 10-30 drops

WOOD BETONY   *Betonica officinalis (Stachys*
officinalis); Labiatae

Energetics: bitter, cool
Meridians/Organs affected: liver, heart

Part used: aerial portions
Active constituents: 15% tannins and several other ingredients
Properties: nervine, sedative, astringent, bitter tonic
Uses: It usually is used as a nervine with special action for diseases of the head. Taken daily with boiled warm milk, it is a good remedy for chronic headaches. It is good for anxiety, hysteria, nervousness, insomnia and often is combined with other nervine herbs.
Dosage: standard infusion or 3-9 gms.; tincture, 10-30 drops

CALIFORNIA POPPY
Eschscholzia california;
Papaveraceae

Energetics: bitter, cool
Meridians/Organs affected: liver, heart
Part used: aerial portions
Active constituents: alkaloids similar to the opium poppy, also flavone glycosides
Properties: nervine, sedative, febrifuge, antispasmodic, analgesic
Uses: It promotes relaxation, countering the effects of nervous tension, anxiety and insomnia. It is used both internally and externally to allay pain.
Dosage: standard infusion or 3-9 gms.; tincture, 10-30 drops

CALMATIVES

These herbs nourish the heart, calm the spirit and are useful for nervous disorders caused by wasting and deficiency, making them especially good for neurasthenia. They possess tonic and nutritive properties and help to increase nerve tissue and cerebro-spinal fluid. They are related to the class of yin tonics and sometimes considered to be yin tonics for the heart. Hence they are often used with tonics or as part of a tonification therapy.

According to Ayurveda such demulcent nervines are better for severe or chronic vata conditions and are safe for long term use. They decrease pitta and increase kapha.

As they tend to be mild in their action, they may not prove strong enough for acute conditions. Other herbs that have nutritive and tonic nervine action include licorice, lily, ophiopogon, ashwagandha and lady's slipper, and such foods as milk and ghee.

ZIZYPHUS   *Zizyphus spinosa; Rhamnaceae*

Energetics: sweet, sour, neutral
Meridians/Organs affected: heart, spleen, liver, gall bladder
Part used: seeds
Active constituents: betulin, betulic acid, jujoboside, jujubogenin, ebelin lactone, others saponins, vitamin C
Properties: nervine, sedative, tonic, astringent
Uses: It treats insomnia, irritability, palpitations, anxiety, spontaneous sweating, nerve weakness, and nervous exhaustion. This is the best of the nutritive sedatives in Chinese medicine. It is safe and effective for children, the weak or the elderly, and should be added to our stock of commonly used herbs.
Dosage: 10-20 gms. in decoction

THUJA (Cedar tree)   *Biotae orientalis and Thuja occidentalis; Cupressaceae*

Energetics: sweet, neutral
Meridians/Organs affected: heart, liver, kidney, colon
Part used: seeds
Active constituents: fatty and essential oils
Properties: nervine, sedative, mild laxative
Uses: It treats nervousness, anxiety, deficient heart blood, palpitations, and insomnia. It is used for constipation in the aged caused by general debility.
Precautions: Avoid using in cases of stagnant mucus in the lungs or diarrhea.
Dosage: 5-15 gms. in decoction; tincture, 10-30 drops

SENECA SNAKEROOT   Polygala senega
Energetics: bitter, spicy, warm
Meridians/Organs affected: lung, heart, kidney
Part used: root

Active constituents: Polygalic acid, pectic and tannic acids, fixed oil, gum, albumen, salts, alumina, silica, magnesia and iron

Properties: It is used in the West as a stimulating expectorant, diuretic and diaphoretic. A nearly identical substance used in Chinese medicine is considered one of the finest heart and mind tonics, being calming to the spirit and promoting positive feelings.

Uses: Here two very similar herbs are used for different purposes by East and West. In the West it is used primarily to aid in the expectoration of mucus in cases of pneumonia and acute bronchial affections. It also is used for croup, whooping cough and the treatment of rheumatic problems, as it has decided blood-moving (emmenagogue) properties. Large doses are emetic and cathartic.

Chinese herbalism uses *Polygala tenuifolia,* of which the root appears to be identical with some Western varieties, to stimulate the flow of energy in the heart, and to treat insomnia, palpitations, anxiety, restlessness and mental instability. It is especially helpful in promoting positive feelings and attitudes in individuals with constrained emotions and depression. It also is used to clear phlegm (mucus) and open the orifices. In this way, according to traditional Chinese medical theory, it benefits the heart and clears the consciousness.

Precautions: The Chinese recognize its emetic and cathartic action and recommend caution in its use.

Dosage: 3-6 gms. Of the tincture, 10-20 drops.

CHAMOMILE   *Anthemis nobilis (Roman), Matricaria chamomila (German); Compositae*

Energetics: bitter, spicy, neutral

Meridians/Organs affected: liver, stomach, lungs

Part used: flowers

Active constituents: essential oil comprised of a blue-colored azulene, also coumarin, flavonic heterosides, tannic acid

Properties: calmative, nervine, antispasmodic, anodyne, diaphoretic, emmenagogue, carminative

Uses: It is used for nervousness, headaches, anxiety, cramps and spasms. It also is beneficial for febrile diseases such as colds and flu. It is frequently used for digestive complaints and taken regularly will gently regulate the bowels. It contains an easily assimilable form of calcium and a tablespoon steeped in a covered cup of boiling water with two slices of fresh ginger is a very effective treatment for menstrual cramps and other pains and spasms. The same tea may be used for minor digestive problems such as acid indigestion and gas.

Dosage: 6-12 gms. in infusion; tincture, 10-30 drops

HERBS FOR REGULATING THE HEART

These are strong herbs with powerful chemical constituents which help regulate heart function. They should be used in the appropriately low doses.

NIGHT-BLOOMING CEREUS   *Cereus grandiflorus,*
                                  Cactus grandiflorus; Cactaceae

Energetics: bitter, warm
Meridians/Organs affected: heart, kidneys
Parts used: flowers and young, tender stems
Active constituents: not available
Properties: sedative, diuretic, cardiac
Uses: It is used for palpitations, anxiety, tachycardia, angina, carditis, pericarditis, arrhythmia, rheumatism, valvular disease, hypertrophy, dyspnoea, mitral regurgitation, pulmonary hemorrhage, and interstitial pneumonia. It is helpful for all cardio-pulmonary diseases.

It also treats cerebral congestion, mental derangements, inflammations of the mucous membranes, prostatic diseases, irritable bladder, renal congestion, dropsy, edematous conditions of the limbs, dysmenorrhea, and chronic bronchitis. It is beneficial for visual defects, tinnitus aurium, exophthalmic goitre, premenstrual syndrome and nervous menstrual defects.

Precautions: Dosage must be carefully regulated. An overdose can aggravate these conditions.

Dosage: Use only one-half to 10 drops of the tincture at a time, two or three times daily

LILY OF THE VALLEY   *Convallaria majalis; Liliaceae*

Energetics: sweet, bitter, neutral, toxic
Meridians/Organs affected: heart, kidney
Part used: leaves
Active constituents: cardiac glycosides, saponins, convallarin and con-
vallaric acid, asparagin, chelidonic acid and various other organic acids
Properties: antispasmodic, cardiac, diuretic, laxative
Uses: It is used for nervous sensitivity, neurasthenia, apoplexy,
epilepsy, dropsy, valvular heart diseases, heart pains and heart diseases
in general. This herb contains glycosides similar to digitalis but milder.
Precautions: Overdose can cause strong stomach and intestinal irri-
tation.
Dosage: 150 mg. of the dried leaf

AROMATIC CONSCIOUSNESS-REVIVING HERBS
(Fragrant Herbs for Opening the Orifices)

Strongly fragrant or aromatic herbs may be used to help restore consciousness in conditions of coma or fainting. Aromatic oils stimulate the
mind and senses and restore brain and heart function.

These herbs may be used for symptoms associated with strokes,
coma, delirium, convulsions and spasms such as locked jaw, clenched
fists, rigid limbs, often with a quickened and flooding pulse. There are
two major categories of this symptomatology:

Hot blockage: irritability, delirium, convulsions, red face, heavy breathing, flooding pulse, high fever and yellow tongue fur. Such symptoms
are called *hot-wind* in Chinese medicine. They are associated with
meningitis, encephalitis, delirium of extreme toxic inflammations, acute
pneumonia, heat stroke, liver disease, uremia and accidents with brain
damage.

Cold blockage: here there will be signs of coldness including coldness of
the body, grayish or pale complexion, white tongue fur and a slow pulse.
There may be a sudden collapse with foaming at the mouth. It usually is
associated with brain injuries and poisoning.

Aromatic herbs that open the orifices may be used similarly to smelling salts if they cannot be taken internally. Because of their dispersing action, they can injure the righteous energy if overused. Making the patient warm is also a very important procedure in such cases and teas for warming the central warmer (maintaining digestion) such as ginger and cinnamon, are helpful.

Other aromatic herbs useful in this way include myrrh, frankincense, sandalwood, black pepper and cloves. For hot blockage conditions, warm aromatic herbs are combined with cold bitter herbs like golden seal or gentian. In India and China, the favorite cooling substance of this category is the gall stone of a cow. It is very effective in febrile diseases that cause a loss of consciousness or delirium.

In Ayurvedic theory, these herbs are used for reviving and stimulating the flow of prana. They are used as part of a system of aroma therapy which includes the use of incense, that is applied in treating most diseases. They reduce vata (air) short term use and decrease kapha (water and phlegm). Those which are warming will increase pitta (fire).

They are generally contraindicated except for the acute conditions they treat.

CAMPHOR   *Cinnamomum camphora; Lauraceae*

Energetics: spicy, bitter, warm, toxic
Meridians/Organs affected: heart, lung, liver
Parts used: crystallized extract, leaves
Active constituents: d-camphora
Properties: stimulant, rubefacient, diaphoretic, parasiticide, analgesic, antiseptic
Uses: It is used for bronchitis and asthma to control hypersecretion, for exhaustion, depression, stomachache and abdominal pain, to stimulate blood and energy circulation, remove excess moisture, and kill insects/worms. It is effective externally against parasites, ringworm, scabies and to stop itch. Camphor is frequently found in oils for external use, as it opens the lungs, relieves congestion and helps to relieve muscle tension and joint pain. It also is used for arthritic and rheumatic pains and pains of trauma and injury (although it should not be applied

directly to open wounds). It is be used as a smelling salt and given internally in small amounts to revive a patient from delirium or coma. A piece of camphor attached to children's underclothing will help to protect them from contagious diseases. As an incense it purifies the air.

Precautions: Contraindicated in pregnancy or low energy conditions. More than one or two gms. can produce harmful side-effects and more than seven may prove fatal. Take only the natural plant extract internally, as the chemically prepared camphor is contaminated with other chemicals.

Dosage: If the leaves are available use about 15-20 gms. infused in a pint of water. The extract is readily available. One teaspoon of the extract can be infused in two cups of water and sipped in teaspoon doses. As a tincture, 5-10 drops may be taken. It may be inhaled to clear the lungs. Of the extract, take only 100-250 mg. internally at a time.

MUSK   *Moschus*

Energetics: spicy, warm
Meridians/Organs affected: heart, spleen
Part used: navel gland secretions of the musk deer
Active constituents: muscone, normuscone
Properties: stimulant, emmenagogue, aphrodisiac
Uses: It revives consciousness, for feverish diseases characterized by convulsions, delirium, stupor and fainting. It also is used to treat blood congestion, arteriosclerosis, toxic sores, boils, energy congestion from injuries, and bruises (externally in a liniment). It helps to move and dissolve tumors and masses, to stimulate menstruation, and to bring down the afterbirth and the fetus of stillborns.
Precautions: For pregnant woman, even inhalation of this substance can cause abortion or miscarriage.
Dosage: 200-375mg.

STYRAX (Storax)   *Liquidamber orientalis;*
                                                             Hamamelaceae

Energetics: sweet, acrid, aromatic, warm
Meridians/Organs affected: heart, spleen

Part used: resin
Active constituents: oleanolic acid, cinnamic ester
Properties: stimulant, emmenagogue, expectorant, irritant, astringent
Uses: It clears blockage of phlegm, opens orifices, clears sinuses and bronchioles. It is applied externally in treating various skin diseases.
Precautions: Do not use during pregnancy.
Dosage: In infusion 1-3 gms. or 10-20 grains

CALAMUS   *Acorus calamus and spp.; Araceae*

Energetics: acrid, slightly warm, aromatic
Meridians/Organs affected: heart, liver, spleen
Part used: rhizomes
Active constituents: essential oil, amino acid, organic acid, sugars
Properties: stimulant, carminative, expectorant, emetic
Uses: It clears nervous tension and dampness of the spleen and stomach, aids digestion, treats dyspepsia and hyperacidity, and regulates gastrointestinal fermentation. It effectively treats poor appetite and gastrointestinal distension. Calamus is highly regarded in Ayurvedic medicine as an herb that promotes wisdom by improving mental focus. In China it is considered a primary herb for restoring the power of speech after a stroke. They also use it to treat insanity, depression and impaired consciousness. In Ayurvedic medicine, the combination of calamus root and gotu kola is a universal tonic for the mind and the nervous system; it increases memory and concentration. Combined with cardamon, it helps the digestion of dairy products.
Precautions: Avoid during pregnancy.
Dosage: standard infusion or 3-9 gms.; tincture, 10-30 drops

BAY   *Laurus nobilis; Lauraceae*

Energetics: spicy, warm
Meridians/Organs affected: heart, spleen
Part used: leaves
Active constituents: essential oil with cineol and pinene, fatty oil with lauric acid, oleic acid, palmitic and linoleic acids
Properties: stimulant, carminative, emmenagogue, diaphoretic, emetic

Uses: Oil of bay is used externally for sprains and bruises. The infused leaves are taken as a tea for hysteria, amenorrhea, gas, colic and indigestion. The berries are used to remove obstructions, to promote abortion and for delayed menses. Four or five moderate doses are said to cure ague (violent fever often associated with malaria).

Dosage: infusion, one level teaspoon in a cup of boiling water; tincture, apply externally for bruises and injuries, and internally use only 5-20 drops; standard dosage in formulas or 3-9 gms.

ANTISPASMODICS
(Herbs for Extinguishing Internal Wind and Relieving Spasms)

The sites of draft or wind diseases, associated with the nervous system, can be internal or external. These conditions may arise as a result of extreme deficiencies (such as kidney and liver yin and blood deficiency) causing hyper-reactivity. They also arise from excess, including high fever or excess liver energy. There are many ways to effectively treat the range of neurological disorders that include functional problems such as Parkinson's disease, nervous depression, pains and itching, and emotional disturbances.

External wind is a superficial disease located on the surface of the skin. It is characterized by fever, chills, itching, aching muscles, runny nose, allergies and floating pulse, and it is treated by diaphoretics. *Internal wind* is treated by antispasmodics. Symptoms of internal wind include dizziness, blurred vision, hypertension, headaches, tinnitus, tremors, muscle twitches, and, in severe cases irritability, vomiting and palpitations. If allowed to progress, these symptoms eventually will lead to such severe conditions as strokes, hemiplegia, aphasia, facial paralysis, epilepsy and loss of consciousness.

It is important to determine first whether the wind symptoms are energetically cool or warm-natured. Then antispasmodics that are cold in nature are chosen to eliminate hot wind conditions, while others that are warm are used to eliminate cold wind conditions.

In all acute conditions, it is good practice to add, as a supporting herb, a small amount of an herbal antispasmodic to help release the tension maintaining the disease process. Chronic neurological conditions such as epilepsy, nervous depression, anxiety and insomnia are difficult to treat because more specific organic imbalances may need to be treated simultaneously by other herbal therapies.

A condition of liver stagnancy can cause a variety of problems classified as *liver-wind* imbalances. The herbs in this category and many nervine herbs are useful for treating this condition. Dredging the liver with cholagogues such as barberry and Culver's root, regulating liver chi with carminatives like tangerine or bitter orange peel, and nourishing liver blood with blood and yin tonics like lycium berries or rehmannia are important fundamental treatments to consider for resolving liver wind imbalances. If there is constipation, an herbal laxative should be used.

There are two distinct subcategories in liver sedation: that of calming liver wind and that of subduing liver yang. Many of the substances used to calm liver wind are insects such as scorpions, centipedes, earthworms, silk worms and grasshoppers. The Chinese extrapolate from the ability of these creatures to crawl on the earth their ability to crawl into the channels and meridians and there relieve spasms.

Liver sedative herbs are used to subdue so-called uprising of liver yang. This condition is associated with a flaring of heat, fits of anger and other uncontrollable emotions. Under such conditions, the yang of the liver tends towards excess while the yin is deficient. Both to subdue the yang with cooling, anti-inflammatory herbs and to nourish the yin with blood or yin tonics is the therapeutic approach in such cases.

Thus the herbs and substances listed under this category are used synergistically with those under the previous categories of nervines, tranquilizers and sedatives. The many preparations and formulas that include animal and insect parts are more strongly antispasmodic. They are more specifically antitremor or anticonvulsive, while Western antispasmodics are a more general category including any herbs that help cramping, gas or muscle tension.

Ayurveda would consider these herbs to calm vata (nervous energy) in acute conditions. Those which are cooling reduce pitta (fire, emotional energy). Many will increase kapha (water) and have a dulling effect upon the mind, as, for example, the insect and animal remedies.

Many of these herbs are toxic and contraindicated in all but the acute conditions they treat, and so should not be used during pregnancy. Some of the safer herbs in this category are caltrops, gambir, wild yam, lobelia and abalone shell. Yet even these should not be used without caution. For deficient types, these herbs must be combined with tonics to guard against their side effects.

ANTELOPE HORN   *Naemorhedis and spp.*

Energetics: salty, cold
Meridians/Organs affected: liver, heart
Part used: the horn (goat horn also can be used)
Active constituents: contains calcium phosphate and kerratin
Properties: antispasmodic, antipyretic
Uses: It is used to subdue liver yang; and for acute cases of severe fever, blurred vision, dizziness, red eyes, headaches, photophobia, spasms, convulsions, childhood convulsions from high fever, delirium, mania, toxins in the blood and fire poison
Dosage: Antelope horn, which is not as readily available, is stronger than goat horn and about half dosage can be used (1-3 gms.). Goat horn should be from 9-15 gms. It should be grated and decocted about 30 minutes before adding any other herb.

GAMBIR   *Uncariae rhyncholphylla; Rubiaceae*

Energetics: sweet, cool
Meridians/Organs affected: liver, heart
Parts used: stem and hooks
Active constituents: alkaloid (rhynchophylline, corynozeine, hirsutine, hirsuteine, isorhynchophulline)
Properties: antispasmodic, anticonvulsant, antipyretic, anti-hypertensive
Uses: This powerful antispasmodic herb used in Chinese herbalism lowers blood pressure. In larger doses it can paralyze the sympathetic nerve endings. It is used to treat high fever, vertigo, nervous and hyper-tensive headaches and hypertension.
Precautions: It is contraindicated for individuals lacking genuine heat and internal nervous tension.
Dosage: 6-15 gms. in mild decoction

CALTROP   *Tribulus terrestris; Zygophyllaceae*

Energetics: acrid, bitter, warm
Meridians/Organs affected: liver, lung
Part used: fruit
Active constituents: kaempferol-3-glucoside, kaempferol-3-rutinoside, tribulo side, saponin, alkaloids, potassium nitrate, essential oil
Properties: antispasmodic, alterative, anodyne
Uses: It relieves spasms, clears the eyes, relieves hypertensive headache and dizziness and chest fullness, and treats mastitis, spermatorrhea, vertigo, itching, hives, skin lesions with severe itching, and vitiligo. It also is effective in treating constrained liver chi with pain and distention in the chest and glands, and deficient mother's milk caused by emotional upset.

Ayurveda classifies it as sweet and cold and uses it as one of its two main diuretic herbs for urinary problems, kidney and lower back pains, urinary tract stones and as an aphrodisiac. Its diuretic action has been confirmed by Chinese research. Found as a common lawn and field weed in this country, it is known as "goat's head" or "puncture vine".
Precautions: It should be used cautiously during pregnancy and for patients with deficient chi and blood.
Dosage: 6-12 gms.

WILD YAM   *Dioscorea villosa; Dioscoraceae*

Energetics: sweet, bitter, warm
Meridians/Organs affected: liver, kidney, spleen
Part used: root
Active constituents: glycoside saponins and diosgenin, which are hormone precursors, especially of progesterone and other cortical steroids that affect the female menstrual cycle and help to reduce pain
Properties: antispasmodic, diaphoretic, diuretic, expectorant, cholagogue
Uses: It treats bilious colic, soothes the nerves in neuralgia and urinary pains, is used for menstrual cramps, is effective for the liver and gall bladder, and for digestive problems associated with an imbalance of

these organs. It is a near-specific for conditions of chronic flatulence and gas.

Precautions: In using, do not confuse oriental tonic wild yams.

Dosage: standard decoction or 3-9 gms.; tincture, 10-30 drops

BLACK HAW   *Viburnum prunifolium; Caprifoliaceae*

Energetics: bitter, cool

Meridian/Organ affected: liver

Parts used: bark and root

Active constituents: amentoflavone, coumarins, scopoletine and aesculetine, arbutin, oleanolic and ursolic acids, sterol

Properties: antispasmodic, analgesic

Uses: It treats all nervous complaints, including convulsions, hysteria and spasms. It is one of the most reliable remedies for menstrual cramps, spasms and pains. It is often combined with false unicorn root *(Helonias)* as a preferred treatment against miscarriage. It also is used to treat asthma, palpitations, heart disease and hysterical fits. It is good for all painful affections, including arthritic and rheumatic complaints.

Cramp bark *(Viburnum opulis)*, usually is used alternately with black haw. Cramp bark is weaker, containing about a third of the resins of black haw.

Dosage: standard infusion or 3-9 gms.

LOBELIA   *Lobelia inflata; Lobeliaceae*

Energetics: bitter, neutral

Meridians/Organs affected: liver, lungs, heart, small intestine

Parts used: seed, leaves and flowers

Active constituents: alkaloids, lobeline, isolobeline, etc., lobelic and chelidonic acid

Properties: antispasmodic, expectorant, stimulant, emetic, alterative, diuretic

Uses: It treats asthma and bronchial spasms, relaxes the respiratory passages, and may be used to lessen the strength of contractions during natural childbirth. It is good for lockjaw and most other spasmodic conditions and is an important herb for poisionous bites and stings. Lobeline is similar to nicotine, and lobelia is used in commercial smoking preparations to counteract the desire for tobacco.

When extracting alkaloids, as with lobelia, prepare an acid tincture using apple cider vinegar. Macerate four ounces of the seeds (the strongest part of this plant), or the entire upper portion of the plant, mix with eight ounces of vinegar, and add to a wide-mouthed jar. After two weeks, strain and bottle for use.

There is conflicting opinion as to the toxicity of lobelia. The author has not found it to be so. On several occasions I have given substantial teaspoonful doses of the tincture, even up to three or four times in succession every ten minutes, to induce vomiting in the treatment of asthma. No side-effects occurred. Instead, the patient felt calm and relaxed.

For a lobelia emetic, I recommend about two quarts of warm mint tea to be taken while administering the lobelia. The late Dr. Christopher prescribed this treatment, advising that it be given when the asthma attack had reached its worst peak. I have followed this several times with good results. Chinese medicine also uses lobelia as a diuretic and regards it as a safe herb.

It is important to recognize that, for some sensitive individuals, this may be an exhausting treatment. The dangers are more from the wrong prescription of emetic therapy than from any special toxicity of the lobelia itself.

Dosage: tincture, 5-15 drops; in infusion, 6-15 gms.

HENBANE   *Hyoscyamus niger; Solanaceae*

Energetics: bitter, warm, toxic
Meridian/Organ affected: liver
Parts used: leaves, seeds
Active constituents: alkaloids including hyoscyamin and atropine, tannin, choline, traces of essential oil
Properties: antispasmodic, analgesic, diuretic, hypnotic
Uses: It stops perspiration, lessens pain, induces sleep, is antispasmodic to the smooth muscle of the gastrointestinal tract, good for hysteria, irritable cough, asthma, gastric ulcer, colitis, and irritable bladder syn-

drome. In the advised small doses, it is a good antispasmodic for many conditions.

Precautions: This herb has figured prominently in literature and folklore throughout the ages as a poisonous narcotic similar to belladonna and datura.

Dosage: powdered leaves, 2-10 grains; alcoholic extract, 2-10 drops

DATURA   *Datura stramonium; Solanaceae*

Energetics: bitter, warm, toxic
Meridian/Organ affected: liver
Parts used: leaves and seeds
Active constituents: stramonium and other alkaloids like henbane
Properties: antispasmodic, analgestic, anaesthetic, sedative, hypnotic, narcotic
Uses: It alleviates pain, stops cough, and relieves asthma and wheezing. It may be externally applied in a liniment for rheumatic aches and pains, boils, ringworm, and as a local anaesthetic. It has been found by the Chinese to be beneficial in the treatment of cancer and is used by them for pain relief.
Dosage: 1/10-5 grains of the powder; fluid extract, 1-3 drops

BELLADONNA   *Belladonna atropa; Solanaceae*

Energetics: bitter, warm, toxic
Meridian/Organ affected: liver
Part used: whole plant
Active constituents: various alkaloids, especially hyoscyamine and scopalamine
Properties: antispasmodic, sedative, diuretic, narcotic
Uses: Its uses are similar to those of henbane and datura, but belladonna is used more for high infectious, feverish conditions with local inflammation and pain. It treats nervous congestion, suppresses the action of the smooth muscles, and is helpful for kidney pains. It is considered a near specific for the relief of colitis. Being a mydriatic, it is used in ophthalmology to dilate the pupils of the eyes.

Belladonna leaves applied externally are used as a treatment and possible cure for cancer by both Western herbalists and in Chinese folk medicine.

Dosage: powdered leaves, 1-2 grains; root, 1-5 grains; alcoholic extract of the leaves 1-3 drops, of the root, -1 drop

EARTHWORM   *Pheretime aspergillum*

Energetics: salty, cold
Meridians/Organs affected: liver, spleen, lung
Part used: whole animal
Active constituents: lumbrofebrine, lumbritin, terrestro-lumbrolysin, hypoxanthine, xanthine, guanine, adenine, guanidine, choline
Properties: antispasmodic, diuretic, alterative
Uses: It opens the bronchioles, meridians and channels of the nervous and circulatory systems. It is used for arthritis, rheumatism, strokes, stiffness of the extremeties, high fever with convulsions and seizures, wheezing caused by lung inflammation, hypertension.
Precautions: Contraindicated during pregnancy.
Dosage: standard decoction or 3-9 gms. They may also be cleaned and macerated in wine to treat arthritic and rheumatic complaints.

ABALONE SHELL   *Haliotidis diversicolor*

Energetics: salty, neutral
Meridians/Organs affected: liver, kidney
Part used: shell
Active constituents: calcium carbonate, with small amounts of magnesium silica, phosphates, iron and chlorides
Properties: antispasmodic, alterative
Uses: It treats diseases of a hot character. It lowers the yang and is good for liver fire with symptoms of dizziness, headache and red eyes. An important Chinese remedy for the eyes, it is used to treat blurred vision, photophobia, pterygium and other visual problems.
Dosage: 9-30 gms. of the crushed shells in decoction

SCORPION
Buthus martensi

Energetics: salty, acrid, neutral, toxic
Meridian/Organ affected: liver
Part used: whole insect
Active constituents: katsutoxin
Properties: antispasmodic, anticonvulsant, alterative
Uses: It treats all spasms, convulsions, tetany, tics, seizures, stroke, facial paralysis, severe headache. It restores the normal flow of energy in the channels and consequently relieves pain. It is used internally or externally for cancer, poisons, and swelling and sores, usually along with centipede.
Precautions: Contraindicated during pregnancy.
Dosage: powder (the usual form of administration) ½-1 gm.; in decoction 2-5 gms.

CENTIPEDE
Scolopendra subspinipes

Energetics: acrid, warm, toxic
Meridian/Organ affected: liver
Part used: whole insect with legs removed
Active constituents: histamine, hemolytic protein, fatty oil, cholesterol, formic acid, hydroxylysine, amino acids
Properties: antispasmodic, anticonvulsant, alterative
Uses: Its uses are similar to those of scorpion, with which it usually is combined. It is particularly good for allergies.

One traditional Chinese form of chemotherapy combines scorpion, earthworm and centipede brewed into a decoction. This is strained and an egg cooked in the tea to make egg drop soup. This is then taken three times a day. It would seem that the cancer cells absorb the protein of the egg along with the toxins of the insects and that this inhibits their growth. This treatment has no harmful side-effects.
Precautions: Contraindicated during pregnancy.
Dosage: 1-3 gms. in decoction; ½-1 gm. in powder

EXPECTORANT AND ANTITUSSIVE HERBS
(Herbs for Dissolving Phlegm and Relieving Cough)

This category is divided into two main groups; expectorant or phlegm-dissolving herbs and antitussive or cough-relieving herbs. In general, however, most expectorant herbs have cough-relieving properties and most cough-relieving herbs tend to aid in the elimination of mucus. The expectorants are in turn divided into two groups according to whether their nature is cooling or warming.

Mucus usually is a by-product of digestion. When digestion is weak an excess of mucus will become apparent in the mucous secreting tissues of the body. These include the lungs, which need extract lubrication to counteract the drying effect of normal respiration; and the reproductive organs, that secrete extract fluid. The bones, joints and connective tissue also need mucoid lubrication. This broad concept of mucus describes a sticky, lubricating secretion found not only in the lungs but in many tissues and organs of the body. This concept corresponds with the definition of the kapha or water humor in Ayurvedic herbalism. Ayurveda concurs with the idea that mucus is a by-product of digestion when it locates the seat of kapha in the stomach.

As mucus accumulates and stagnates, it becomes a toxic substance called *ama*. The accumulation of *ama* is a serious problem, giving rise to congestion throughout the organs and systems of the body. This is the cause of most degenerative diseases, including artheriosclerosis, cancer, arthritis, senility, asthma and emphysema.

Herbs that have a warming and diuretic property, such as pepper, cinnamon and ginger, are very helpful in preventing, drying and eliminating excess mucus. Warming stimulants support the *ministerial fire* of the spleen-pancreas, which is called *agni* in Ayurveda. *Agni* has a much broader meaning as well, referring to the fundamental life-force of the body. When one eats poorly, weakening the capacity to digest and eliminate food, the digestive fire weakens. This causes an accumulation of fluids, usually in the abdomen first and then in the hips and throughout the body.

Other herbs to improve digestion can help in reducing phlegm. As mucus is a product of dampness, according to Chinese medical theory, herbs to eliminate dampness usually have expectorant action. Carminatives prevent dampness and phlegm by stimulating peristalsis. Tonics prevent phlegm by maintaining the general hormonal and metabolic levels of the body.

Phlegm in the lungs can cause coughing, wheezing, shortness of breath and costal or rib pains. Improving digestion is the major strategy in eliminating mucus and sinus congestion. The use of antitussive and expectorant herbs are a symptomatic approach to clearing the channels of mucus and eliminating it from the lungs, bronchioles and sinuses.

Mucus in the stomach can give rise to symptoms of nausea, vomiting, loss of appetite, distended stomach and sometimes a shallow cough. Here the aim of treatment is to harmonize the stomach, using carminative and diuretic herbs that transform mucus.

Mucus or phlegm also can block the nerve channels of the body (described as acupuncture meridians). This in turn can cause lymphatic swellings, goiter and scrofula. For this we use herbs, like seaweeds, that dissolve phlegm and soften hard masses. These are combined with carminative and diuretic herbs that transform and eliminate mucus.

Still another kind of phlegm is called "invisible phlegm obstructing the heart and consciousness". This may not be obvious as a mucus condition. It causes such disorders as senility, mental disorders, heart problems, stroke, coma and seizures. Some expectorant herbs such as fritillary are used as adjunctive herbal therapy for this condition, in conjunction with other properties appropriate to the individual case.

Clear or white phlegm means that the condition is caused by cold

If it is yellow or blood-tinged, the condition is one of heat and stagnation. Cooling or warming expectorants are prescribed according to whether the symptoms indicate a condition caused by hot or cold.

In terms of Ayurveda these are the principal herbs for treating kapha (water) disorders.

COOLING EXPECTORANTS
(Herbs that Cool and Dissolve Hot Phlegm)

Cooling expectorants are used for hot and dry phlegm. They are indicated for dry cough, difficult expectoration, swollen lymph glands, lung or breast abscesses and bleeding from the lungs. Many are demulcent and possess moistening properties. As such, they are related to yin tonics, which may be similarly used as expectorants. Most Western demulcent expectorants, like comfrey or chickweed, fall in this category. Their taste usually is sweet, salty or bitter. Some are good for goiter, scrofula and cancer.

In Ayurvedic terms, these herbs reduce pitta (fire) and vata (air). They increase or liquify kapha (water) and facilitate its passage out of the body.

As many of these herbs are sweet and sticky, they are contraindicated in conditions of cold or damp phlegm and weak digestion.

FRITILLARY (Mission bells) *Fritillaria spp.; Liliaceae*

F. thunbergii is the variety commonly but not exclusively used in Chinese medicine. The many varieties found in North America include *F. pudica* and *F. atropurpurea,* both of which are edible. *F. meleagris,* commonly found in European rock gardens and said to be quite poisonous, contains a heart-depressant alkaloid.

Energetics: bitter, sweet, cool
Meridians/Organs affected: lung, heart
Part used: bulb
Active constituents: the Chinese variety contains various alkaloids including verticin, fritillin and fritillarin
Properties: expectorant, antitussive, tonic
Uses: It treats chronic tracheitis, bronchitis, bronchial asthma, yin defi-

cient coughs (tuberculosis) and other coughs. It also is used to reduce swollen thyroid gland and dissolve hard lymphatic lumps and nodules and lung or breast abscesses, and to treat cancer of the lungs. Traditionally it was considered incompatible with aconite, but research has not so far shown this to be true.

Precautions: It is contraindicated for patients with low energy and weak digestion.

Dosage: 3-9 gms.

KELP   *Fucus versiculosis; Laminariaceae*

Energetics: salty, cool
Meridians/Organs affected: liver, stomach
Part used: whole plant
Active constituents: iodine, calicium, iron, alginic acid, mannitol, carotene, protein, riboflavin, vitamin C
Properties: expectorant, demulcent, emollient, alterative, diuretic
Uses: It soothes irritated throat and mucous membranes, soothes coughs, dissolves firm masses such as tumors, treats enlarged thyroid, lymph node enlargement and swollen and painful testes, and reduces edema. Many species are used. These include *L. Japonica* (called kombu), *L. angusta, L. cichorioides, L. religiosa, L. longipedalis.* and many other varieties of edible seaweed.
Precautions: Generally contraindicated for patients with a weak, cold digestion (cold deficient spleen and stomach).
Dosage: 3-15 gms.

COMFREY   *Symphytum officinale; Boraginaceae*

Energetics: bitter, sweet, cool
Meridians/Organs affected: lungs, stomach
Part used: aerial portions
Active constituents: allantoin, tannins, mucilage, starch, inulin
Properties: expectorant, antitussive, demulcent, alterative, astringent, vulnerary
Uses: It moistens the lungs, helps dissolve and expel mucus, soothes the throat, lowers fever, relieves cough, and treats asthma. It is applied

externally as a poultice and taken internally to promote healing of injured tissues and bones.

Dosage: standard infusion or 3-9 gms.; tincture, 10-30 drops

CHICKWEED   *Stellaria media; Caryophyllaceae*

Energetics: bitter, sweet, cool
Meridians/Organs affected: lungs, stomach
Part used: aerial portions
Active constituents: saponins
Properties: expectorant, demulcent, emollient, antitussive, antipyretic, alterative, vulnerary
Uses: It moistens and aids the expectoration of phlegm from the lungs, relieves sore throat, lowers fevers, and treats stomach and duodenal ulcers. Externally applied as an oil, ointment or poultice, it relieves dryness and irritation, promotes healing and softens the skin.
Chickweed oil (page 60) has similar, though milder anti-itch, anti-psoriasis and anti-irritant properties to cortisone creme without the long term harmful side effects.
Dosage: 6-15 gms.

SOW FENNEL   *Peucedanum palustre; Umbelliferae*

In Europe a species known as Masterwort, *P. ostruthium* is similarly used. Various *Peucedanums* are found in North America. Some, such as *P. ambiguum, montanum, scopularum* and *utriculatum,* are said to have been used by the Native Americans both as food and medicine. Others, such as *P. grayii* and *platycarpum,* are suspected to be poisonous. The Chinese species (*P. praeruptorum*) is highly regarded for treating phlegm, cough and inflammatory lung diseases. Some of the non-Chinese species have similar properties.

Energetics: spicy, bitter, cool
Meridians/Organs affected: lungs, stomach, colon
Part used: root
Active constituents: 95% terpenes (pinene, phellandrene, limonene), oxypeucedanine, othol and a furanocoumarin
Properties: expectorant, antitussive, diaphoretic, diuretic, stomachic, emmenagogue
Uses: It is used for asthma, cough, flatulence, dyspepsia, epilepsy, colic, amenorrhea, dysmenorrhea, apoplexy and palsy. These uses accord with Chinese practice. They say that it lowers excess energy, stops

cough and settles the stomach, and can be used for colds, headache, coughs, asthma, dyspnea and chest tightness.
Dosage: standard infusion or 3-9 gms.

TRICHOSANTHES
Trichosanthes kirilowii; Cucurbitaceae

Energetics: sweet, bitter, cold
Meridians/Organs affected: lung, stomach, colon
Part used: fruit
Active constituents: triterpenoid saponins, fatty oil, resins
Properties: expectorant, antitussive, emollient
Uses: It is used for inflammation of the respiratory organs and irritated coughs, and to soften and dissolve nodules in the lungs and chest that cause constriction, lung and breast abscesses. Externally it is used as a poultice for swollen and inflamed sores and abscesses. The root is anti-inflammatory and demulcent.

Although uses given above are for the Chinese species, there are many related North American members of this family that may have similar properties and uses, for example, *Cucurbita foetidissima* known as "buffalo gourd", which grows on dry ground throughout the midwest and southwest. The seeds may be ground and eaten as a mush. Both the whole gourd and the root were crushed in water and used by the early settlers to clean their hands, indicating that they probably contain saponins.
Precautions: Contraindicated for individuals with cold, damp phlegm with weakness of digestion and stomach.
Dosage: 9-30 gms.

BAMBOO
Phyllostachys spp.; Graminae

Energetics: sweet, cool
Meridians/Organs affected: varies depending on part used
Parts Used and Properties: The leaves are diuretic. The root is astringent, styptic and antipyretic. The epidermis or shavings of the young stems are sedative, antiemetic, antipyretic, stop cough and clear the heart of invisible phlegm. The tabasheer or siliceous secretions are spe-

cifically anti-inflammatory and tonic for the lungs. Specifically, this part of the bamboo enters the heart, liver and gall bladder.
Active constituents: silicone, potassium hydroxide
Uses: It is used to treat lung inflammation and phlegm that is difficult to expectorate. It also is used to stop spasms, convulsions caused by phlegm and heat, strokes with phlegm obstructing the breathing passages, and childhood convulsions. It is especially useful for treating children's coughs and mucus.

In Ayurvedic herbalism it is considered a lung tonic. With one part cinnamon, two parts cardamon and four parts black pepper, eight parts bamboo tabasheer are ground into a powder with sixteen parts raw sugar. This makes *sitopaladi churna,* used for the treatment and prevention of colds, coughs, bronchitis and asthma.
Dosage: 3-12 gms.

EUPHORBIA (Pill-bearing spurge) (Chinese), (Europe and N. American);

Euphorbiae helioscopia
E. pilulifera
Euphorbiaceae

Energetics: acrid, bitter, cool, slightly toxic
Meridians/Organs affected: colon, spleen, lung, large intestine
Part used: entire plant
Active constituents: resin, calcium, wax, calcium malate, lignin, bassorin, volatile oil
Properties: expectorant, diuretic, anti-inflammatory
Uses: It is used for asthma, chronic inflammation of the respiratory ducts, chronic bronchitis, and emphysema. It is also given for the common cold and hay fever allergies.

Studies were conducted in China in which 20% preparations of the neutral saponins from this herb were injected intramuscularly for the treatment of cancer of the esophagus. More than half of the 64 patients studied either were completely cured or markedly improved. Results usually were noted within five days of this treatment. Even the patients whose esophageal tumors remained unreduced in size were able to swallow food more easily. This indicates that the tumors may have been softened by the saponins in the herb.

Precautions: Many poisonous spurges resemble each other, making positive identification important. The Western and Chinese varieties mentioned here seem to be nearly equivalent to each other in their properties, and their toxicity levels are negligible.
Dosage: 3-15 gms. in decoction internally

HOREHOUND   *Marrubium vulgare; Labiatae*

Energetics: bitter, cool
Meridians/Organs affected: lung, spleen, liver
Part used: leaves
Active constituents: a bitter principle called marrubine, an essential oil and tannin
Properties: expectorant, bitter tonic, diaphoretic, diuretic
Uses: Horehound is used for coughs, lung problems, hoarseness and typhoid fevers, especially those with accompanying liver imbalances. It calms the heart, relieves palpitations and restores normal glandular secretions. It often is taken as a syrup with honey. A tea of the leaves is used to treat skin eruptions.
Dosage: standard infusion or 3-9 gms.

CLAM SHELLS   *Meretricix meretrix*

Energetics: bitter, salty, neutral
Meridians/Organs affected: lung, kidney
Part used: crushed shells
Active constituents: calcium carbonate, chitin
Properties: expectorant, demulcent, anti-inflammatory, astringent, tonic
Uses: It clears inflammation from the lungs and dissolves congested and inflamed lung phlegm. It also inhibits sweating and diarrhea, incontinence of seminal fluid, menorrhagia, leucorrhea, and urinary dribbling. It is useful for treating edema, softening tumors and masses, thyroid lump and lymphatic congestion. The powder may be freely applied externally for the treatment of burns.
Dosage: 9-30 gms. in decoction. This should first be cooked alone and then strained before adding herbs to the decoction.

PUMICE   *Pumex*

Energetics: salty, cold
Meridian/Organ affected: lung
Part used: the finely powdered stone
Active constituents: aluminum, potassium, calcium, sodium and silicon dioxide
Properties: expectorant, antitussive, sedative, alterative, diuretic
Uses: It is used for inflammation and congestion of the lung with thick phlegm that is difficult to expectorate. It helps soften lymphatic nodules and goiter. It helps remove excess fluid from the genito-urinary tract by promoting urine and inhibits leucorrhea. The charred powder is be taken for stomach pains and hyperacidity.
Precautions: It usually is contraindicated for individuals with chronic low energy and metabolism with feelings of coldness.
Dosage: 9-15 gms. in decoction, boiled alone before adding other herbs.

WARMING EXPECTORANTS
(Herbs that Warm and Dissolve Cold Phlegm)

All herbs in this category have a spicy-warm nature and enter the lungs or spleen. The major indications for their use is clear, whitish phelgm, coldness and pale complexion. They treat cough, vomiting, asthma and other mucous conditions, including phlegm blocking the channels, that may cause epilepsy, stroke or paralysis. These herbs are mostly carminatives and expectorants and eliminate the accumulation of mucus by improving digestion. They may be supported by combination with other carminative, stimulant, chi or yang tonics, as individual cases indicate.

According to Ayurveda, they decrease kapha (water) and vata (air) and increase pitta (fire).

They are contraindicated for dry cough and inflammatory conditions.

YERBA SANTA   *Eriodictyon spp.; Hydrophyllaceae*

Energetics: spicy, warm
Meridians/Organs affected: lungs, spleen
Part used: leaves
Active constituents: eriodictyol, homoeriodictyol, chrysocriol, zan-thoeridol and eridonel. Also free formic and other acids, glycerides of fatty acids, a yellow volatile oil, a phytosterol, resin and glucose.
Properties: expectorant, carminative, alterative
Uses: It counteracts both hot and cold phlegm, and is an excellent expectorant, especially when combined with grindelia. It also pro-motes salivation and aids digestion. Externally it is used to treat rashes, especially poison oak or ivy rashes.
Dosage: standard infusion or 3-9 gms.; tincture, 10-30 drops

GRINDELIA (Gumweed)   *Grindelia spp.; Compositae*

Energetics: bitter, pungent, warm
Meridians/Organs affected: lung, kidneys
Parts used: dried leaves and flowering tops
Active constituents: up to 21% amorphous resins, tannin, laevoglucose and volatile oils
Properties: expectorant, antispasmodic, sedative, demulcent
Uses: It is used for colds, nasal congestion, bronchial irritation, coughs including spasmodic coughs and whooping coughs, and for asthma. It usually is combined with yerba santa as a syrup. Used externally, it is one of the best treatments for burns, rashes, blisters, poison oak and ivy dermatitis. A fomentation of grindelia may be applied to the affected areas a few times a day.
Precautions: Grindelia may take up selenium compounds from the soil and store them. This makes large doses mildly toxic. Further, because of its high resin content, it is considered hard on the kidneys and for this reason usually is used only for acute ailments. Small doses of grindelia are thought to lower the heart rate.
Dosage: infuse one teaspoon of the flowering tops and leaves in a cup of boiling water covered until cool enough to drink. In combination with other herbs use 3-6 gms.; tincture, 5-30 drops.

ELECAMPANE
Inula helinium; Compositae

Energetics: pungent, bitter, warm
Meridians/Organs affected: lungs, spleen
Parts used: root, flower
Active constituents: essential oil, bitter principles, inulin, resin
Properties: expectorant, stomachic, antiemetic
Uses: The flowers are used by the Chinese to lower the chi, bring up and dissolve phlegm, stop coughs, wheezing, hiccoughs, nausea and vomiting. Both the flowers and the roots are good for weakness of digestion with damp accumulation (damp spleen), bloating abdomen and gas. (See root under chi tonics, pg.298)
Dosage: standard infusion or 3-9 gms.; tincture, 10-30 drops

JACK IN THE PULPIT
Arisaema triphyllum,
A. maculatum; Araceae

Energetics: acrid, warm, toxic
Meridians/Organs affected: lung, liver
Part used: root
Active constituents: triterpenoid saponins, benzoic acid
Properties: expectorant, diaphoretic, carminative, antispasmodic
Uses: It is used to dry phlegm (very drying), for hoarseness, aphonia (loss of voice), feelings of burning and constriction in the throat with throat, mouth and tongue sore and sensitive. It is used for asthma, croup, whooping cough, chronic laryngitis, stomatitis, colic, and flatulence. It opens the channels and meridians and treats associated dizziness, numbness, facial paralysis, strokes, seizures, lockjaw, and spasms of the hands and feet. It is used externally as a poultice or liniment for sores, ulcers, boils and swellings caused by trauma and injuries; also for tinea capitis (scalp eruptions), tumors, and as a gargle for sore throat from excessive speaking.
Dosage: one teaspoon infused in a cup of boiling water; in formulas, 1-6 gms.; tincture, 10-20 drops

SUNDEW   *Drosera rotundifolia; Droseraceae*

Energetics: acrid, warm
Meridian/Organ affected: lungs
Part used: aerial portions
Active constituents: naphthoquinone derivatives, plumbagin and hydroplumbagin, flavonoids, enzymes, organic acids and traces of essential oil
Properties: expectorant, antispasmodic, demulcent, alterative
Uses: It is used for all respiratory diseases, coughs, asthma, whooping cough and bronchitis. It is an alterative and tonic against arteriosclerosis and for promoting longevity. A tea was considered to have aphrodisiac and rejuvenative properties. Externally, the fresh juice is directly applied to warts and corns to stimulate their removal. It was also used to help curdle milk.
Dosage: only one teaspoon of the dried herb steeped in a pint of boiling water. Throughout the day a total of up to one to two cups are taken in small mouthful doses. It is best sweetened with honey. Of the tincture, 3-6 drops.

BLOODROOT   *Sanguinaria canadensis; Papaveraceae*

Energetics: bitter, acrid, hot, toxic
Meridians/Organs affected: lung, heart, liver
Part used: root
Active constituents: alkaloids including whelidonine, berberine, chelerythrine, sanguinarine
Properties: expectorant, alterative, stimulant, diuretic, febrifuge, sedative, emetic in larger doses
Uses: It is used internally as an expectorant for acute and chronic respiratory tract affections, sinus congestion, laryngitis, sore throat, asthma with cold thick phlegm, and croup. Most effective for pneumonia are 1 to 2 drop doses repeated frequently throughout the day. It combines well with wild cherry bark, eucalyptus and honey in a syrup. A syrup may also be made with garlic and bloodroot tincture.

The tincture is directly applied externally for the treatment of fungus, eczema, cancers, tumors, and other skin disorders. It is a good remedy for athlete's foot and rashes. An ointment of bloodroot alone or in combination with other herbs is directly applied to venereal sores, tinea capitis, eczema, ringworm, scabies and warts.

Dosage: As a stimulant, expectorant or alterative use ¼-½ teaspoon of the powdered root or ½-1 gm. in decoction; tincture, 5-20 drops

Bloodroot and Bayberry Snuff Powder

The powders of bloodroot and bayberry may be combined to make snuff. A pinch is snuffed into each nostril to heal nasal polyps, rhinitis and other nasal affections.

EUCALYPTUS
Eucalyptus globulis and spp.;
Myrtaceae

Energetics: spicy, warm
Meridians/Organs affected: lungs, kidneys
Part used: leaves
Active constituents: essential oil with cineole, ellagic and gallic acid, bitter principle, resin, antibiotic properties, tannin
Properties: expectorant, stimulant, antibiotic, antiseptic, rubefacient
Uses: A tea made from the leaves is a good treatment for coughs, colds, flu, croup, pneumonia and asthma.

The oil is one of the most powerful antiseptics. It may be combined with olive or sesame oil. As an ointment, rub it directly on the chest or back to relieve congestion in the lungs. The steam is inhaled for the same purpose. An emulsion is made by combining equal parts of the oil with powdered slippery elm or gum arabic and water. After being well shaken, the mixture is taken internally in teaspoon doses for tuberculosis and other infections and inflammations of the lungs.

The oil is rubbed over aching muscles or trauma sites to stimulate circulation and relieve pain and blood congestion. A simple external ointment or balm is made by mixing the oil with heated paraffin and sufficient melted bee's wax to harden to the desired consistency.

Precautions: Eucalyptus oil should be used infrequently since it is difficult to eliminate through the kidneys.

Dosage: standard infusion of the leaves, 3-9 gms.; oil, ½-5 drops. For local application to sores, injuries and ulcers, mix one ounce of the oil in a pint of lukewarm water and apply. The ointment may be applied freely as needed.

THYME   *Thymus vulgaris and spp.; Labiatae*

Energetics: spicy, warm
Meridians/Organs affected: lungs, liver, stomach
Parts used: leaves, flowers
Active constituents: essential oil with thymol, cavacrol, cymol, linalool, borneol, bitter principle, tannin, flavanoids, triterpenic acids
Properties: expectorant, antitussive, antispasmodic, carminative, stimulant, emmenagogue, diuretic, antiseptic
Uses: It is used for acute and chronic respiratory affections, cough, asthma, colds, flu, spasmodic coughs, whooping coughs, sore throat. It also is used for stomach weakness and digestive problems. Taken before sleeping, it is a remedy against nightmare. It has both stimulant and relaxant properties so that it tends to regulate the system as needed. It is a commonly used condiment in cooking.
Dosage: standard infusion or 3-9 gms.

PLATYCODON   *Platycodon grandiflorum; Campanulaceae*

Energetics: bitter, acrid, neutral
Meridians/Organs affected: lung, stomach
Part used: root
Active constituents: saponins, inulin, platycodigenin
Properties: expectorant, demulcent
Uses: It loosens phlegm, stops cough in both hot and cold conditions, aids the elimination of pus in the upper parts of the body, is effective for sore throat, lung abscess, and loss of voice. It has an ascending energy and is sometimes added in small amounts to formulas to direct the therapeutic action of other herbs to the upper parts of the body. It is grown in many parts of this country as an ornamental bellflower.
Dosage: standard decoction or 3-9 gms.

MUSTARD SEEDS   *Sinapsis alba; Brassicae*

Energetics: spicy, hot
Meridians/Organs affected: lung, stomach
Part used: seed
Active constituents: sinalbin, sinapine, myrosin
Properties: expectorant, carminative, stimulant, analgesic
Uses: It dispels phlegm, stops cough, warms the lungs, alleviates body and joint pain, treats watery, oozing, chronic sores (yin boils), warms the center and improves digestion. It usually is used externally as an oil or plaster for its pain and tension relieving properties.
Precautions: Contraindicated in any heated condition.
Dosage: standard decoction or 3-9 gms.

ANTITUSSIVE HERBS
(Herbs for Relieving Cough and Asthma)

Herbs in this category possess specific cough-sedating properties. They are used primarily for this specific action, often regardless of whether the condition is hot or cold, excess or deficient. Their use is largely symptomatic; hence they usually are combined with other herbs that treat the causes. Sometimes, however, they are used in a more energetic manner. They are antispasmodic, antiasthmatic and bronchodilators, and work well with herbs from the two previous categories which are more fundamental in their actions. For colds and flu they often are used with surface-relieving (diaphoretic) herbs. Most of them also help stop vomiting.

In Ayurvedic terms they reduce kapha (water). Their action on the other humors is mixed. They have no special contraindications other than their restriction to symptomatic use.

WILD CHERRY BARK (Chokecherry)   *Prunus virginiana, P. serotina; Rosaceae*

Energetics: acrid, astringent, warm, slightly toxic
Meridians/Organs affected: spleen, lung
Part used: bark

Active constituents: hydrocyanic glycoside, isoamygdaline, organic acids, tannin

Properties: antitussive, pectoral, astringent, carminative

Uses: It calms the respiratory nerves and allays cough and asthma. It also is an outstanding remedy for weakness of the stomach with irritation, such as ulcers, gastritis, colitis, diarrhea and dysentery. It is helpful combined in digestive tonics with such herbs as licorice, ginseng, cyperus, anise and tangerine peel. These herbs are macerated for two weeks to six months in rice wine. They are then strained and the resultant tincture is taken in teaspoonful doses before meals. The Native Americans employed the sedative properties of this plant to assist in relieving the pains of labor. The bark, collected in the fall, is one of the best herbs for respiratory complaints and cough.

Precautions: Hydrocyanic acid is toxic in sufficient amounts and this seems especially true of the wilted leaves known to poison livestock. The toxicity appears in all members of the *Prunus* genus, including almonds, peaches, apricots and cherries. All contain amygdalin which in water hydrolizes into hydrocyanic acid. The degree of toxicity depends on a number of factors. Removal of the outer coat of the seed, cooking and combining with sugar or licorice lessens the potential toxic aspects. (See apricot seed, below)

Dosage: Normal dose in hot or cold infusion (boiling destroys the amygdalin that is the main active constituent). In formulas, 3-9 gms.; tincture, 10-15 drops.

APRICOT SEED   *Prunus armenica; Rosaceae*
(Bitter almond)

Energetics: bitter, warm, slightly toxic

Meridians/Organs affected: lung, colon

Part used: kernel of fruit

Active constituents: amygdalin (which yields hydrocyanic acid, glucose and benzaldehyde)

Properties: antitussive, expectorant, laxative

Uses: It treats cough, bronchitis, asthma, emphysema, and both cold and hot coughs. It is especially good for dry coughs, owing to its oily nature. More demulcent than wild cherry bark, apricot seeds are a mild laxative for dryness in the colon.

Laetrile is derived from apricot seeds and has been used with success in Mexico and Germany for the treatment of cancer. The Chinese use the related peach seeds for dissolving tumors and, in some cases cancer.

Precautions: They are contraindicated for diarrhea (wild cherry bark is then used in its place).

Hydrocyanic (prussic) acid is a general protoplasmic poison even at a dose of 2.5 grams. Lethal doses for adults have been reported at around 50-60 kernels, for children it is as few as 10. The Chinese use the bark of the apricot tree or the bark of the root as an antidote. Licorice or jujube taken with it also helps as an antidote. This also applies to the use of wild cherry bark or peach seed.

Dosage: standard infusion or 3-9 gms. of the crushed seeds. (see precautions)

MULLEIN   *Verbascum thaspus; Scrophulariaceae*

Energetics: bitter, astringent, cool
Meridians/Organs affected: lungs, stomach
Parts used: leaf, flower, root
Active constituents: saponins, mucilage, two flavonoids (hesperidin and verbaside), aucubin, traces of essential oil
Properties: expectorant, demulcent, antispasmodic, antitussive, astringent, anodyne, vulnerary
Uses: It is used for cough, hoarseness, bronchitis, phlegm, and whooping cough. The flowers are specifically sedative and anti-inflammatory. An oil made from them (see medicated oils, pg.59) is used for otitis media and earaches. The leaves are smoked, alone or with coltsfoot and yerba santa, to soothe the throat and as a substitute for tobacco. The root treats eye inflammations, is a vulnerary, and is good for cramps and diarrhea. It also is good for bleeding from the lungs or from the gastrointestinal tract.

Dosage: standard infusion or 3-9 gms.; tincture, 10-30 drops

COLTSFOOT   *Tussilago farfara; Compositae*

Energetics: bitter, sweet, neutral
Meridian/Organ affected: lung
Part used: leaves, flowers
Active constituents: flowers contain mucin, two flavonoids (rutin and hyperin), triterpenoid saponins, taraxanthin, tannin, phytoserols arnidiol and faradio, essential oil. Leaves contain mucin, abundant tannin, sitosterol, saltpeter, inulin, a glycosidal bitter principle.
Properties: antitussive, expectorant, demulcent, anti-inflammatory, astringent
Uses: It sedates cough reflex, resolves wheezing, is used for colds, hoarseness, bronchitis, sore throat, shortness of breath, and dry cough. The crushed leaves are applied to relieve insect bites and stings. The tea helps stop diarrhea.
Dosage: standard infusion or 3-9 gms.; tincture, 10-20 drops

LOQUAT   *Eriobotrya japonica; Rosaceae*

Energetics: bitter, neutral
Meridians/Organs affected: lung, stomach
Part used: leaves
Active constituents: amygdalin, neroldiol, farnesol
Properties: antitussive, expectorant, anti-inflammatory
Uses: It lowers chi, stops cough and vomiting, clears inflammation from the lungs, expels phlegm, clears stomach heat, treats hiccoughs and belching. This native Chinese plant is a common ornamental in this country.
Dosage: 6-15 gms. in infusion

MULBERRY   *Morus alba; Moraceae*

Energetics: sweet, cold
Meridian/Organ affected: lungs
Part used: bark of root
Active constituents: carotene, succinic acid, adenine, choline, amylase
Properties: antitussive, expectorant, anti-inflammatory, diuretic

Uses: It is anti-inflammatory to the lungs and bronchioles, quiets cough and wheezing in asthma and emphysema. It is used when inflammation of the lungs inhibits perspiration, causing swelling of the extremities facial edema, fever, thirst, difficult urination and a floating pulse.

Dosage: 6-15 gms. in decoction

ASTER (Red stalked aster)

*Aster tartaricus,
Compositae*

Energetics: spicy, slightly warm
Meridian/Organ affected: lung
Part used: root
Active constituents: saponins, shiionon, quercitin, anthole, arabinose, oleic acid and aromatic acid
Properties: antitussive, expectorant
Uses: It is very effective in inhibiting cough and eliminating phlegm, for chronic coughs, cold and damp coughs with abundant or occasionally blood-streaked phlegm.

The various North American asters include *A. aestivus* and *A. cordifolius,* which have not been used as expectorants. Since *A. puniceus* has diaphoretic and antispasmodic properties, it possibly can be used similarly to the Chinese variety.

Dosage: standard decoction or 3-9 gms.

LUNGWORT

Pulmonaria officinalis; Boraginaceae

Energetics: astringent, sweet, mildly bitter, cool
Meridians/Organs affected: lungs, stomach
Part used: aerial portions
Active constituents: mucilage
Properties: expectorant, demulcent, antitussive, astringent, tonic
Uses: It is used for cough, irritated throat, bleeding from the lungs, and dysentery. As a poultice, it helps enlarged thyroid, burns and tumors, and reduces swelling and inflammation from injuries and bruises. It is related to comfrey and similar to it in properties and potential use as a yin tonic.

Dosage: standard decoction or 3-9 gms.; tincture, 10-30 drops

STICTA (Pulmonaria)   *Sticta pulmonaria; Lichenes*

Energetics: sweet, mildly bitter, cool
Meridians/Organs affected: lungs, stomach
Part used: whole lichen
Active constituents: stictic acid, similar to cetraric acid found in Iceland moss
Properties: expectorant, antitussive, nutritive, tonic, demulcent, antiinflammatory
Uses: It is used for irritated cough, shoulder and neck pains, hay fever, catarrhal asthma, whooping cough, and croup

One variety grows on the trunks of coniferous trees in the forests of the Pacific Northwest. According to King and Scudder, it acts specifically on the base of the brain and the vagus nerve and all bodily parts affected by them. Thus it is particularly good for pulmonary, shoulder, occipital and neck pains. It also is used for flu, sinus congestion, night sweats and summer influenza. Like Iceland moss, it is a nutritive, yin tonic.
Dosage: in decoction 3-15 gms.

HONEY LOCUST   *Gledista triacanthos; Leguminosae*

Energetics: acrid, bitter, warm
Meridians/Organs affected: lung, colon
Part used: pods
Active constituents: saponins, tannin, sitosterol
Properties: antitussive, expectorant, aromatic, stimulant
Uses: It clears the lungs, relieves phlegm, and revives consciousness in strokes and seizures. A suppository of honey locust is inserted into the rectum at night for the treatment of roundworms.
Precautions: Contraindicated during pregnancy.
Dosage: 1-3 gms. in pill or powder form only.

SUBSTANCES FOR TOPICAL APPLICATION

These substances are mainly toxic minerals and herbs used topically for parasites, swelling, pain, injuries, bleeding, inflammation and the healing of skin lesions. They are applied in ointments, powders or external fomentations. Some may be taken internally but since most are poisonous it is preferable not to do so. Internal use is especially contraindicated for weak and sensitive individuals, pregnant women and young children.

Many herbs are good for external application. Generally, an herb will be good externally for what it does internally. Astringents are particularly useful for promoting the healing of wounds and sores. Demulcents may be applied for their soothing action. Heat-clearing herbs may be applied for their anti-inflammatory action. The herbs and minerals listed here are limited to external and topical application. As they are used locally and symptomatically their humoral predominance is not important.

Minerals are an important part of the herbalist's pharmacopoeia and are integral to the oriental systems. They are particularly useful applied externally.

ALUM   *Potassium aluminum sulphate*

Energetics: sour, astringent, cold, toxic
Meridians/Organs affected lung, spleen, stomach colon
Properties: styptic, astringent, hemostatic, parasiticide, expectorant, antibiotic

Uses: It destroys external parasites, relieves itching, and is used as an external fomentation for ringworm, scabies, itch and damp rashes. Used as a styptic, it stops bleeding. It is an astringent for chronic diarrhea. It dries phlegm and dampness and may be used as an adjunctive treatment to prevent excessive salivation in epilepsy. It treats leucorrhea, trichomonas, jaundice and hepatitis. Alum makes an effective mouthwash for swollen or bleeding gums and is good topically for hemorrhoids. It is one of the best substances for healing ulcerative sores on the skin or the mucous membranes.

Dosage: 100-1000 mg. of the powder internally, 3-6 gms. externally

BORAX   *Sodium borate*

Energetics: sweet, bitter, salty, cold, toxic
Meridians/Organs affected lung, stomach
Properties: astringent, expectorant, antiseptic, ophthalmic (eye wash)
Uses: Topically applied for wounds and injuries, it prevents putrefaction. It is a major ingredient in eye wash medicines
Precautions: Internally it is quite toxic, although it has been used to dispel phlegm from the lungs.
Dosage: 200-1000 mg. of the powder internally, 3-6 gms. externally

SULPHUR   *Sublimated sulphur*

Energetics: sour, hot, slightly toxic
Meridians/Organs affected kidney, spleen, pericardium
Properties: laxative, alterative, yang tonic, anti-rheumatic
Uses: It is used externally as an ointment against scabies, tinea infection and other skin diseases especially when combined wth calomelas, mylabris and borneol. It kills parasites, tonifies fire, strengthens yang and reduces yin-cold. Internally, it is used for cold yin patterns associated with deficient yang including rheumatism, aching lower back, impotence, and constipation caused by lack of peristaltic strength in the colon. It also is used to treat asthma caused by internal coldness. It may be baked with tofu (soybean curd) before taking internally.

Precautions: It is contraindicated during pregnancy or in wasting fever-ish diseases.
Dosage: internally, 1-3 gms.; externally, use as needed

CALOMELAS   *Mercurious chloride*

Energetics: acrid, cold, toxic
Meridians/Organs affected liver, kidney, bladder
Properties: parasiticide
Uses: It is externally applied as a powder to treat parasites such as sca-bies and tinea. It also is used externally as a wash for neurodermatitis and syphilitic sores. Although it has been used as a diuretic for edema and decreased bowel movements, internal use should be avoided.
Precautions: Calomelas is a toxic substance that contains mercury. Overdose can cause degeneration of the intestinal walls, kidney dam-age and acute nephritis. In case of contact, wash the mouth out with water to prevent inflammation.
Dosage: no more than 100-200 mgs. internally

REALGAR   *Arsenic disulfide*

Energetics: bitter, cold, toxic
Meridians/Organs affected liver, colon
Properties: anti-parasitic, antifungal
Uses: It is used externally for dermatomycoses, ringworm, scabies and damp rashes. It is applied as a soak for any type of itching skin condi-tion, including parasites, abscesses, ulcerations, and venomous bites and stings. Internally it is effective for intestinal parasites, especially round-worm. Combined with borneol as a tincture, it may be applied topi-cally for herpes zoster; with alum for nasal polyps; and with borax for ulcerations of the mouth, tongue or throat. Combined with golden seal and borneol, it can be made into an ointment and applied externally for scabies and ringworm.
Precautions: It is contraindicated during pregnancy and for individuals with a deficient yin or blood condition or wasting disease.
Dosage: 200-400 mgs. internally

MINIUM   Red lead oxide

Energetics: acrid, salty, cool, toxic
Meridians/Organs affected heart, spleen, liver
Properties: disinfectant, anti-inflammatory, antiseptic
Uses: It expels poisons and generates agglutination of tissue. Generally, it is used topically only for swelling and ulcers, since it decreases pus and promotes healing.
Dosage: no more than 100 mg. internally; best to use externally only

CAMPHOR (see aromatic herbs for opening the orifices, pg. 361)

BUTTERCUP (Crowfoot)   *Ranunculus bulbosus and spp.; Ranunculaceae*

Energetics: acrid, hot, toxic
Meridian/Organ affected heart
Parts used: juice of leaves and flowers
Active constituents: protoamemonin
Properties: rubefacient, counterirritant
Uses: It is directly applied to remove warts. The juice is topically applied to rheumatic and gouty joints to relieve these conditions. A tincture may be both externally applied and taken internally to treat shingles and sciatica.
Precautions: External application may cause blisters and lead to ulceration with prolonged use. Internal overdose may cause gastroenteritis.
Dosage: of the tincture, 6-8 drops (internally)

TULIP   *Tulipa edulis; Liliaceae*

Energetics: sweet, cold, toxic
Meridians/Organs affected liver, spleen
Part used: bulbs
Active constituents: colchicine, alkaloids, in some species, glucomannan
Properties: antipyretic, anti-inflammatory, antitumor
Uses: The bulb is made into a paste and topically applied for lymphatic cancers, nodules, sores, ulcers, boils, and toxic swellings.

Precautions: It is a slow-acting poison and should not be taken internally.
Dosage: in formulas for internal usage 1-6 gms. in decoction

DELPHINIUM (Larkspur)

Consolida regalis;
Ranunculaceae

Energetics: bitter, acrid, hot, toxic
Meridians/Organs affected kidney, heart
Part used: aerial portions
Active constituents: a poisonous alkaloid, calcatrippine, which is the same as aconitine
Properties: parasiticide
Uses: It is made into a lotion or tincture for topical application to kill lice, crabs and other parasites.
Precautions: Do not use internally.

DAFFODIL

Narcissus pseudo-narcissus;
Amaryllidaceae

Energetics: bitter, acrid, hot, toxic
Meridian/Organ affected liver
Part used: bulb
Active constituents: two alkaloids, narcissine and lycorine
Properties: astringent
Uses: The crushed bulb mixed with toasted barley flour is topically applied to dissolve hard swellings and draw out slivers. The bulbs boiled in oil are applied externally to treat discoloration of the skin and to relieve chafed heels, burns, stiff or painful joints, and other local affections. The juice of the bulb mixed with honey and tincture of myrrh make drops to relieve earache and to dispel pus or wax from the ear. An ointment for external application to sore and bruised parts has been made from this herb since ancient times.
Precautions: There have been many cases of daffodil poisoning resulting in death because they were mistaken for onions. The poison seems very stable and resistant to heat. Do not use internally.

PARASITICIDES

These herbs kill or expel internal and external parasites. It is easier to remedy a problem caused by excess than one caused by deficiency and wasting. In excess conditions, fasting and the taking of bitter, eliminative and detoxifying herbs often is all that is necessary to eliminate most parasites, including intestinal ones. In cases of deficiency, however, it is necessary to help the body develop the internal strength to fight off the parasites, also using tonic foods and herbs. Specific antiparasitical herbs are combined with digestive chi tonics.

Parasites flourish in an environment created by eating too much of sweets and starchy food. They usually are repelled and destroyed by herbs and foods with a bitter taste. Hence very bitter herbs like wormwood or golden seal are effective against parasites. Hot spicy herbs like cayenne also help burn up parasites and are used in tropical areas partly for this reason. Acid fruit, like sour plums, can help weaken them or reduce their motility. However, some antiparasitical herbs, like pumpkin seeds, have a bland or sweet taste, and act more by specific constituents or special potency (*prabhava*) than by energetics.

Substances that repel or expel worms are called vermifuges, while those that destroy them are called vermicides. Anthelmintic is a generic term for either.

Dietary therapy is essential in the treatment of parasites. Fasting or eating lightly is recommended during the first day or two of the treatment. This is especially so for those with normal to excess constitutions. Sweets, sugar, juices, fruit, rich, greasy foods and white flour products are to be avoided. One folk remedy for the treatment and prevention of parasites is to take two or three tablespoons of uncooked rice first thing each morning. This is a particularly valuable remedy for humid, tropical climates where parasites are a major problem. It might also be good to take a teaspoon or two of a strong bitter herb. Garlic and the seeds of mango and papaya also have been used as folk remedies for parasites.

Antiparasitical herbs should be used with purgatives like rhubarb or aloe, which help expel the worms from the body. Herbal enemas also are helpful.

In terms of Ayurveda, these herbs decrease kapha (water) and increase vata (air). Their action on pitta (fire) determined by whether their nature is heating or cooling. Most (except garlic) are regarded as depleting to sexual vitality.

Cautions and contraindications are mainly for deficient types, as this is a mildly strong form of reducing therapy. Anthelmintics should be avoided during pregnancy.

GARLIC This is an important anthelmintic herb and also a good yang tonic. (See section on yang tonics, pg.305)

PUMPKIN SEEDS   *Curcubita moschata; Curcubitae*

Energetics: sweet, neutral
Meridians/Organs affected: colon, stomach
Part used: seed, husk
Active constituents: The seed contains an isoprenoid compound with anthelmintic properties, as well as a high mineral content.
Properties: anthelmintic, nutritive, vermifuge, diuretic
Uses: It is used for tapeworm and round worm. A handful of the seeds should be eaten three times a day while fasting for a period of several days. It is helpful to accompany this with other anthelmintic treatments, like garlic tea enemas. Pumpkin seeds also are useful for nausea, motion sickness and swollen prostate.
Dose: 30-60 gms. eaten or in decoction

WORMSEED (Levant)
Artemisia cina,
A. santonica; Compositae

Energetics: bitter, aromatic, warm
Meridians/Organs affected: colon, liver, stomach
Part used: oil from herb or seeds
Active constituents: essential oil, a glycoside and a bitter principle
Properties: anthelmintic, carminative, stomachic, emmenagogue, narcotic
Uses: Most of the *Artemesias* are good for parasites. These include wormwood, southernwood and mugwort. They also are good for dysentery and have antifungal properties. This variety is more specific but not necessarily more powerful than the others. It is used for tape, round, thread, seat or pin worms. Take 3-10 drops of the oil mixed with honey three times a day for three or four days. Alternatively, the whole seeds can be crushed and taken in half-teaspoonful doses mixed with honey. This should be followed by an herbal laxative such as cascara bark.

American wormseed, *Chenopodium ambrosioides var. anthelminticum,* an unrelated plant, may be used in the same way.
Dose: 6-15 gms. in infusion

PINK ROOT
Spigelia marilandica; Loganiaceae

Energetics: bitter, pungent, cold, toxic
Meridians/Organs affected: colon, stomach
Parts used: whole plant, root
Active constituents: spigeline, a poisonous alkaloid, tannin, resin, wax, fat, albumen, myricin, mucilage and a bitter principle
Properties: anthelmintic, vermifuge, narcotic
Uses: This very effective treatment for expelling tapeworms and roundworms was used by the Native Americans. If given in the proper dosage it is safe for children, and should be followed by a purgative such as magnesium sulphate (epsom salts).
Precautions: If the laxative salts are not taken immediately after the herb, there can be toxic side-effects, including blurring vision, dizziness, spasms and palpitations. In large doses there can be depression of both

respiration and circulation and possible death from convulsions.

Dose: of the powdered root, 1-2 tsps. for adults, ¼-½ tsp. for children, taken morning and evening for three or four days, each time followed by a purgative. An infusion is made with one-half ounce of the root in a pint of boiling water. For children, one tablespoon of the infusion is given morning and evening, for adults, one cup, to be followed by a laxative such as senna with fennel and ginger.

MALE FERN
*Aspidum filix-mas,
Dryopteris felix-mas; Polypodiaceae*

Energetics: bitter, cold, toxic
Meridians/Organs affected: colon, stomach, liver
Part used: rhizome
Active constituents: aspidinol, albaspidine, phloraspine and filicinic acid
Properties: anthelmintic, vermifuge, alterative, astringent
Uses: It stuns and paralyzes, without killing, tapeworms, round worms and hookworms. It also is good for sores, boils, carbuncles, swollen glands and epidemic flu. It inhibits bleeding of a hot nature and is combined with cedar leaves for uterine bleeding. With other alteratives like honeysuckle, forsythia and dandelion it treats toxic blood conditions. Like pink root and other toxic anthelmintics, it should be taken with a saline purgative (magnesium sulphate) or a strong laxative like castor oil, to prevent poisoning.
Precautions: No alcohol or oil should be taken during this treatment, as they would increase the absorption of the toxic principle.
Dose: as an anthelmintic, take 1-4 teaspoons of the liquid extract or the powdered rhizome in capsules in the evening while fasting, followed with a purgative. As an alterative, standard decoction is used or 3-9 gms.

POMEGRANATE
Punica granatum; Punicaceae

Energetics: sour, astringent, warm, slightly toxic
Meridians/Organs affected: colon, stomach, kidney
Parts used: bark, root bark, peel of fruit

Active constituents: an alkaloid, pelletierine, 20% tannin, inulin, mannitol, malic acid, calcium oxalate
Properties: anthelmintic, astringent
Uses: It stops diarrhea due to cold and deficiency, and kills and expels tape worms and round worms. The root bark is considered the superior anthelmintic, the peel a safer astringent. Ayurveda considers the fruit to be an excellent blood tonic and anti-pitta (fire) remedy.
Precautions: As with the other toxic anthelmintics, do not mix with alcohol, oils or fats.
Dose: standard decoction or 3-9 gms., follow with a laxative

BRUCEA   *Brucea javanica; Simarubaceae*

Energetics: bitter, cold, toxic
Meridian/Organ affected: colon
Part used: seeds
Active constituents: an alkaloid, brucamarin, a glycoside, dosamine and formic acid
Properties: anthelmintic, astringent
Uses: In Chinese herbalism this is a near specific for amoebic dysentery, and also is effective for nematodes and tapeworms. The seeds are split open and taped over warts or other excrescences to stimulate their removal. They are good internally, or externally as a douche for trichomonas vaginitis.
Precautions: It is a gastrointestinal irritant and contraindicated for individuals with digestive weakness, nausea, or vomiting. It is contraindicated during pregnancy and to be used with great caution for children.
Dose: 7-15 seeds with the shell removed. They may be taken whole or with jujubes.

BETEL NUT   *Areca catechu; Palmae*

Energetics: acrid, bitter, warm, mildly toxic
Meridians/Organs affected: spleen, stomach, colon
Part used: seeds

Active constituents: arecoline, which is closely related to pilocarpine. (It stimulates peristalsis and at the same time causes bronchial constriction, is antidoted by atropine or epinephrine), 14% fixed oil, mannosan and galactans

Properties: anthelmintic, vermifuge, carminative, diuretic, astringent

Uses: It moves chi downward and removes food stagnation, helps digestion and eliminates all worms including tapeworms, pinworms, roundworms and body flukes. It has mild toxic properties and should be taken with a purgative such as castor oil. One method is to take 30 grams of betel nut powder (less for children) before breakfast. Expulsion of the worms should occur within nine hours. If not, a purgative should be taken. It also is good to use pumpkin seeds simultaneously throughout the day. The pericarp of the nut is used in Chinese medicine as a carminative and thought to be very effective for gas, bloating and constipation. Both parts of the betel palm are good diuretics for treating edema.

Precautions: Avoid during pregnancy.

Dose: 6-12 gms. in decoction; 30 gms. for tapeworm

PART THREE

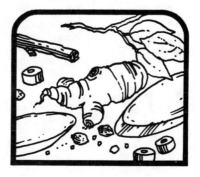

Appendices

Appendix A
THE CHEMISTRY OF HERB ENERGETICS
by Christopher Hobbs

The tastes and colors of medicinal plants are important indicators of their therapeutic properties. These properties are known collectively as "herb energetics" and form an integral part of ancient healing systems such as Traditional Chinese Medicine and Ayurveda.

One area that has been little explored in the literature of botanical medicine is the possible connection between the tastes and colors of herbs and the known physiological effects of the chemicals that create these energetic principles. For instance, consider an herb that has a bitter taste. In Traditional Chinese Medicine, bitter herbs are placed into a particular therapeutic category because of this taste. This herb will obviously contain chemical constituents that, when isolated, are bitter—but do the observed pharmacological effects of these constituents correspond with that of the whole herb?

These observable connections form the basis for an interesting approach in the continuing validation of traditional medicines using modern scientific methods. While this process is worthwhile, consider the possibility that ancient and highly evolved medical systems, such as Traditional Chinese Medicine, might also be validating scientific medicine simultaneously.

THE NEI CHING

In Traditional Chinese Medicine, one of the oldest and influential of the medical texts is the *Nei Ching*. This text describes the ancient system called the "five elements", in which various bodily parts, aspects of human nature (including the emotions), the seasons, and other universal influences are integrated to emphasize their effects on each other, and on the whole. The "whole" is defined here as encompassing the whole environment in which we live, the whole world, the whole body, and encompasses other influences that may come to bear on us. Thus there are five colors, five flavors, five seasons and five viscera as follows:

VISCERA	ELEMENT	COLOR	FLAVOR
liver	wood	green	sour
heart	fire	red	bitter
spleen	earth	yellow	sweet
lungs	metal	white	pungent
kidneys	water	black	salty

TASTE

Although the Chinese have ascribed certain physiological effects to the flavors, it must be remembered that the five flavors in relation to their system and culture may differ in meaning from our own perception of them. The determination of flavor is a very subjective experience, especially when one considers that the sense of smell is intimately linked to, and very much influences, our perception of taste.

This is one reason why it is important for herbalists and researchers delving into herbal energetics to taste and smell the actual herbs for themselves, developing their own sense (if you will) of these properties, and how they relate to their physiological effects.

In the following sections I will attempt to establish correlations between the activity of herb tastes as indicated in Chinese texts (principally the *Nei Ching*)—and both the accepted activity of the tastes in Western herbology and the pharmacology of constituents that have been studied to support these actions.

Sour

In the *Nei Ching* it is said that "Sour substances are astringent and prevent or reverse the abnormal leakage of fluids and energy." Sour is widely accepted in Chinese medicine to "drain" the liver.

In Western herbalism, lemon juice has been long known as a "liver cleanser" and detoxifying agent. It increases saliva flow[1], which aids digestion, easing the work of the liver. These acids also show antibacterial and antiviral activity[2]

The sour flavor in plants is mainly due to soluble carboxylic and dicarboxylic plant acids,[3] such as citric, maleic and oxalic acids. Ascorbic acid also has a sour taste. The sources of some of these are:

ACID	SOURCE
lactic	common in roots and germinating seeds
oxalic	beets, dock, oxalis spp.
citric	lemons, blackberries
malic	apples

Because of their acid nature, these compounds can cleanse and detoxify by changing the polarity of certain fat-soluble toxins,[4] rendering them more water-soluble, easily excreted by the kidneys. This possibly takes strain off the liver, the organ that bears the burden of detoxifying these compounds with its enzyme systems.

Tissues that come into contact with acids will react by contracting, for the acids increase the contractability of muscles by affecting the pH and ion balance. They also have an astringent action in precipitating proteins, similar to gallic acid.[5] One pharmacology text, notes that "acids dry up the secretion [of the lungs] . . . "[6]

A further interesting point is that when acid substances (such as lemon juice) enter the stomach, the hydrochloric acid secretion is inhibited. By reflex, the amount of acid entering the duodenum is smaller, so less bicarbonate-rich fluids from the liver are required to neutralize the acid.[7] Thus, the liver is protected from "abnormal leakage of fluids" (*Nei Ching*) that may occur due to stress. Studies have also shown that pancreatic secretions and bile are increased by acids,[8] additionally aiding the liver.

Another effect of adding weak acid to the daily diet is an increase in the excretion of ammonia. This may have a favorable effect on the body, for ammonia, a by-product of protein digestion, can be toxic in even small amounts.

A Chinese herb that is sour and has been well documented for its liver protective ability[9] is *Schizandra chinensis.*

Bitter

In the *Nei Ching,* it is said that "Bitter substances drain and dry." The major target organ is said to be the heart, but bitter is also of importance to clear and open the upper respiratory tract. In Western herbology, bitter has a long history of use as an important activator of the digestive system. Bitter drugs, such as gentian have been shown in scientific studies to stimulate digestive secrections, increase the strength of the peristaltic waves, mixing and moving the food more effectively.[10] Many of these studies have been performed in Germany and other parts of Europe, where bitters are popular. Of great interest, too, is a recent study showing that bitters stimulate immune system function![11]

Many bitter herbs are used by Western herbalists to treat congestion of the lungs.[12, 13] These include squill, lobelia, ipecauana, quassia and senega. According to Traditional Chinese Medicine, bitter disperses obstruction and increases the flow of air in the lungs. It is interesting to note that one authoritative Western medical writer feels that the bitter herbs mentioned above "may act through sympathy between the gastric and bronchial mucous membranes."[14]

There are several important bitter plant medicines that affect the heart. The most famous is digitalis, which contains bitter cardiac glycosides, among them, digitoxin.[15] In fact, most of the active heart medicines are bitter tasting—including *Convallaria majalis, Scilla maritima,* and *Apocynum cannabinum.*[16]

Among the major constituents in plants that impart a bitter flavor to them are sesquiterpenes[17] and alkaloids.[18] Additionally, some glycosides,[19, 20] such as getiopicroside in gentian are extremely bitter.

Sesquiterpenes are a class of terpenoid compounds that have fifteen carbon atoms, are a "heavy note" in essential oils, and have boiling points over 200 degrees centigrade. These compounds are especially abundant in the *Compositae,* and impart a bitter flavor to such herbs as mugwort, wormwood, chamomile, coltsfoot, boneset and feverfew.[21] The anti-inflammatory, antispasmodic and antibacterial activity of many of these plants is well documented.[22]

The bitter substances in other classic "bitter tonics" are alkaloids, such as berberine in barberry root.

One has also to take "temperature" into account. Some bitters are cooling, some warming. The sesquiterpenes mentioned above usually are warming, in that they occur along with the monoterpenes and resins in resinous and essential-oil bearing plants, such as elecampane. This could be confusing, for many of the isolated sesquiterpenes, such as bisabolol from chamomile, are anti-inflammatory.[23] Since these substances are not in their pure state when they are used in clinical application, it is important to look at the action of the whole complex.

Alkaloid-bearing bitter herbs, such as barberry, golden seal and coptis usually are considered cooling. They contain berberine, hydrastine, coptine and other alkaloids that are anti-inflammatory, (affect the nervous ennervation of the microcirculation in the mucous membranes; are tonic and cooling to the mucous membranes)[24] and are known to be antibacterial.[25]

Thus, one could make a case for "bitter drains and dries" (*Nei Ching):* the secretions of the liver (including the bile) and other organs are increased, helping to move toxins out of the body. The drying effect results from excess secretions being expelled, and lessening of inflammation which lower exudation.

It is good to remember that all taste therapies work within a tonic-excess balance. Tonic (small to moderate) amounts will be beneficial for most people; but excess quantities will have a deleterious or opposite effect to the therapeutic one that is desired.

Sweet

In Traditional Chinese Medicine, sweet is considered tonic. Herbs with this taste nourish the stomach and spleen-pancreas, and these in turn are said to strengthen the flesh. "Sweet" obviously relates to sugars—most notably glucose, sucrose and fructose. Plants contain hundreds of different sugars, including the long chains that form starch, cellulose, insulin and other materials.[26] Plants create sugars from sunlight, carbon dioxide, and water. Besides fulfilling structural and energy needs, sugars also are attached to many secondary metabolic products in order to make them more water-soluble and transportable. The large, diverse group of plant constituents known as glycosides are of this type.

In Western medicine, although there is not the same emphasis on sweet tonics, to strengthen the energy or vitality of the body, the concept is not unknown. Sweet foods and roots, such as yams, barley, tapioca, and treacle (molasses) are all known as strengthening foods. They can be recommended when a person is recovering from illness, especially when the digestion is weak and inefficient, in which case they are combined with an aromatic bitter tonic.[27] This relates to the Chinese practice of taking ginseng, a root thought to be both a bitter tonic and a Chi tonic.[28]

Simple sugars are more readily assimilated and utilized by the body as nourishment. The brain, muscles and all the tissues of the body feed on glucose. When glucose is readily available, the digestive tract does not have to work as hard and vital energy is preserved. In natural tonic foods this works well, but when foods are refined, and the simple sugars are taken in their purified form, the results can be undesirable.[29] (Note, however, that in both Ayurvedic medicine and Traditional Chinese Medicine, refined sugar is considered a medicine for some constitutional types.[30])

Traditional Chinese Medicine recognizes different categories of tonic herbs all of which are sweet in nature. Some herbs are for deficient Chi patterns, such as ginseng, codonopsis, astragalus, dioscorea, atractylodes, zizyphus and licorice.[31]

When one studies the modern research on some of these herbs, two effects predominate: immune system tonification and adaptogenic qualities. In a recent American study, astragalus, codonopsis, ginseng and atractylodes were administered orally to AIDS patients (people who demonstrate profound deficiency) to relieve symptoms, increase energy and strengthen their immune systems.[32] These herbs have been well-studied for their immune-activating effects.[33,34,35,36] Some herbs of this tonic class are soaked in honey and stir-fried to make them even sweeter.

A major class of compounds, heteropolysaccharides (giant sugar molecules, with a molecular weight in the range of 25,000 to 250,000), contained in many herbs that strengthen immune system (i.e. astragalus[37]) has been well studied[38] and shown to markedly strengthen various aspects of immune function.

Recently, Western herbalists have been investigating the possibility of similar tonics in use in Western medicine are sweet and contain immune strengthening properties. Since, almost without exception, the tonics in question are made entirely from roots, it would seem wise to look among the Western materia medica for immune-tonifying roots, possibly some that were used by Western American Indians for increasing vitality and restoring health.

Obviously much work needs to be done in this area, but the author can make some suggestions. Such blood tonifying roots as burdock, American ginseng, dandelion, wild angelica and desert parsley (*Lomatium*) should be explored. Various species of *Lomatium and Ligusticum* (lovage) have large, sweet roots, and were extensively used as an important food source,[39] and regarded as among the most important of medicines[40] by Native American Indians . They are quite sweet-tasting in the spring, especially after roasting. Also, the more than 90 species from the genus *Astragalus* growing in the Western U.S., some of which were used for medicine and food by the Native Americans[41] would merit study.

Pungent

This flavor is also referred to as acrid. It supplements the functions of the liver and nourishes the lungs. The *Nei Ching* says that "It has a dispersing and moving effect" (especially where there is congestion and stagnation).

According to Tierra,[42] a study done in India[43] found that spicy tasting herbs such as black pepper and ginger intensify and prolong the effects of other herbs, and also of chemical drugs such as antibiotics. They do this by inhibiting the liver's tendency to neutralize them when their biochemical components enter the liver through the bloodstream. This may demonstrate the validity of the universal practice of herbalists in adding to some preparations a small amount of a spicy tasting herb such as pepper, ginger or prickly ash bark as a catalyst. This is done on the principle that it helps to concentrate and deliver the primary action of the other herbs in the formula.

Stress is one major cause of congestion. It stimulates the sympathetic nervous system,[44] which causes the muscles to tense, readying them for "flight or fight." When this stimulation becomes chronic, organs and other parts of the body can become quite "congealed." Cold also can have this effect.

Acrid herbs are used for similar conditions in Traditional Chinese Medicine and Western herbalism. Chinese herbs such as ginger, cinnamon, cnidium (*Ligusticum*), dong quai, *Asarum* and citrus all contain essential oils and resins which slightly irritate the mucosa, increasing the flow of blood. Some of these constituents are absorbed into the small intestine and enter the blood, warming the interior organs and stimulating metabolic functions. Finally, they may be excreted by the mucosa in the lungs, urinary tract, or other parts of the body, in the process having a warming, dispersing, and stimulating effect.[45] Because they increase the flow of blood, it is easy to see why they are considered to have a dispersing effect.

In Western medicine, two types of acrid, stimulating herbal actions are commonly mentioned, local and remote stimulation. Local stimulation refers to irritants, such as wintergreen oil (Tiger Balm falls into this category). In bringing blood to the surface they relieve aching joints, muscles, and perhaps relieve stagnancy in bruises or even prolapsed veins. The remote action functions as a "counter-irritant", working from the local irritation through nerve reflex action, opening up, or slowing down the blood circulation in an interior part of the body. For instance, the application of a mustard poultice on the chest increases breathing and removes congestion.[46]

Some of the best-studied plant constituents that create this stimulation or irritation on (and in) the body include resins, oleo-resins, volatile oils, and isothiocyanates (mustard oils).[47] Examples of resinous plants are poplar buds (balm of gilead), propolis, and pine or fir products, such as pitch.

Plants containing volatile oils are extremely common and useful for warming and dispersing congestion, though they usually do not penetrate as deeply as the resinous plants (they are often used for dispersing congestion at the surface). Plant families that contain essential oils are the *Umbelliferae* family (parsley), which includes the Chinese herbs dong quai, ligusticum and fennel; the mint family, comprising all the mints and rosemary and lavender; and the eucalyptus family, the laurel Family, and several other tropical families.

Oleo-resins are the active principle of cayenne pepper, black pepper and long pepper[48], which are used world-wide for their stimulating and warming properties. Mustard oils are, of course, found in many members of the mustard family, such as horseradish, radish, black mustard and watercress, and many members of the onion family, such as garlic and leeks.

In the West, acrid is not considered to be a taste, as is, for example, salty, but rather a warming sensation. For this reason, it is hard to make a case for herbs with this taste having an affinity for any particular organ, though they do have a propensity to affect the mucous membranes, primarily of the lungs, digestive tract and urinary tract, when ingested.

Salty

According to Traditional Chinese Medicine, salty herbs nourish the kidneys, make the heart pliable and strong and have a general "softening effect."

In the late 20th century, one doesn't hear much about the beneficial or therapeutic properties of salt. After years of societal abuse, salt is now generally regarded as a substance to be avoided. There is probably some wisdom in this attitude, for excess refined salt in the diet has been implicated as a major factor in high blood pressure, which affects millions of Americans each year.

In some earlier societies, salt was a luxury and treasure. So it is not surprising that herbs that had a salty taste were considered therapeutic, an estimate still sustained in pharmacology books of the early years of this century. For instance, weak salt solutions were understood to have a tonic and moisturizing effect on tissues, for "Dilute solutions of chloride of sodium . . . disolve both albumins and globulins."[49] This moisturizing effect is known also in Chinese Medicine. When there is too high a concentration, however, salt has a very irritating and drying effect. An increased salt intake is known to stimulate the excretion of urea, a waste product of protein metabolism.[50]

One of the most interesting effects of salt is sodium's influence over the other mineral ions, such as potassium, calcium, phosphorus. The ratio of various mineral ions in bodily fluids is extremely important, and maintains a delicate equilibrium. They affect the moisture balance of all the cells, and especially the quality and strength of the nerve impulse.

Salty herbs are not well known therapeutically in Western herbalism. However, many salty flavored herbs, such as celery and parsley (parsley root is a well-known diuretic) are available. Seaside plants also are rich in salt, and Native American Indians called some desert plants "saltbush", because the ash tasted salty, and used them to flavor food and replace body salt lost in the high heat.[51]

In Traditional Chinese Medicine, salty is probably the least commonly used of the flavors. Looking through the *Materia Medica,* one sees few plants that contain that taste; rather, most of the salty substances mentioned are seaweeds, seashells and animals. The therapeutic categories in which it is more commonly found are "Substances that settle and calm the spirit," "herbs that tonify the yang," (In macrobiotics, salt is considered the most yang substance, even though in Traditional Chinese Medicine it is considered cold) and "herbs that invigorate the blood."[52] These categories are not surprising, for the amount of salt in the body affects the nerves and the consistency of the blood.

In Traditional Chinese Medicine, salty herbs also are said to "nourish" the kidneys. Salt strongly affects the excretion or retention of potassium from the body, and the kidneys are the major organs that work with the balance of these ions.[53]

THE ENERGETICS OF COLOR

In addition to tastes and smells, color is considered an important indicator of the therapeutic quality of herbs. Most ancient healing systems, beginning with the Greeks, have related colors to healing. In Traditional Chinese Medicine, colors are a part of the 5-element theory, though their importance has diminished somewhat in recent years.

The correspondences between color and function given in the *Nei Ching*[54] are as follows:

"**Green**: pervades and strengthens the liver," relates to sour.

"**Red**: retains the essential substance of the heart," relates to bitter.

"**Yellow**: strengthens the spleen," relates to yellow.

"**White**: strengthens the lungs," corresponds to pungent.

"**Black**: strengthens the kidneys," its taste is salty.

Can any connections be made between the pharmacological actions now ascribed according to the coloring pigments in plants and the above correspondences?

The coloring pigments in plants fall into several general categories, and these are related to the colors named above:

Green: chlorophylls **Red**: carotenoids, anthocyanins and phycobiliproteins **Yellow**: flavonoids, carotenoids **White**: lack of pigments **Black**: quinones, allomelanin, charcoal

An analysis of the action of the above color pigments follows:

Green

The pigments we usually associate with green are the chlorophylls, especially chlorophyll a and b. In modern natural therapy, chlorophyll is known for its purifying and blood-building properties, and chlorophyll clearly has antiseptic properties.[55] Because one of the liver's main functions is the detoxification of the blood, chlorophyll may assist and support the liver in this major job.

Red

The main red and orange pigments are the carotenoids, anthocyanins and phycobiliproteins. Red seaweeds are an excellent source of these compounds.

An example of a common carotenoid is β-carotene. This compound has been studied for its ability to protect against aging and cancer,[56] and demonstrates anti-oxidant properties.

It is known that when brain or heart ischemia (lack of oxygen) occurs, free-radicals are generated (superoxide, hydroxyl radicals). These, in turn, react with membrane -SH structures, resulting in intracellular potassium ion loss, damaging cells. This may be one of the primary mechanisms for heart muscle damage in heart attack. By acting as strong free-radical scavengers, the carotenoids may protect the heart.

Yellow

Flavonoids are the compounds that most commonly cause yellow light to be reflected from plants (flavus = yellow). They have a wide range of physiological effects on the human organism, these include: steroidal, anti-inflammatory, antispasmodic and antifungal activity; and free-radical scavenging ability.

In Chinese medicine, many tonic herbs are yellow, as, for example, astragalus and licorice. These herbs are often stir-fried in honey, enhancing their yellow nature. They are considered to be strengthening to the spleen-pancreas, removing nutritional and immune deficiencies.

White

Pungent herbs that reflect the entire visual spectra, creating white include horseradish and daikon radish. Both of these herbs are known to clear the airways, acting as expectorants, and to be especially tonifying to the lungs.

Black

Phytomelanin and other nitrogen-containing melanin-like compounds in plants are found in seed coats and in roots and root bark. Certain herbs that have been heated or charred contain high amounts of activated charcoal, which is used in medicine as an absorptive and as an antidote to toxins.[57] This ability of carbon to counteract toxins could provide support and protection to the kidneys, which have to purify the blood, excreting toxic wastes. Processed rehmannia is a black herb that is used as a kidney tonic.

As may be seen from the above, there are connections, both obvious and oblique between the therapeutic activity of the flavors and what is known in the West about the pharmacological effects of the constituents they contain. This is not surprising, for Traditional Chinese Medicine is very much an exact science, refined over several thousand years. Body chemistry, and the ways biochemical harmony is maintained and restored when that harmony is lost, is one process, whether East or West.

It is the hope of the author that work in this area will continue to be of interest to researchers, and many more connections between the two medical cultures will become clear. For that will enhance our opportunities to learn more about the disease process; and about health, both personal and planetary, and how best to maintain it.

REFERENCES

1 Larghi, O. P. et al. 1979. *Perception 8:* 339-46.

2 Pangborn, R. M. et al. 1975. *Rev. Assoc. Argent Microbiol.* 7: 86-90.

3 Robinson, Trevor. 1980. *The Organic Constituents of Higher Plants* (Amherst, Cordus Press).

4 Solomons, T.W. 1980. *Organic Chemistry,* 2nd ed. (NY, John WIley & Sons), pp. 245-247.

5 McGuigan, Hugh Alister. 1928. *A Text-Book of Pharmacology and Therapeutics* (Philadelphia, W.B. Saunders Co.), p. 509.

6 Brunton, T. Lauder. 1893. *A Text-Book of Pharmacology, Therapeutics and Materia Medica* (NY, Macmillan), p. 253.

7 Vander, Arthur J. et al. 1980. *Human Physiology,* 3rd ed. (NY, McGraw Hill Book Co.), p. 425.

8 Sollman, Torald. 1936. *A Manual of Pharmacology* (Philadelphia, W.B. Saunders), p. 908.

9 Gengtao, Liu. 1985. "Hepato-Pharmacology of *Fructus Schizandrae* ", ed. Chang H. M. et al., *Advances in Chinese Medicinal Materials Research* (Philadelphia, World Scientific), p. 257.

10 [Author missing]. 1986. *Zeitschrift Phytotherapie* 7: 59-64.

11 *ibid.*

12 Wood, George B. 1856. *A Treatise on Therapeutics and Pharmacology* (Philadelphia, J. B., Lippincott and Co.), p. 213, p. 290.

13 Brunton, *op. cit.,* p. 253-255.

14 Wood, George B., *op. cit.,* vol. II, p. 648.

15 Movitt, Eli Rodin. 1946. *Digitalis and other Cardiotonic Drugs* (NY, Oxford University Press).

16 *ibid.*

17 Burnett, William C., Samuel B. Jones, & Tom J. Mabry, 1977. *The Role of Sesquiterpene Lactones in Plant-Animal Coevolution* (Dept. of Botany, U. Georgia, n.p.).

18 McGuigan, *op. cit.,* p. 498.

[19] Sancin, Pietro et al. 1981. Acta Pharm. Jugosl. 31: 39.

[20] Leung, Albert Y. 1980. *Encyclopedia of Common Natural Ingredients* (NY, John Wiley & Sons), p. 180-181.

[21] Heywood, V.H. and J.B. Harborne 1977. *The Biology and Chemistry of the Compositae* (NY, Academic Press), 2 vols.

[22] Wagner, H. & P. Wolff, ed. 1977. *New Natural Products and Plant Drugs with Pharmacological, Biogical or Therapeutical Activity* (NY, Springer-Verlag), p. 157-176.

[23] *ibid.*

[24] Martinet, *op. cit.,* p. 62.

[25] Henry, Thomas Anderson. 1949. *The Plant Alkaloids* (London, J. & A. Churchill), p. 345.

[26] Robinson, *op. cit.,* pp. 13-21.

[27] Fernie, W.T. 1905. *Meals Medicinal* (Bristol, John Wright & Co.), p. 607.

[28] Hou, Joseph P. 1978. *The Myth and Truth About Ginseng* (NY, A.S. Barnes & Co.).

[29] Dufty, William. 1975. *Sugar Blues* (NY, Warner Books, inc.).

[30] Jolly, Julius. 1951. *Indian Medicine* (Poona, India, C.G. Kahikar).

[31] Bensky & Gamble, *op. cit.*

[32] Dharmananda, Subhuti. 1987. Swanson Health Shopper, Aug.-Sep.

[33] Wenbin, Chen et al. 1983. J. of Trad. Chinese Med. 3: 63-68.

[34] James, John S. 1987. A.I.D.S. Treatment News 25, February 13.

[35] *Proceedings of the 4th International Ginseng Symposium.* 1984. (Daejeon, Korea, Korea Ginseng & Tobacco Research Institute).

[36] James, John S., *op. cit.*

[37] Huang, Qiaoshu et al. 1982. *Jaoxue Xuebao* 17: 200; CA 96(21) 177998q.

[38] Wagner, H. et al. 1985. "Immunostimulatory Drugs" in *Economic and Medicinal Plant Research* (NY, Academic Press).

[39]   Mead, George R. 1972. *The Ethnobotany of the California Indians* (U. of N. Colorado, Museum of Anthropology), pp. 120-121.

[40]   Turner, Nancy. 1980. *Ethnobotany of the Okanagan-Colville Indians* (n.p, n.p.), p. 66.

[41]   Hellson, John C. & Morgan Gadd. 1974. *Ethnobotany of the Blackfoot Indians* (Ottawa, National Museums of Canada, paper no. 19).

[42]   Personal Communication, February 23, 1988.

[43]   Atal, C. K. et al. 1981. Journal of Ethnopharmacology 4: 229-232.

[44]   Sealy, Hans. 1976. *The Stress of Life,* revised ed. (NY, McGraw-Hill).

[45]   McGuigan, *op. cit.,* p. 311-320.

[46]   Wood, *op. cit.,* II, p. 741.

[17]   Sollmann, *op. cit.,* pp. 191-203.

[48]   Leung, Albert Y. 1980. *Encyclopedia of Common Natural Ingredients* (NY, John Wiley & Sons).

[49]   Brunton, *op. cit.,* pp. 600-601.

[50]   Brunton, *op. cit.,* p. 601.

[51]   Bean, Lowell John & Katherine Siva Saubel. 1972. *Temalpakh: Cahuilla Indian Knowledge and Usage of Plants* (Morongo Indian Reservation, Malki Museum Press).

[52]   Bensky and Gamble, *op. cit.*

[53]   Vander, *op. cit.,* p. 377-380.

[54]   Veith, Ilza. 1949. *The Yellow Emperor's Classic of Internal Medicine* (reprinted: Berkeley, University of California Press,1972).

[55]   *Merck Index.* 1976. 9th ed. (Rahway, Merck Co.), p. 275.

[56]   Cutler RG. 1984. "Carotenoids and retinol: Their possible importance in determining longevity of primate species", Proc. Nat. Acad. Sci. 81: 7627.

[57]   *Merck Index.* 1976. 9th ed. (Rahway, Merck Co.), p. 230.

Appendix B
HERBAL SUPPLEMENTS FOR VEGETARIANS
by Michael Tierra

One of the most significant recent socio-biological trends has been the rise in vegetarianism. This single practice alone significantly alters body chemistry and, thus, the body's overall energetic balance. For vegetarians we certainly must consider the first principle of traditional Chinese medicine which is "first tonify the deficiency," instead of viewing every disease as a symptom of toxicity requiring cleansing and eliminative therapies.

In traditional healing systems, such as Chinese and Ayurvedic medicine, food is considered the first and best tonic. Traditional cultures in which little or no meat is eaten develop an understanding of the use of certain nutritive tonic herbs that may be substituted for meat. Thus, in Ayurvedic medicine, herbs are combined and prepared into pastes (avelehas), while Chinese tonic herbal preparations use rich roots, barks and berries all of which resemble powerful "meaty" flavors and textures that seem to provide deep sources of supportive nutritive energy.

As it is important to know what foods to eat and how to prepare them according to individual needs and climatic regions, it is also valuable for vegetarians to learn how wisely to incorporate such powerful herbal substances into the diet.

Indian cooking uses a wide variety of spices and special curry-like substances, especially in the preparation of grains, beans and vegetables. While these appeal to the senses, their deeper purpose lies in enhancing digestive capabilities for successful assimilation of the complex carbohydrates of vegetable foods. While Indian cuisine often is debased by the overuse of such hot spices, the original blends tended to combine a variety of spices together in a balanced way to promote digestion and health.

The basis of Indian curry is three important spices: cumin seed which is heating and carminative and has a strong spicy flavor; coriander seed which has a cooler energy and milder spicy flavor; and turmeric root which is pleasantly bitter and only slightly spicy-tasting, imparts a golden color to food, and has liver detoxifying, blood moving and digestive properties. These three spices used together are balanced within themselves and are most important in promoting optimal digestion and assimilation of complex carbohydrates.

In addition, various local regions add different spices according to climate and geography. Cayenne pepper, black pepper and ginger are added to food in cold weather and climates. Asafoetida is added as a substitute for garlic and to help prevent and eliminate gas and bloating. Spices such as cinnamon, cloves and nutmeg are used for sweeter dishes, which include fruit.

A basic digestive formula in powder form, sprinkled directly on food or taken after meals to eliminate gas and bloating is "hingashtak" (named for the major herb in the formula, asafoetida). There are various traditional hingashtak blends of which a basic one is composed of asafoetida, caraway seeds, long pepper, black pepper, cumin seeds, omum seeds and rock salt, all in equal parts. A North American version includes wild yam and dandelion roots combined with the traditional herbs of the gland, as given above.

"Draksha" is a liquid preparation in which various heating spices are freshly ground into a fine powder, extracted in some spirits, and then added to formulas at about 10% alcohol to grape juice. This is taken before meals to stimulate enzymes and digestive secretions and impart strength through better digestion and assimilation. The most important spices for draksha are long pepper and black pepper, but others, such as ginger, cloves and cinnamon, also are incorporated in some formulas.

Another formula, used especially in cold damp climates, is "trikatu". Trikatu is a basic warming herbal stimulant of which there are many variations. The most important of these includes equal parts black pepper, long pepper and ginger. One that is milder and better suited for children substitutes two parts of powdered anise seed for the long pepper. Trikatu is often used for allergies, for warming and drying effects and clearing mucous secretions. These powders often are mixed with honey to form a paste and a little is taken each morning and at other times through the day as needed. It is very effective for use in cold, damp climates, situated near water and for allergies caused by coldness.

"Sring bhasma" is a natural substance used by yogis and others in the Himalayas. It is made by calcining (heating to a high temperature) deer antlers (that are naturally shed each year). This is ground to a fine white powder and added to a small amount of whey while chanting a mantra. One-quarter teaspoon of this mixture is taken once or twice a day throughout the cold season to counteract coldness and help stimulate body heat.

"Chyavanprash" is an ancient Ayurvedic tonic that is made from approximately 20 to 60 ground herbs, of which the primary ingredient is amla. This is then combined with whole jaggury, derived from the pure unrefined juice of the sugar cane, ghee, sesame oil, and sometimes honey, to form a delicious herb food that has powerful rejuvenative and strengthening powers. Chyavanprash is used for many of the same purposes that the Chinese use ginseng, but is more nutritive. It may be taken alone or mixed with warm water as a nutritive tonic, followed with a cup of boiled warm milk.

The Chinese have a large number of tonic herbs that are used seasonally, and especially by Taoist priests, as a substitute for meat. Of these, ginseng is considered the king of tonics. There are many varieties of ginseng, of varying grades and quality. Ginseng works by augmenting the ATCH or energy- generating hormone from the pituitary gland. It is specifically indicated for deficient conditions, ranging from low energy and chronic fatigue to digestive weakness, lung weakness, anemia and general debility.

Wild, uncultivated ginseng, considered the finest, is extremely rare and expensive. Short of that, one should be sure to purchase roots that are at least seven years old. At that age the ginsenosides are sufficiently developed. Chinese or Korean ginseng is either naturally white or, as the result of a special steaming process, red. White ginseng is neutral to warm in energy, while red is definitely warming. Thus it is better for a person with high metabolism, or one who lives in a warmer climate, to use the cooler, white variety. For people who have a lower metabolism with coldness, or live in cold climates, the red ginseng is better.

American ginseng (*Panax quinquefolium*) is more bitter than the Chinese and considered to be generally cooler and better suited for use as a blood tonic. It is best to use it for women; when one is more highly stimulated or eats more meat; or lives in warm climates. It seems that American ginseng is now preferred by American Chinese to the Chinese or Korean varieties.

Ginseng is a chi tonic and maintains stamina, strength and overall immune potential. It may be taken once or twice a day if needed, or once or twice a week to maintain adequate energy levels.

There are a variety of ways in which to take ginseng:

1. Chew a piece each day.
2. Slowly simmer or steam the root and use the liquid as a tea.
3. Simmer and chop a whole root and use the stock to make soup.
4. During the cold seasons, leave a root to macerate in a pint of quality grain spirits such as vodka. Take a teaspoon once or twice daily.

In addition, ginseng is often combined with other traditional Chinese tonic herbs such as atractylodes, astragalus, poria mushroom, licorice, dong quai, lycii berries and with deer antler to augment its tonic effects.

As beneficial as it is, it is possible to overuse ginseng. This can create conditions of "stagnant chi," because the energy that is being generated cannot properly circulate. Stagnant chi symptoms can include bloating; gas, chest or abdominal pains; and even moodiness. One then would use carminative and digestive herbs, such as ginger root or citrus peel, to help move chi through the system. Ginseng may be more suitably used during the colder seasons or when one is weak than in hot weather or when one is overly strong or constipated.

Codonopsis pilosula, "Dan sen," is an acceptable, cheaper substitute for ginseng. It is considered to have half the strength of ginseng. Being milder, it is better suited for use on a year-round basis.

Astragalus membranicus, or "huang chi" in Mandarin and "bok kee" in Cantonese dialect, is a major herb for tonifying the immune system. It has been demonstrated to be clinically effective to offset the negative side effects of chemotherapy and radiation therapy used for cancer victims. It is an excellent herb to use as a tonic throughout the year for aiding digestion as well as promoting immunity.

Dong quai *(Angelica sinensis)* is sometimes called "women's ginseng" because it is to the blood what ginseng is to the energy of the body. Women generally need blood tonics while men more often need energy tonics such as ginseng. There are, of course, many occasions when each can benefit from the other or from a combination of both. It is a specific for all gynecological disorders of women. Like ginseng, astragalus and codonopsis, dong quai is made into a tea, soup or wine. It is more bitter than those substances, so the amount used in soups should be carefully adjusted. Traditional Chinese families buy a pound of either ginseng or codonopsis, a pound of astragalus, and for women a pound of dong quai, to be used in soups on a weekly basis for the entire family throughout the year.

These are some of the tonic herbs that should be used by vegetarians on a fairly regular basis to help create the extra yang energy that one might derive from eating meat. They are especially helpful in colder climates. In appropriate amounts and frequencies, they may be used throughout the year.

Generally when using these tonic herb foods, one should limit or avoid intake of cold, raw foods and sweet or sour fruits soon after taking the herbs. This is because their more extreme yin energy tends to weaken and counteract the effects of the tonic herbs.

---

[1] Medical doctors should realize, that energetically speaking, antibiotics are extremely cooling and may not be nearly as effective for vegetarians as for carnivores in overcoming inflammatory conditions. Because vegetarians are metabolically and energetically cooler, antibiotics will tend to create imbalance, and consequent adverse reactions, in vegetarians. Antibiotics are at best only temporarily effective for them, with the infection recurring later or in another area.

This is also true of other so-called natural anti-inflammatory substances such as vitamin C. The answer is to combine some kind of tonification therapy, whether it be rich proteinaceous broths such as miso and seaweeds, or tonic herbs in small amounts, such as ginseng and astragalus, to offset the negative effects of the antibiotics.

[2] An important study of the harmful effects of meat-eating and of the meat industry is *Diet for a New America* by John Robbins (Stillpoint Press). This well-documented book discusses the range of negative effects of excessive meat-eating: the moral issues involving the killing of animals; health issues; the practices of an industry that seems to foster gross insensitivity and cruelty to animals; and the key role animal husbandry plays in the destruction of forests and other natural environments for grazing.

Appendix C
AYURVEDA AND CHINESE MEDICINE
A COMPARATIVE VIEW
by David Frawley

In our presentation of traditional natural healing systems, the two most enduring and comprehensive are those of India and China. Both remain alive today, having survived the influences of Western imperialism and allopathic medicine. What follows is a comparison of the basic concepts which show that the two systems have much in common. There are many exceptions and variations on these fundamental principles as both systems are intricate and many sided. It should, however, give us much food for thought and further study.

Chinese medicine is based upon the meaning of yin and yang. These are two basic forces of the cosmos—light and dark, firm and yielding, active and passive, masculine and feminine. On a physical level, health is the balance between yin and yang in the body; disease is the imbalance.

Ayurveda, the traditional medicine of India, also views health as the balance of primary forces and ill-health as the imbalance. While the Chinese system essentially follows a binary symbolism, the dualities of yin and yang, the Ayurvedic system employs a triplicity of forces. The three biological humors of Ayurveda are the "doshas" of vata, pitta and kapha. "Dosha" means "that which causes or produces darkness and decay,"—so when the body/mind is imbalanced, the biological humors initiate the disease process.

The biological humors reflect the five elements, just as in the Chinese system yin and yang are related to a five element sequence. Vata, primarily the element of air, means literally in Sanskrit, "that which blows". Pitta, what cooks or digests things and is primarily the element of fire, is also called "agni", which specifically means fire. Pitta also means bile. Kapha, the element of water, literally translates as "that which sticks or clings". It is also called "phlegm". Air, fire and water are the mobile or animating principles of the five elements and are therefore primary in determining the life process.

Yet each humor is composed of a second element as well, as each of these active elements requires a passive medium for it to be contained in the static physical body.

Water, exists in the medium of earth, which contains it. Hence, kapha, containing earth, abides in the body largely in congealed form.

Fire exists in the body in the medium of water (oil); it cannot exist directly in the body without destroying it. Hence, pitta also contains an aspect of water.

Air exists in the body in the medium of ether, the defined space in which it operates.

Just as yin and yang are part of an intricate and comprehensive cosmic symbolism, so are the three doshas. Vata, the air humor, relates to the God Brahma, the cosmic creator and law giver. Kapha, the water humor, reflects the God Vishnu, the force of divine love, the cosmic maintainer from whom come the saviors or avatars who guide humanity. Pitta, the fire humor, relates to Shiva, the cosmic destroyer and god of knowledge, who takes us beyond the illusion of the phenomenal world to the eternal reality beyond. The three humors reflect the divine trinity on the physical level.

While the two systems differ in orientation, the Chinese towards a dualistic cosmic thinking and the Ayurvedic towards a trinity of forces, their approach and manner of thinking is of the same order.

YIN AND YANG AND THE THREE HUMORS

Yin and yang can be related more specifically to the three humors. Yin is also defined as water in Chinese medicine and is much like the water humor, kapha. Moist, heavy and cold, it makes up the body fluids, just like kapha. Yang, similarly, is like the fire humor, pitta. Both are hot, dry and light and govern body function, digestion and circulation.

The concepts of yin and yang are much like biological humors. Therefore, we can also view the Chinese as a two humor system and the Ayurvedic as a three humor system. (Older Western and Greek medicine, still used today in some Islamic cultures, is a four humor system.) Naturally, on some level, it should be possible to translate one in terms of the others.

The third of the humors, vata, the air humor, relates to the Chinese concept of "chi". Chi is the life-force or the air principle behind yin and yang. Vata, also called "prana" or life-force in Sanskrit, similarly moves pitta and kapha, fire and water. Vata or chi is said to govern the flow of energy through the channels and meridians ("srotamsi" in Ayurveda). Both systems view the human body as a network of these different channels and the disease process as a wrong energy flow within them. Both discriminate different types of chi or prana governing the different nervous activities in the human body.

We see that the three humors of vata, pitta and kapha are equivalent to the Chinese principles of chi, yang and yin. With the addition of chi we get something in Chinese medicine like the three humors of Ayurveda.

Ayurveda and Chinese medicine add a fourth principle: the blood. The Chinese relate blood to yin and chi to yang—as lesser degrees of the same force. In Ayurveda the blood is usually under pitta, fire. This is because the blood suffers mainly through damage from excessive heat, fire or toxins, which generally come from pitta.

The terms "wind", "fire", and "phlegm" also exist in Chinese medicine as defining various pathogenic influences of the disease process. In Chinese medicine we refer to "wind", disorders or "fire" diseases. In Ayurveda the humors can also refer to different kinds of disease. The Chinese concept of wind disorders, like that of vata or wind disorders in Ayurveda, refers primarily to diseases of the nervous system. Much of the understanding of wind disorders in Chinese medicine will therefore be helpful in understanding vata disorders in Ayurveda (and vice versa). Similarly, pitta diseases are most of the typical heat and fire disorders in Chinese medicine and Kapha diseases are water toxin, dampness and phlegm. The treatment methods for these conditions in both systems of healing are closely related.

THE DISEASE PROCESS

In the treatment of disease both Ayurveda and Chinese medicine employ similar forms of "differential diagnosis". These typically include examination of pulse, tongue, abdomen. Other signs and symptoms and the questioning of the patient are also used.

Ayurveda is based upon ascertaining of individual constitutional types according to the three humors. The disease process tends to follow the predominant humor in the constitution. Hence, it is first of all necessary to determine the nature or constitution of the individual. This requires an extensive examination of constitution ("prakriti pariksha"). Ayurvedically, we speak of individuals as vata or air types; pitta or fire types; and kapha or water types, in different combinations and to different degrees. The nature of an illness is thus examined relative to all of the above considerations.

Chinese medicine, on the other hand, is based more primarily on examining the nature and development of the disease as yin or yang. First of all in Chinese medicine we determine the stage of the disease. This may be done according to the eight principles of yin/yang, hot/cold, excess/deficient, surface/interior (used more commonly in acupuncture), according to the six meridian syndromes (the three yang, three yin stages of disease of the Shang Han Lun, used more extensively in herbal medicine) or other such systems.

Chinese medicine does contain the concept of constitutional types as yin and yang but it is not as developed, nor is it given such emphasis as in Ayurveda. Ayurveda similarly does examine the stage or nature of the disease, but does not give it as much primary emphasis as Chinese medicine. It is possible to use one system to cross reference the other; Ayurveda for its constitutional view and Chinese medicine for its analysis of disease.

CONSTITUTIONAL TYPES

Pitta or fire types are essentially yang types in Chinese medicine. They are hot in constitution, they tend to be vehement, aggressive and ambitious. They are also prone to anger, they like being leaders, they have a ruddy complexion, strong digestion, good circulation, and usually suffer from inflammatory or infectious diseases. In Chinese medicine these are the individuals who usually suffer from liver disorders, excess liver fire, excess liver yang, or some deficiency style heat.

Kapha or water types are similar to yin types. They tend to be emotional, romantic, receptive, loyal, prone to attachment, slow in movement and action. They have a white, moist complexion, tend to hold excess phlegm, water or fat. In Chinese medicine they would often suffer from diseases of phlegm, dampness, water toxin and cold.

Vata or air types have no direct correspondence in Chinese medicine, but they could be called "chi" types; not in the sense of possessing large amounts of chi (usually they are deficient in this regard) but in suffering mainly from chi disorders. These include lack of strength, poor stamina, shortness of breath, weak or variable digestion, intestinal gas and poor circulation. Air types are nervous, changeable, indecisive, dominated by fear and anxiety, have a darkish or brownish tinge to their complexion, are thin, dry, excitable and move quickly. They tend to suffer from nervous disorders, insomnia, arthritis and chronic, wasting diseases.

Some of the characteristics of vata come under yang. For example, air types are light, mobile, adaptable and articulate. Others come under yin. They tend to be sensitive, lacking in self-confidence and may be easily influenced.

EXCESS AND DEFICIENCY PATTERNS

In the language of Ayurveda, treatment is usually referred to as reducing the aggravated or excess humor. Conditions are thought of according to the elevated dosha that produces them. Insomnia, for example, is usually owing to high vata, too much air and ether in the system, inhibiting the calm and groundedness necessary for sleep. It is recognized that a humor which is too low may be productive of disease. Yet it is the one that is too high which is considered to be the main causative factor, and the one most specific for treating the disease.

In the language of Chinese medicine, however, treatment is usually referred to as strengthening or tonifying the underlying deficiency. The most primary deficiencies are yin and yang, with those of chi and blood relative to these. Deficiency conditions are regarded as the root or radical cause of most diseases. The Chinese also speak of reducing excesses but these are considered more as external pathogens than internal forces.

For this reason, the languages of Ayurveda and Chinese medicine are often opposite in form. What is high pitta or high fire in Ayurveda may be defined as deficiency of yin, lack of water or vital fluids in Chinese medicine. Similarly, high kapha in Ayurveda, manifested, perhaps, as severe edema along with poor circulation and chronic chills, may be regarded as deficiency of yang, lack of primary fire in Chinese medicine.

Vata or air types often suffer from deficiency generally and so can develop any deficiency or any combination of deficiencies. In Chinese terms they would tend towards deficiency of both yin and yang. They would suffer from both cold and dehydration.

Why is it that some patients develop a yin deficiency, others a yang deficiency while others develop both? An Ayurvedic constitutional analysis would show us this predisposition.

Kapha types are likely to develop a deficiency of yang, with internal accumulation of cold and dampness. Similarly, they will often have a deficiency of chi, (as chi and yang go together) and may also suffer from lack of strength, shortness of breath or poor digestion. They will be least likely to suffer from a deficiency of yin. However, they may develop a deficiency of blood, because excess mucus in the body and excess plasma in the blood may inhibit red blood cell production and cause anemia.

Women who suffer from deficiency of blood along with water retention are usually kapha types (such as those treated by Tang kuei and Peony combination, Dang gui shao yao san).

Pitta types will be the least likely to develop deficiency of yang. Similarly, they do not often develop deficiency of chi, as their yang fire will be able to support the chi. They will, however, tend more towards chi than yang deficiency. Pitta types commonly develop deficiency of yin along with internal heat or deficiency of fire (such as treated by the famous Rehmannia 6 formula, Liu wei di huang wan). They can also develop deficiency of blood, with bile and heat damaging and thinning the blood.

Vata types tend to become deficient in both yin and yang. They most commonly tend towards deficiency of yin (dehydration), as the main property of vata is dryness. Yet this yin deficiency will usually not involve any heat symptoms. It will often be found with deficiency of yang, cold extremeties and degenerated metabolism (such as treated by

Rehmannia 8, Jin gui shenn qi wan). They will similarly tend to suffer from both chi and blood deficiency at the same time.

Through a better understanding of constitutional types we will be able to better understand what herbs and therapies may cause side effects in long term usage.

STAGES OF DISEASE

In Chinese medicine disease is regarded as progressing from yang to yin stages. Yang conditions generally involve heat, occur on the surface or exterior of the body (which may also include the gastrointestinal tract) and involve a pattern of excess. The invading pathogenic factor is strong, the intrinsic energy of the body is strong and the symptoms tend to be acute.

Yin conditions, opposite to this, generally involve cold, occur in the interior of the body, in the organs themselves and involve a pattern of deficiency. The pathogen and the intrinsic energy of the body are weak and the symptoms are chronic.

In Ayurveda disease is usually not classified as progressing from one humor to another. Yet a similar concept exists in terms of the stages of time.

The first phase of life, childhood, is dominated by the water humor. Water is the formative element and we can see that most diseases of childhood are of a kapha or phlegm nature. They involve excess mucus and respiratory system disorders.

The second portion of life, middle-age, starting at puberty, is dominated by pitta, fire. Most diseases of this time period involve heat, fever, inflammation, infection and toxic blood conditions.

The last stage of life is dominated by vata, air. Most of the diseases of aging are air disorders such as loss of teeth and hair, wrinkles, dryness of skin, depletion of body fluids, failure of sight and hearing. Most diseases of aging in Chinese medicine are vata diseases in Ayurveda.

This pattern of three stages also occurs in the disease process itself. The initial stage of disease, called "Greater Yang" in Chinese medicine, mainly involves a cold and damp invasion of the lungs and the body surface, as in the common cold and flu. This is like the kapha stage of disease. The next two stages of disease in Chinese medicine are called

"Lesser Yang and Sunlight Yang". These are mainly heat syndromes, fevers and infectious diseases and they could be correlated to the pitta stage of disease in Ayurveda.

The last three stages of disease in Chinese medicine, the yin phases, involve cold, dehydration, chronic weakness and debility, and the problems of aging. These are mainly vata disorders, or the vata stage of disease. However, the last stage of disease in the Chinese system, called "Absolute Yin", involves the separation of yin and yang and the derangement of the five elements. It resembles the last phase of disease in Ayurveda when all three humors are aggravated at once.

For this reason in Ayurveda kapha diseases are the most mild and vata diseases are the most severe. Similarly, kapha diseases are the fewest in number and vata diseases are the most in number, with pitta falling in between.

PATTERNS OF TREATMENT

Chinese medicine follows a basic treatment pattern of two stages. First the excess is cleared; then the deficiency is tonified. Excesses are pathogenic accumulations which may be heat, cold, wind, damp, stagnations of chi, blood and water, or other factors. Deficiencies are of yin, yang, chi and blood.

Without first clearing the excess, which may be anything from a common cold to an acute infection, it is not possible to treat the deficiency. Herbs that build up deficiencies also tend to feed excesses and will aggravate excess conditions. However, to some degree, excess and deficiency may be treated at the same time. The situation may be complicated or the patient may be too weak to take the stronger clearing therapies. This, however, should only be done when necessary.

Ayurvedic treatment follows three stages. The principle is the same in that first toxins are cleared and then tonification is given. The clearing therapy, however, is divided into two parts. The first stage is the clearing of "ama", a term denoting accumulated toxins or waste materials from poor digestion. This usually involves normalizing digestion and elimination and clearing the tongue of any coating. It also commonly involves clearing fever and dispersing stagnation.

The second stage involves clearing the excess dosha or biological humor of vata, pitta or kapha. This involves special methods for each humor. Whereas in Chinese medicine disease is usually treated as an external force entering into the body, in Ayurveda it is regarded as being caused by an excess of humors in the body itself. Hence, in Ayurveda, cleansing therapy has two stages: one for the external factor or ama and the other for the internal factor, the dosha.

The third stage is tonification or rejuvenation, rebuilding the body. Tonification is also relative to the particular humor and the kinds of deficiencies it creates.

METHODS OF TREATMENT

In Chinese medicine the appropriate therapeutic means are used for clearing excesses and strengthening deficiencies. Herbs stimulate different actions to eliminate toxins from the body. Diaphoretics promote their dispersal through sweat; purgatives through elimination; diuretics through urination; emetics through vomiting; expectorants through discharge of phlegm and so on. Heat-clearing herbs directly kill pathogens. Tonic herbs similarly are employed relative to which of the four entities of chi, blood, yin and yang that they rebuild.

Therapies are usually given relative to disease manifestations. Diaphoretics are given during colds and flu, purgatives during fever and constipation, etc. Tonification is given in chronic conditions or between acute attacks.

PANCHA KARMA

Ayurveda employs the same therapeutic methods and also uses them during active stages of the disease. However, in Ayurveda, clearing methods may be used for internal cleansing or disease prevention purposes even when there is no disease manifestation. This again is relative to the concept of clearing the doshas, which as internal forces can be corrected any time, not just when they produce an active disease. For example, while Chinese medicine applies the purgation method for the acute stage of fever or infection, Ayurveda uses it as part of a process of detoxification in eliminating excess pitta from the body.

This usage of therapeutic methods for internal cleansing purposes is specific to Ayurveda. It is called "pancha karma", "the five actions", according to the five main methods used. Patients undergo systematic massage, sweating, and other detoxifying methods to eliminate the root of disease in the aggravated humor.

Prior to this treatment the patient should follow a special diet along with herbs to improve digestion for a period of weeks to months. This is to clear the ama, or the toxins that inhibit the system. Without clearing ama first, the pancha karma treatment cannot be effectively done. Usually the patient must have a certain strength to undergo pancha karma therapy. It is not generally given during acute stages of disease. Most diseases must be returned to milder symptoms before pancha karma can be safely done; and this is part of its proper preparation.

Pancha karma then begins with the preliminary treatment ("purva karma"). This process usually involves daily oil massage with special medicated oils (usually prepared with sesame oil) and sweating therapies (which may use various herbs to help stimulate the process). Both therapies may be whole body or focus on certain parts of the body. Medicated oils, for example, may be applied in steady drops to the forehead, or a special cap is employed to allow the whole head to be soaked in oil for an extended period. Different kinds of sweating apparati may be employed, including hoses for local application of medicated steam. This preliminary cleansing process allows the humors to be brought into the gastrointestinal tract for elimination from the body. It is given for a period of one week to a month, or more.

Following this treatment comes the five main purification processes. These are therapeutic emesis ("vamana") for kapha, purgation ("virechana") for pitta and medicated enemas ("basti") for vata. The waste material is then examined to determine the amount of the humor that has been expelled from the body. Additional methods are therapeutic release of toxic blood ("raktamoksha"), mainly for pitta, and nasal medications ("nasya"), mainly for vata. Raktamoksha involves a therapeutic bleeding of the patient at special sites on the body. Nasya involves applying oils or decoctions taken through the nose to directly cleanse or nourish the brain and the nervous system.

This whole process may have to be done for extended periods of time, or repeated periodically for severe diseases. It is only after this is accomplished that radical tonification or rejuvenation can effectively proceed through the use of special powerful herbs, like ashwagandha (*Withania somnifera*) or certain mineral preparations.

However, the same therapies can be done in a milder way or combined to some extent for less severe conditions. This is like the simultaneous use of tonification and reduction methods in Chinese medicine. For example, for vata types, this may involve daily oil massage, occasional medicated enemas and tonic herbs. Consistency is important. Mild therapies done regularly over long periods of time will be more effective than radical therapies done partially, or done once, followed by a return to the normal, usually disease inducing, life-style.

Ayurveda emphasizes establishing a life-style in harmony with the individual constitution. This involves not only diet and herbs but also oil massage, exercise, meditation, appropriate work, sleep and other stabilizing life- patterns. Without the right life-style, mild natural remedies of herbs and diets may not be effective. Hence we need not only use herbal therapies to treat manifest diseases. We can also use them strategically to prevent them from manifestation. That is one of the special gifts of the Ayurvedic system.

USE OF HERBS

Both Ayurveda and Chinese medicine rely heavily on the use of herbs. Ayurveda, however, uses more mineral preparations than Chinese medicine. Ayurvedic medicine is still largely alchemical and uses specially humanized forms of minerals like mercury and sulfur, gold and silver. It also uses precious gems: diamonds, rubies, and others, either with herbs, or by themselves. These are used to treat severe conditions.

The same therapies that can be brought about through herbs can be brought about through humanized minerals, which are thought to possess stronger heating or cooling energies. The process of humanization of minerals is often elaborate, however, without such exactitude, such substances, if taken internally, are toxic or even deadly. (Unfortunately, the F.D.A. will not allow these alchemical preparations to come into this country for commercial sales.

About one-third of the herbs used in Ayurveda are the same as in Chinese medicine. These include common spices like cinnamon, ginger and turmeric, but many others as well. The uses are, in all but exceptional cases, the same.

However, each system uses many major tonics that are not in use in the other, even though some of these may grow in the other country. Ginseng was not used in Ayurvedic medicine until recently. Ashwagandha seems to be unknown to the Chinese. Bala (*Sida cordifolia*), an important Ayurvedic tonic, is used in China as a minor heat-clearing herb.

Chinese medicine is more purely an herbal medicine. As such it is the most developed pure herbal system in the world. Ayurveda, however, has a more comprehensive grasp of the healing properties of all the different kingdoms of nature.

THE FIVE ELEMENTS

Both Chinese and Ayurvedic medicine employ a sequence of five elements but the two sequences differ. Ayurveda has the same scheme as the ancient Greeks—earth, water, fire, air and ether. The Chinese use the first three but add wood and metal.

However, a study of the *I Ching*, the source book of Chinese culture and the origin of the five element theory, shows a correlation. The element of wood is represented by the trigrams of thunder (chen) and wind (sun), which can thereby also be seen to represent the element of air in its yin and yang phases. Wood, like air, is also the life- force. The element of metal is represented by the trigrams of heaven (chien) and the lake or valley (tui), which similarly can be correlated to the element of space in its yin and yang phases (expansion and contraction).

The basic Chinese five element sequence derives from the "Sequence of Later Heaven or the Inner World Sequence" of the *I Ching* (Shuo kua, Discussion of Trigrams), thought to show the movement of forces in time. This sequence places the trigrams for wood in the east, fire in the south, metal in the west and water in the north (see Wilhelm/Baynes translation of *I Ching*, pg. 269). Earth is said to be in the center.

There is a second sequence for the trigrams, the "Primal Arrangement or Sequence of Earlier Heaven" (often the Sequential Arrangement is drawn as placed within the Primal Arrangement). The Primal Arrangement places the trigrams for fire in the east, heaven (space) in the south, water in the west and earth in the south (ibid. pg. 266). Air could thereby be placed in the center.

The primal arrangement can thus be correlated to the five element sequence of the Hindus and Greeks. It is thought to show the ideal state of forces behind the manifestation of time. While the ordinary Chinese five element pattern of the Sequential Arrangement shows the terrestrial order, the Primal Arrangement can be said to reflect the cosmic order. Hence we see that both five element sequences were known in ancient China. It may not be possible to simplistically interchange their Ayurvedic and Chinese forms but they do have more in common than appears at first; and a common origin may exist.

HISTORICAL CONTENTS

There have been many contacts between India and China throughout the centuries that have brought their healing traditions into proximity. In ancient times, up to the Tang dynasty (7th century century A.D.), Chinese medicine used more alchemical and mineral preparations and employed such methods as therapeutic vomiting, which are more typical of Ayurveda today.

Much of this contact came through Buddhism. Buddhism originated in the Indian cultural and scientific matrix and included many aspects of it. This was not only the use of the Sanskrit language and the practice of yoga but also included Ayurveda, Hindu astrology and other forms of the knowledge developed in India since the time of the ancient seers or rishis. Prominent Buddhist teachers like the sage Nagarjuna were Ayurvedic doctors and wrote commentaries on traditional Ayurvedic texts. They often added much to the science and their works are still revered and used today.

Buddhist medicine in Tibet, Sri Lanka and other Buddhist countries is still primarily Ayurvedic at the root; uses the same terminology and most of the same medicines and therapies as the Ayurveda practiced in India today. Yet when Buddhism came to China, a highly evolved system of medicine already existed. Hence, Buddhism in China adapted itself to the indigenous medicine. However, some evidence of interchange exists.

Certain Chinese formulas, particularly those in the "Aromatic

Orifice-opening" category, resemble Ayurvedic formulas. This category of formulas treats nervous system disorders and uses alchemical ideas. Styrax formula (Su he xiang wan), for example, reflects a probable Indian influence. It uses many indigenous Indian herbs and more commonly used Ayurvedic ones: *Terminalia chebula, Piper longum,* sandalwood, aquilaria, olibanum, cinnabar and so on. Styrax formula[1] also uses gold and silver, pearl, musk, cow's gall bladder stones, calamus and cloves and other Ayurvedic medicines, not as commonly used in Chinese medicine.

Chinese medicine, however, does not have the sophisticated process of detoxifying the mineral substances that we find in Ayurveda.

Other evidence of interchange predates the Buddhist period. Both Taoist and Hindu sources speak of an earlier golden age ruled by the sages, who also formulated their systems of medicine. Foremost of these for both cultures were the mythical seven seers identified with the stars of the Big Dipper. Both cultures employed an astrology of 27 or 28 lunar constellations that mark largely the same groups of stars. They both start with the constellation that marks the Pleiades, where the vernal equinox occured 1500-2000 B.C. showing some communication around that time.

It may well be that this ancient enlightened culture spoken of in both cultures was the same. Both Indian and Chinese mythology appear to look for it in arctic regions. In this regard Lao-Tzu may be correct in regarding what we call civilization as a disease, a fall from an earlier state of grace in which humanity lived a simple life in harmony with nature and in communion with the Gods.

The medical systems were part of a system of spiritual science, including astrology and meditation, which both the Chinese and the Indians saw at the origins of human civilization. It is to that integral spiritual science that as a culture we need to return to today. Both Chinese medicine and Ayurveda give us a basis for reformulating that in a global context.

---

[1] and other similar Chinese formulas

Appendix D/LATIN GLOSSARY

Acanthopanax gracilistylus and spp.	Rheumatism ginseng, Wu jia pi
Achillea millefolium	Yarrow
Achryanthes bidentata	
Aconitum aconite, A. Napellus	Aconite, Monkshood
Acorus calamus and spp.	Calamus
Aesculus californica	California buckeye
Aesculus hippocastanum	Horse chestnut
Agastache rugosa	Patchouli
Agnus castus	Chaste tree
Agrimonia eupatori	Agrimony
Agropyron repens	Couchgrass
Alchemilla vulgaris	Lady's mantle
Aletris farinosa	True unicorn root
Allium fistulosum	Scallions
Allium macrostemon	Chinese chive
Allium sativum	Garlic
Alisma plantago	Water plantain
Aloe barbadensis-officinalis	Aloe
Alpinia offinarum	Galangal
Althea officinalis	Marshmallow
Amaranthus hypochon-driacus and spp.	Amaranth
Amoracia lapathifolia	Horseradish
Anemone pulsatilla	Pulsatilla
Anemopsis californica	Yerba mansa
Anethum graveolens	Dill
Angelica archangelica and A. brewerii	Angelica
Angelica pubescens	Tu huo
Angelica sinensis and A. polymorpha	Dong quai
Anthemis nobilis	Roman chamomile
Apium graveolens	Celery
Aralia racemosa, A. californica, A. nudicaulis and A. quinquefolia	Spikenard
Arctium lappa	Burdock
Arctostaphylos uva ursi	Uva ursi
Areca catechu	Betelnut
Arisaema triphyllum and A. maculatum	Jack in the pulpit
Artemisia abrotanum	Southernwood
Artemisia apiacea	Wormwood
Artemisia cina, A. santonica	Wormseed (Levant)
Artemisia vulgaris	Mugwort
Asarum canadensis and spp.	Wild ginger
Asclepias tuberosa	Pleurisy root
Asparagus officinalis	Asparagus
Aspidium filix-mas	Male fern
Aster tartaricus, A. puniceus and spp.	Aster, Red stalked aster
Astragalus mongolicus, A. membranaceus and A. hoantchy	Astragalus, Yellow vetch
Atractylodes alba	Atractylodes
Atropa mandragora	Mandrake
Balsamodendron mukul	Guggul
Baptisia tinctoria	Baptisia
Barosma betulina	Buchu
Belladonna atropa	Belladonna
Berberis vulgaris	Barberry
Betonica officinalis	Wood betony
Betula alba or	*B. lenta* Birch
Biotae orientalis	Thuja, Cedar tree, Chinese arbor vitae
Borago officinalis	Borage
Boswellia carterii	Frankincense
Brucea javanica	Brucea
Bryonia alba and B. dioica	White Bryony
Bubalus bubalis	Water Buffalo horn
Bupleurum falcatum	Bupleurum, Chai hu
Buthus martensi	Scorpion
Cactus grandiflorus	Night-blooming cereus
Calamus craco	Calamus
Calcium sulfate	Gypsum
Calendula officinalis	Calendula
Cannabis sativa	Marijuana
Capsella bursa-pastoris	Shepherd's purse
Capsicum frutescens	Cayenne
Carthamus tinctorius	Safflower
Carum carvi	Caraway
Carum copticum	Ajwan, Omum
Caryophyllus aromaticus	Cloves
Cascara amarga	Honduras bark
Cascara sagrada	same
Cassia acutifolia	Senna
Caulophyllum thalictroides	Blue cohosh

Ceanothus americanus	Ceanothus, Red root
Celosiae argentea and C. cristata	Cockscomb, Celosia
Centella asiatica	Gotu kola
Cereus grandiflorus	Night-blooming cereus
Cetraria islandica	Iceland moss
Chaenomelis lagenariae	Quince
Chamaelirium luteum	False Unicorn root
Chelidonium majus	Greater celandine
Chenopodium ambrosioides var. anthelminticum	American wormseed
Chimaphila umbellata	Pipsissewa
Chionanthus virginicus	Fringetree
Chondrus crispus	Irish moss
Chrysanthemum balsamita	Costmary
Chrysanthemum parthenium	Feverfew
Chrysanthemum morifolium	Chrysanthemum
Chrysanthemum vulgare	Tansy
Cimicifuga racemosa	Black cohosh
Cinchona succirubra;	Cinchona
Cinnabaris	Cinnabar
Cinnamomum camphora	Camphor
Cinnamomum cassia	Cinnamon
Cistanches salva	
Citrullus vulgaris	Watermelon
Citrus aurantium	Bitter orange
Citrus reticulata	Mandarin orange, Chen pi
Clematis spp.	Clematis
Codonopsis pilosula	Codonopsis, Dang shen
Coix lachryma	Coix seed
Collinsonia canadensis	Collinsonia
Convallaria majalis	Lily of the valley
Commiphora myrrha	Myrrh
Consolida regalis	Delphinium, Larkspur
Coriandrum sativum	Coriander
Coriolus versicolor (also Trametes v. and Polyporus v.)	Shelf mushroom
Cornu cervi	Deer antler
Cornus officinalis	Dogwood
Corydalis formosa and spp.	Corydalis, Turkey corn
Corynanthe yohimbe	Yohimbe
Crataegus spp.	Hawthorn
Crinis carbonisatus	Calcined human hair
Crocus sativus	Saffron
Croton tiglium	Croton

Cucumis sativus	Cucumber
Cucurbita foetidissima	Buffalo gourd
Cucurbita moschata	Pumpkin
Cucurbita sativus	Watermelon
Cuminum cyminum	Cumin
Curcuma longa	Turmeric
Cuscuta chinensis, C. europaea and C. japonica	Dodder
Cydonia oblonga	Quince
Cynoglossum officinale	Hound's tongue
Cyperus spp.	Sedge, Cyperus
Cypripedium pubescens	Lady's slipper
Cytisus scoparius;	Scotch broom
Daemonorops draco	Dragon's blood
Datura stramonium	Datura, Thorna
Daucus carota	Wild carrot
Dioscorea batata and D. japonica	Dioscorea
Dioscorea villosa	Wild yam
Diospyros kaki	Persimmon
Dipsacus sylvestris and spp.	Teasel
Drosera rotundifolia	Sundew
Dryopteris felix-mas	Male fern
Echinacea spp.	Echinacea
Eclipta alba and E. prostrata	Eclipta
Eletarria cardamomum	Cardamon
Eleutherococcus senticosus	Siberian ginsen§
Emblica officinalis and E. ribes	Amla, Emblic myrobalans
Ephedra sinica	Ma huang
Ephedra spp.	Ephedra
Epimedium grandiflorum and spp.	Epimedium
Erythraea centaurium	Centaury
Equisetum spp.	Horsetail
Epigea repens	Gravel root
Eriobotrya japonica	Loquat
Eriodictyon californica and spp.	Yerba santa
Eschscholzia california	California popp
Eucalyptus globulis and spp.	Eucalyptus
Eugenia jambolanum	Jambul
Euonymus atropurpureus	Wahoo, Burnin§ and E. europoeu:

Euphorbiae helioscopis and E. pilulifera	Euphorbia, Pill-bearing spurge
Euphrasia officinalis	Eyebright
Eupatorium purpureum	Gravel root
Ferrum	Iron
Ferula asafoetida	Asafoetida
Filipendula ulmaria	Meadowsweet
Floritum	Fluorite
Foeniculum officinalis	Fennel, and F. vulgare
Forsythia suspensa	Forsythia
Fremontia californica	(Calif. sp. similar to slippery elm)
Fritillaria thunbergii and spp.	Fritillary, Mission bells
Fucus versiculosis	Kelp
Fumaria officinalis	Fumitory
Galium aparine	Cleavers, Bedstraw
Ganoderma lucidum	Ling zhi mushroom
Garcinia hanburyi	Gamboge
Gardenia florida	Gardenia
Gastrodia elata	
Gaultheria procumbens	Wintergreen
Gekko gekko	Gecko lizard
Gentiana lutea;	Yellow gentian
Gentian officinalis	Gentian
Geranium maculatum	Cranesbill
Ginkgo biloba	Ginkgo
Gledista triacanthos	
Glycyrrhiza glabra	Licorice
Gossypium herbaceum	Cotton
Grifola umbellata	Grifola
Grindelia spp.	Grindelia, Gumweed
Guiacum officinalis	Guaicum
Hamemelis virginiana	Witch hazel
Haemititum	Hematite
Haliotidis diversicolor	Abalone
Harpagophytum procumbens	Devil's claw, Grapple plant
Hedeoma pulegoides	Pennyroyal
Helonias dioica	False unicorn
Heuchera americana	Alum root
Hibiscus rosa-sinensis	Hibiscus
Hordeum vulgaris	Barley
Humulus lupulus	Hops
Hydrangea arborescens	Hydrangea
Hydrastis canadensis	Golden seal

Hydrocotyle asiatica	Gotu kola
Hyoscyamus niger	Henbane
Hypericum perforatum	St. Johnswort
Hyssopus officinalis	Hyssop
Illicium anisatum	Star anise
Impatiens palida	Impatiens, Jewelweed
Inula helinium	Elecampane
Ipomoea jalapa	Jalap, Morning glory
Iris versicolor	Blue flag
Isatis bryonia	
Isatis tinctoria	Woad
Jeffersonia diphylla	Jeffersonia
Juglans cinerea	Butternut
Juglans regia	Walnut
Larrea divaricata	Chaparral
Leonorus cardiaca	Motherwort
Leptandra virginica	Culver's root
Lewisia rediviva	Bitterroot
Ligusticum levisticum	Lovage
Ligusticum lucidum	Privet
Ligusticum off.	Lovage
Ligusticum porteri	Osha
Ligusticum wallichi	
Lilium tigrinum	Tiger lily
Linum usitatissimum	Linseed, Flaxseed
Liriosma cupana	Muira-Puama
Lithospermum arnebia, L. rudrale	Gromwell
Lobelia inflata	Lobelia
Lonicera japonica	Honeysuckle
Lophatheri gracilis	Dwarf bamboo
Lycium chinensis and spp.	Lycium, Wolfberry, Matrimony vine
Lycoperdon solidum	Tuckahoe mushroom, Fu ling
Lycopus virginicus	Bugleweed
Lythrum sallicaria	Loosestrife
Magnolia lilifora and M. officinalis	Magnolia
Mahonia repens	Oregon grape
Mandragora spp.	Mandrake
Marrubium vulgare	Horehound
Matricaria chamomila	German chamomile
Mel	Honey
Melissa officinalis	Lemon balm
Mentha arvensis	Poleo
Mentha piperita	Peppermint

Mentha pulegium	Pennyroyal
Mentha virides	Spearmint
Meretricix meretrix	Clam
Mirabilitum	Sodium sulphate
Monarda punctata	Horsemint
Morinda officinalis	
Morus alba and	Mulberry
M. microphylla	
Moschus	Musk
Myrica cerifera	Bayberry
Myristica fragrans	Nutmeg
Naemorhedis and spp.	Antelope horn
Narcissus pseudo-	Daffodil
narcissus	
Nasturtium officinalis	Watercress
Nelumbium nuciferae	Lotus
Nelumbium luteum	Yellow water lily
Nepeta cataria	Catnip
Nephelium longana	Longan berries
Notopterygium	
Nymphea ordorata	White pond lily
Ocimum basilicum	Basil
Olea europea	Olive
Ophiopogon japonicus	Ophiopogon
and spp.	
Oplopanax horridum	Devil's club
Origanum marjorana	Marjoram
Origanum vulgare	Oregano
Oryza sativa	Rice
Os draconis	Dragon bone, ossified bones of pre-historic mammals
Ostrea gigas	Oyster shell
Paeonia moutan	Moutan peony
Paeonia alba	Peony
Paeonia suffruticosa	Tree peony
Panax ginseng	Ginseng
Panax quinquefolium	American ginseng
Panax pseudoginseng	Tienchi ginseng
Parrietoria officinalis	Pellitory of the wall
Passiflora incarnata	Passion flower
Pausinystalia yohimbe	Yohimbe
Petroselinum spp.	Parsley
Peucedanum ostruthium	Masterwort
Peucedanum palustre and spp.	Sow fennel, Marsh parsley
Peumus boldus	Boldo
Pfaffia paniculata	Suma, Brazilian ginseng

Pharbitis hederacea	Jalap, Morning glor
Phaseolus calcaratus	Azuki or aduki bea
Phaseolus munginis	Mung bean
Pheretime aspergillum	Earthworm
Phragmites communis	Reed grass
Phyllostachys spp.	Bamboo
Phytolacca spp.	Pokeroot
Picramnia antidesma and spp.	Cascara amarga
Pimento officinalis	Allspice
Pimpinellum anisum	Anise
Pinellia ternata	
Pinus sylvestris	Scotch or Norway
Pinus tabulaeformis	
Piper cubeba	Cubeb
Piper longum	Pippli long pepper,
Piper methysticum	Kava kava
Piper nigrum	Black pepper
Plantago psyllium	Psyllium
Plantago spp.	Plantain
Plastrum testudinis	Turtle
Platycodon grandiflorum	Platycodon
Podophyllum peltatum	Mandrake
Pogostemon cablin	Patchouli
Polygala senega	Seneca snakeroot
Polygonatum officinale	Solomon's seal
Polygonum aviculare	Knotweed
Polygonum bistorta	Bistort
Polygonum multiflorum	Fo-ti
Polypodium vulgare	Polypody fern
Polyporus tuberaster	Tuckahoe mushroo Fu ling
Populus balsamifera	Balsam poplar
Populus fremontii	Fremont cottonwo
Populus nigra	Black poplar
Populus tremuloides	Quaking aspen
Poncirus trifolata	Bitter orange
Poria cocos	Poria mushroom
Portulaceae oleracea	Purslane
Prunella vulgaris	Self-heal
Prunus Armenica	Apricot
Prunus persica	Peach
Prunus virginiana and P. serotina	Wild cherry, Chokecherry
Pseudostellaria heterophylla	
	Prince's ginseng
Psoralea corylifolia, P. esculenta and spp.	Psoralea, Scurfy pe
Pteria margaritifera	Pearl
Puerariae lobata et thunbergiana	Kudzu, Kuzu
Pulmonaria officinalis	Lungwort
Punica granatum	Pomegranate
Pyrola rotundifolia and spp.	Pyrola

Quercus alba and spp.	Oak
Ranunculus bulbosus and spp.	Buttercup, Crowfoot
Raphanus sativus	Radish
Rehmannia glutinosa	Rehmannia, Chinese foxglove
Rheum palmatum	Rhubarb
Rhamnus cathartica	Buckthorn
Rhus glabra	Sumac
Rhus toxicodendron	Poison ivy, Poison oak
Ribes rubrum	Black currant
Ricinus communis	Castor bean
Rosa spp.	Rose
Rubiae cordifoliae and R. tinctoria	Madder
Rubus ideaus	Raspberry
Rubus villosus	Blackberry
Rumex crispus	Yellow dock
Ruta graveolens	Rue
Sacharum granoram	Barley malt or rice syrup
Salix alba and S. nigra	Willow
Salvia milthiorrhiza	
Salvia officinalis	Sage
Sambucus canadensis	Elder bark
Sambucus nigra	Elder flowers
Sanguinaria canadensis	Blood root
Sanguisorba officinalis	Burnet
Santalum album	Sandalwood
Sassafras albidum	Sassafras
Satureja hortensis	Savory
Satureja douglasi	Yerba buena
Saussurea lappa	Costus
Schizandra chinensis and S. sinensis	Schizandra
Schizonepeta	
Scolopendra subspinipes	Centipede
Scrophularia nodosa	Figwort, Carpenter's square
Scutellaria lateriflora and S. laterifolia	Scullcap
Sabal serrulata	Saw palmetto
Sesamum indicum	Sesame
Sida cordifolia	Bala
Silybum marianum	Milk thistle
Sinapsis alba	Mustard
Smilax officinalis	Sarsaparilla
Solanum dulcamara	Bittersweet
Spigelia marilandica	Pink root

Spirodela polyrhiza	Duckweed
Stachys palustris	Hedge nettle
Stellaria media	Chickweed
Stephania tetandra	
Sticta pulmonaria	Sticta, Pulmonaria
Stillingia sylvatica	Stillingia
Stachys palustris	Wood betony
Succinum	Amber
Symphytum officinale	Comfrey
Symplocarpus foetidus	Skunk cabbage
Syzygium cumini	Jambul
Tabevulia	Pau d'Arco, Taheebo
Tanecetum vulgare	Tansy
Taraxacum officinale	Dandelion
Terminalis belerica	Beleric myrobalans
Terminalia chebula	Chebulic myrobalans, Haritaki
Thuja occidentalis	Thuja, Amer. arbor vitae, White cedar
Thymus vulgaris and spp.	Thyme
Trachelospermum jasminoides	Star jasmine
Tribulus terrestris	Caltrop, Gokshura, Puncture vine
Trichosanthes kirilowii	Trichosanthes
Trientalis borealis	Starflower
Trifolium pratense	Red clover
Trigonella foenumgraecum	Fenugreek
Trillium pendulum	Trillium
Triticum vulgare	Wheat
Tulipa edulis	Tulip
Turnera aphrodisiaca	Damiana, Turnera
Tussilago farfara	Coltsfoot
Typhus spp.	Cattail
Ulmus fulva	Slippery elm
Unicaria rynchophylla	Gambir
Urtica urens	Nettles
Usnea barbata	Bear lichen
Vaccinium myrtillus and spp.	Huckleberry, Bilberry
Valeriana officinalis	Valerian
Verbascum thapsus	Mullein
Verbena hastate	Blue vervain
Verbena officinalis	Vervain
Viburnum opulis	Cramp bark
Viburnum prunifolium	Black haw
Viola tricolor	Pansy, Heartsease
Vitex agnus-castus	Chaste tree
Vitex vinifera	Grape

Withania somnifera	Ashwagandha
Xanthium strumarium	Cocklebur
Xanthoxylum americanum	Prickly ash
Yucca spp.	Yucca
Zea mays	Corn
Zingiber officinale	Ginger
Zizyphus sativa	Jujube dates
Zizyphus spinosa spp.	Zizyphus

Appendix E/MEDICAL GLOSSARY

Abortifacient   causes induced abortion

Alterative   tending to restore normal health; cleanses and purifies the blood; alters existing nutritive and excretory processes gradually restoring normal body functions

Amenorrhea   absence or suppression of menstruation

Analgesic   relieves pain when taken orally

Anhydrotic   stops sweating

Anodyne   relieves pain when applied externally

Anthelmintic   helps destroy and dispel parasites (includes vermicides and vermifuges

Antibacterial   destroying or stopping the growth of bacteria

Antibilious   reduces biliary or jaundice condition

Antibiotic   inhibits growth of or destroys microorganisms

Antiemetic   lessens nausea and prevents or relieves vomiting

Antifungal   destroying or preventing the growth of fungi

Antigalactagogue   prevents or decreases secretion of milk

Anti-inflammatory   counteracting or diminishing inflammation or its effects

Antioxidant   inhibits oxydation

Antiparasitical   destructive to parasites

Antiperiodic   relieves malarial-type fevers and chills; prevents regular recurrances

Antiphlogistic   relieves inflammation

Antipyretic   dispels heat, fire and fever

Antiscorbutic   effective against or a remedy for scurvy

Antispasmodic   relieves spasms of voluntary and involuntary muscles

Antitussive   prevents or relieves coughing

Antiviral   inhibits a virus

Aperient   a mild laxative

Aphasia   inability to express oneself properly through speech or loss of verbal comprehension; sensory and motor areas may be involved

Aromatic	herbs which contain volatile, essential oils which aid digestion and relieve gas
Ascaris	roundworm (also called maw-worm and eelworm) found in the small intestine causing colicky pains and diarrhea, especially in children
Ascites	excessive accumulation of serous fluid in the peritoneal cavity
Asthenia	lack or loss of strength, usually involving muscular system
Astringent	firms tissues and organs; reduces discharges and secretions
Bactericide	destroys bacteria
Bitter tonic	bitter herbs which in small amounts stimulate digestion and otherwise help regulate fire in the body
Bolus	a suppository injected into the rectum or vagina
Calmative	soothing, sedative action
Cardiac	heart tonic or restorative
Carminative	relieves intestinal gas, pain and distention; promotes peristalsis
Cataplasm	another name for poultice
Cathartic	strong laxative which causes rapid evacuation
Cholagogue	promotes flow and discharge of bile into intestine
Chorea	nervous disorder marked by muscular twitching or arms, legs and face
Counterirritant	external application of an irritating substance to relieve pain in another more deep-seated part or to speed healing from increased circulation of the area
Cystitis	inflammation of the urinary bladder
Demulcent	soothes, protects and nurtures internal membranes
Demulcent febrifuge	reduces heat while building bodily fluids
Deobstruent	removes body obstructions
Depurative	cleanes or purifies blood by promoting eliminative functions
Dermatomycoses	skin infection caused by fungi

Detergent	cleansing to wounds, ulcers or skin itself
Detoxicant	removes toxins
Diaphoretic	causes perspiration and increases elimination through the skin
Digestant	contains substances (i.e. ferments, acids) which aid in digestion
Diuretic	promotes activity of kidney and bladder and increases urination
Drastic	a very active cathartic which produces violent peristalsis
Dropsy	generalized edema
Dyskinesia	defect in voluntary movement
Dysmenorrhea	painful or difficult menstruation
Dyspnea	sense of difficulty in breathing, often associated with lung or heart disease
Emetic	induces vomiting
Emmenagogue	helps promote and regulate menstruation
Emollient	soothes, softens and protects the skin
Enteritis	inflammation of the small intestine
Enterorrhagia	hemorrhage from the intestine
Enuresis	involuntary urination
Ephidrosis	abnormal amount of sweating
Epigastric	upper middle region of abdomen
Eructations	belching
Erysipelis	an acute disease of skin and subcutaneous tissue with spreading inflammation and swelling
Exanthema	any eruption of the skin accompanied by inflammation
Exophthalmic	protrusion of the eyeball
Expectorant	promotes discharge of phlegm and mucus from lungs and throat
Febrifuge	reduces fever
Fistula	abnormal tubelike passage from a normal cavity or tube to a free surface or to another cavity
Galactagogue	promotes secretion of milk
Gastralgia	pain in the stomach

Gastroenteritis	inflammation of the stomach and intestinal tract
Gastroptosis	condition in which stomach occupies an abnormally low position in the abdomen
Gleet	mucous discharge from urethra in chronic gonorrhea in the urine
Hemiplegia	paralysis of one half of the body
Hemostatic	stops the flow of blood; type of astringent that stops internal bleeding or hemorrhaging
Homeostasis	equilibrium of internal environment
Hydragogue	promotes watery evacuation of bowels
Hyperch-lorhydria	excess of hydrochloric acid in gastric secretion
Hypnotic	powerful nervine relaxant and sedative that induces sleep
Hypochondriac	upper lateral region on each side of the body and below the thorax; beneath the ribs
Intercostal	between the ribs
Laxative	promotes bowel movements
Lithotriptic	dissolves or discharges urinary and biliary concretions
Menorrhagia	excessive bleeding during menstruation
Monoplegia	paralysis of a si ngle limb or a single group of muscles
Mydriatic	dilates the pupil
Narcotic	depresses central nervous system, thus relieving pain and promoting sleep
Nephritis	inflammation of the kidney
Nervine	strengthens functional activity of nervous system; may be stimulants or sedatives
Neurasthenia	severe nerve weakness; nervous exhaustion
Neurodermatitis	inflammation of skin with itching that is associatted with emotional disturbance
Nutritive	increases weight and density; nourishes the body
Opthalmic	healing to disorders and diseases of the eyes
Osteomyelitis	inflammation of the bone, especially the marrow
Oxyuris	genus of nematode intestinal worms which includes pinworms (also called threadworm and seatworm)

Parturient	stimulates uterine contractions which induce and assist labor
Pectoral	healing to problems in the broncho-pulmonary area
Phagocytosis	ingestion and digestion of bacteria and particles by phagocytes
Plethora	overfullness of blood vessels or of the total quantity of any fluid in the body
Portal	concerning entrance to an organ, especially that through which blood is carried to liver
Prophylactic	agent which wards off disease
Pruritis	severe itching
Pterygium	opaque triangular thickening of tissue extending from inner canthus to border or cornea with apex toward pupil
Purgative	causes watery evacuation of intestinal contents
Puerpural	period following childbirth
Pyelitis	inflammation of the pelvis of the kidney and its calices
Refrigerant	reduces body temperature and relieves thirst
Rhinitis	inflammation of nasal mucosa
Rubefacient	with local application stimulates capillary dilation and action, causing skin redness
Scorbutic	concerning or affected with scurvy
Scrofula	variety of tuberculous adenitis
Sedative	calms or tranquilizes by lowering functional activity of organ or body part
Septicemia	presence of pathogenic bacteria in the blood; blood poisoning
Sialogugue	promotes secretion and flow of saliva
Specific	a remedy having a curative effect on a particular disease or symptom
Spermatorrhea	abnormally frequent involuntary loss of semen without orgasm
Spondylosis	abnormal immobility and fixation of vertebral joints

Stimulant	increases internal heat, dispels internal chill and strengthens metabolism and circulation
Stomachic	strengthens stomach function
Styptic	externally applied will arrest local bleeding by contracting blood vessels
Subcostal	beneath the ribs
Sudorific	stimulates production and secretion of perspiration
Tetters	skin disease with pimples or blisters such as herpes, ringworm, or eczema
Tinea capitis	fungal skin disease of the scalp
Tinnitus	ringing or tinkling sound in the ear
Tonic	stimulates nutrition and increase systemal tone, usually in the absence of illness
Vasodepressant	lowers blood pressure by dilatation of blood vessels; having a depressing influence on circulation
Vasodilator	causes relaxation of blood vessels
Vermifuge	expels or repels intestinal worms
Vermicide	destroys worms
Vulnerary	assists in healing of wounds by protecting against infection and stimulating cell growth

BOTANICAL INDEX

GENERAL INDEX

BIBLIOGRAPHY

EARLY EUROPEAN HERBALISM

Culpepper, Nicholas. *CULPEPPER'S COMPLETE HERBAL.* W. Foulsham and Co. A reprint of the original seventeenth century copy.

Macer. *MACER'S VIRTUE OF HERBS.* Hemkunt Press. A republication of a popular medieval herbal that describes herbs energetically.

NORTH AMERICAN

Christopher, Dr. John R. *SCHOOL OF NATURAL HEALING.* Provo, UT: Biworld, 1976.

Courtenay and Zimmerman. *WILDFLOWERS AND WEEDS.* Cincinnati, New York, Toronto, London, Melbourne: Van Nostrand Reinhold. A book useful for its many outstanding photographs of wildflowers and weeds, many of which are used medicinally.

Foster, Steven. *EAST-WEST BOTANICALS.* Ozark Beneficial Plant Project, HCR Box 3, Brisey, MO, 65618. A cross-reference of medicinal herbs between North America and China.

Grieve, Mrs. M. *A MODERN HERBAL.* New York, NY: Dover, 1971. A two volume reprint of the work originally published in 1931.

Hobbs, Christopher. *CHINESE HERBS GROWING IN THE WESTERN U.S.* Botanica Press, P.O. Box 742, Capitola, CA 95010. Presenting a cross-reference of a number of North American plants with similar species found growing in China (many plants different from Foster, above).

Hoffmann, David. *THE HOLISTIC HERBAL.* Findhorn Press. An excellent presentation of the British Herbal Association.

Law, Donald. *THE CONCISE HERBAL.* St. Martin's Press. A good introductory herbal for the layperson. Includes the making of herbal wines.

Lust, John. *THE HERB BOOK.* Bantam. An excellent introductory book on herbal medicine for the layman.

Millspaugh, Charles F. *AMERICAN MEDICINAL PLANTS.* New York, NY: Dover, 1974. Republication of the work published by John C. Yorston & Co. in two volumes under the title *Medicinal Plants.*

Moore, Michael. *MEDICINAL PLANTS OF THE MOUNTAIN WEST.* Santa Fe, NM: Museum of New Mexico Press, 1979. An excellent book on Western medicinal herbs.

Nickell's, J. M. *J. M. NICKELL'S BOTANICAL READY REFERENCE.* P.O. Box 23096, Los Angeles, CA 90023: M. L. Baker. An indispensible reference for herb identification, listing some 2,465 herbs.

Priest and Priest. *HERBAL MEDICATION, A CLINICAL AND DISPENSARY HANDBOOK.* Fowler. An authoritative presentation of the clinical usage and principles of the British Institute of Medical Herbalists.

Rose, Jeanne. *HERBS AND THINGS.* New York, NY: Grosset and Dunlap. An introduction to self-healing with herbs.

Schauenberg and Paris. *GUIDE TO MEDICINAL PLANTS.* Keats. A materia medica that organizes herbs according to their biochemical constituents.

Schultes, Richard. *MEDICINES FROM THE EARTH.* San Francisco, CA: Harper and Row, Alfred van der Marck, dist. A compendium of medicinal herbs, authoritatively presented with up-to-date biochemical constituents and beautiful illustrations.

Shook, Edward E. *BEGINNING AND ADVANCED TREATISE IN HERBOLOGY.* Republished by Trinity Center Press, P.O. Box 335, Beaumont, CA and CSA Press, Lakemont, GA 30552.

Stuhr, Ernst T. *MANUAL OF PACIFIC COAST DRUG PLANTS.* Reprinted by Botanica Press (see Hobbs). A republication of a work first published in 1933 describing the medicinal uses of plants of the Pacific Northwest.

Tenney, Louise. *TODAY'S HERBAL HEALTH.* Hawthorne Books, P.O. Box 62, Provo, UT 84601. An introductory herbal that describes the combination of micronutrients with herbs.

Tierra L.Ac., Lesley. *THE HERBS OF LIFE, HEALTH AND HEALING USING WESTERN AND CHINESE TECHNIQUES*, published by Crossing Press.

Tierra, Michael. *THE WAY OF HERBS.* Simon and Schuster. Introducing the principles of self-help and herbal therapy.

Tierra L.Ac., OMD, Michael (editor). *AMERICAN HERBALISM: Essays by members of the American Herbalists Guild*, published by Crossing Press.

Tierra L.Ac. OMD, Michael and Cantin, Candis, *THE SPIRIT OF HERBS, GUIDE TO THE HERBAL TAROT*, published by US Games.

Vogel, A. *THE NATURE DOCTOR.* Bioforce-Verlag, Teufen, Switzerland. A collection of Swiss folklore and healing.

Weiss MD, Rudolf Fritz, *HERBAL MEDICINE*, published by AB Arcanum, Gothenburg, Sweden, Beaconsfield Publishers LTD, Beaconsfield, England. Distributed by medicina biologica, 4830 N.E. 32nd Ave.. Portland, OR 97211.

Willard, Terry, Ph.D. *HELPING YOURSELF WITH NATURAL REMEDIES.* CRCS Publications. P.O. Box 208950, Reno, NV 98515. An excellent practical book on herbal self-treatment by the author of *Wild Rose College of Natural Healing.*

ANTHROPOSOPHICAL MEDICINE

Bott, Victor, M.D. *ANTHROPOSOPHICAL MEDICINE.* Thorsons. Introducing the principles of Anthroposophical medicine with its unique energetic description of diseases and herbs based upon the teachings of the great pragmatical mystic, Rudolph Steiner.

NATIVE AMERICAN

Hutchens, Alma R. *INDIAN HERBOLOGY OF NORTH AMERICA.* Merco, 620 Wyandotte East, Windsor 14, Ontario, Canada, 1969. A study of Anglo-American, Russian and Oriental literature on Indian medical botanics of North America.

Moerman, Daniel E. *MEDICINAL PLANTS OF NATIVE AMERICA.* Ann Arbor, MI: University of Michigan Museum of Anthropology. A two volume work on medicinal plants used by the Native Americans.

Mooney, James. *THE SWIMMER MANUSCRIPT OF CHEROKEE SACRED FORMULAS AND MEDICINAL PRESCRIPTIONS.* First published by the U.S. government in 1932, reissued by Botanica Press, Capitola, CA. This is an important early document that is a first-hand account of the high art of Cherokee herbal medicine.

Vogel, Virgil J. *AMERICAN INDIAN MEDICINE. University of Oklahoma Press. A good historical presentation of the various herbal remedies used by tribes throughout the U.S.*

AYURVEDA

Dash, Bhagwan and Junius. *A HANDBOOK OF AYURVEDA.* New Delhi, India: Concept Publishing. A good presentation of the principles of Ayurvedic medicine with many of the traditional herbs and preparations outlined.

Dash, Bhagwan. *AYURVEDIC TREATMENT FOR COMMON DISEASES.* Delhi Diary 1/172, Jore Bagh Market, N. Delhi, India. An outline of basic diseases with treatment using Ayurvedic herbs and preparations.

Dastur, J. F. *EVERYBODY'S GUIDE TO AYURVEDIC MEDICINE.* D. B. Taraporevala Sons and Co. Private LTD. 210, dr. D. Naoroji Road, Fort, Bombay-1, India. A repertory of therapeutic prescriptions based on the indigenous systems of India.

Frawley, David and Lad, Dr. Vasant. *THE YOGA OF HERBS.* Twin Lakes, WI. Lotus Press, 1986. Describes the use of Western herbs energetically, incorporating them into the system of Ayurveda.

Jain, S. K. *MEDICINAL PLANTS.* India: National Book Trust. A description of a number of medicinal herbs used by the people of India.

Lad, Dr. Vasant. *AYURVEDA, THE SCIENCE OF SELF HEALING.* Twin Lakes, WI. Lotus Press, 1984. An excellent introduction to the principles of tridosha and Ayurvedic medicine.

Murthy, Dr. N. Anyneya and Pandey, D. P. *AYURVEDIC CURE FOR COMMON DISEASES.* Vision Books, Madarsa Road, Mashmere Gate, Delhi-110006, India. An outline of diseases and Ayurvedic preparations used to treat them. One of the problems with this book is that the preparations are not generally available anywhere except in India.

Ojha, Divakar and Kumar, Ashok. *PANCHAKARMA- THERAPY IN AYURVEDA.* Chaukhamba Amarabharati Prakashan, Varanasi, India. A presentation of the five external methods of purification therapy used in Ayurvedic medicine.

Sharma, Prof. P. V. *INTRODUCTION TO DRAVYAGUNA (Indian Pharmacology).* Varanasi, India: Chaukhambha Orientalia. A good reference on the principles of Ayurvedic pharmacy.

Thakkur, Chandrashekhar G. *AYURVEDA FOR YOU.* Ancient Wisdom Publications. Available from Popular Book Depot, Grant Road, Bombay, India; New Book Co. Pvt. Ltd., 188090 dr. D.N. Road, Bombay-1, India; D.B. Taraporevala 210, dr. D.N. Road, Bombay-1, India. Presenting a number of home cures, treatment of specific diseases, and herbs found both in other parts of the world and some of the more important herbs found in India. It is an Ayurvedic doctor's presentation of aspects of his clinical experience.

Thakkur, Chandrashekhar G. *INTRODUCTION TO AYURVEDA.* Ancient Wisdom Publications (see above for distributors). A good presentation of the basic theoretical principles of Ayurvedic medicine.

ECLECTICS

KING'S AMERICAN DISPENSATORY. Portland, OR: republished by Eclectic Medical Publications. The outstanding two volume 2,200 page materia medica first published during the latter part of the last century. A landmark work on Eclectic Medicine and the clinical use of North American herbs.

Scudder, Dr. *STUDY OF DISEASE AND SPECIFIC MEDICINE.* Portland, OR: republished by Eclectic Medical Publications. It is a two volume work outlining the principles of holistic diagnoses and treatment that was being evolved by the Eclectics. There is much in common with principles of traditional Chinese and Ayurvedic medicine although these systems were not widely known at the time.

HERBAL HISTORY

Griggs, Barbara. *GREEN PHARMACY, A HISTORY OF HERBAL MEDICINE.* New York, NY: Viking Press, 1982. A fascinating history of herbal medicine which includes a history of Samuel Thompson and the North American eclectics.

Hand, Wayland D., ed. *AMERICAN FOLK MEDICINE.* Berkeley, Los Angeles, London: University of California Press. Based on a series of individual presentations by professors and ethnobotanists throughout the country that took place at a conference on American Folk Medicine in December of 1973.

CHINESE

A BAREFOOT DOCTOR'S MANUAL. Cloudburst Press, revised and enlarged edition. The manual used by the barefoot doctors of China. It lists over 520 herbs, and mineral and animal derived substances used for medicine, many that are common with species and plants found in the West and other parts of the world.

Bensky and Gamble. *CHINESE HERBAL MEDICINE.* Eastland Press. A materia medica of Chinese medicinal herbs.

Cheung, Dr. *DIALECTICAL DIFFERENTIAL DIAGNOSIS AND TREATMENT.* Traditional Chinese Medical Publishes, 2400 Geary Boulevard, San Francisco, CA. 94115. An excellent introduction for the acupuncturist and herbal practitioner on the principles of Chinese diagnoses and herbal therapy.

Connelly, Dianne M. *TRADITIONAL ACUPUNCTURE: THE LAW OF THE FIVE ELEMENTS.* Columbia, MD: The Centre for Traditional Acupuncture Inc. Presents an in-depth description of the fascinating system of Chinese five element theory.

Hsu, Dr. Hong-yen and Preacher, Dr. William G. *CHINESE HERB MEDICINE AND THERAPY.* Los Angeles, CA: Oriental Healing Arts Institute. An introduction to the principles of Chinese herbology.

Hsu, Dr. Hong-yen. *COMMONLY USED CHINESE HERB FORMULAS WITH ILLUSTRATIONS.* Los Angeles, CA: Oriental Healing Arts Institute. A comprehensive description of traditional Chinese formulas which would be suitable for clinical use except for a few minor flaws in the description of the parts of the herbs intended for use and as to whether they are processed or not.

Hyatt, Richard. *CHINESE HERBAL MEDICINE.* Schocken. An introduction to the principles of Chinese herbal medicine.

Kaptchuk, Ted. *THE WEB THAT HAS NO WEAVER.* St. Martins Press. A wonderful presentation of the fundamental principles of Chinese medicine.

Keys. *CHINESE HERBS.* Tuttle. A materia medica of Chinese herbs emphasizing their Western therapeutic properties and not their energetics.

Leung, Albert Y. *CHINESE HERBAL REMEDIES.* New York, NY: Universe Books. An in-depth, fine presentation of Chinese home remedies using herbs that are commonly found growing in the West.

ORIENTAL HEALING ARTS INTERNATIONAL BULLETIN. Oriental Healing Arts Inst., 1945 Palo Verde Ave., Suite 208, Long Beach, CA 90815. A quarterly journal on Chinese herbal medicine, including case studies, scientific investigations and clinical experiences of Chinese and occidental practitioners.

Perry. *MEDICINAL PLANTS OF EAST AND SOUTHEAST ASIA.* Cambridge, MA and London, England: Mit Press. A large, scholarly volume on the herbs of that region.

THE JOURNAL OF THE AMERICAN COLLEGE OF TRADITIONAL CHINESE MEDICINE. Vol. 3, 1983. Traditional Chinese Medical Publisher (see Cheung). This journal outlined the Chinese pharmacopoeia which formed the basis for the categorization which was followed in creating the present volume. It is a quarterly publication with outstanding contributions from Chinese and occidental practitioners of Traditional Chinese Medicine.

Tierra, Michael and Tierra, Lesley. *CHINESE- PLANETARY HERBAL DIAGNOSES.* East-West Herb School, Box 712, Santa Cruz. CA 95061. A concise handbook for the clinical application of Chinese diagnostic principles. Some reference to the use of special herbs, foods and Planetary formulas.

Yeung, Him-che. *HANDBOOK OF CHINESE HERBS AND FORMULAS.* Self-published and available from the author in West Los Angeles or from Redwing Distributors in Boston, MA. A two volume materia medica and formulary on Chinese herbalism, highly practical and useable in a clinical practice.

NUTRITION

Ballentine, Rudolph. *DIET AND NUTRITION, A HOLISTIC APPROACH.* Honesdale, PA: Himalayan International Inst., 1978. An important and comprehensive presentation on aspects of nutrition incorporating the traditional principles of Ayurveda with Western nutrition.

Colbin, Annemarie. *FOOD AND HEALING.* Ballantine Press. An excellent presentation of the principles of macrobiotic food therapy and beyond by the author of *Book of Whole Meals.*

Flaws, Bob and Wolfe, Honora. *PRINCE WEN HUI'S COOK, CHINESE DIE-TARY THERAPY.* Blue Poppy Press. A presentation of the principles of dietary therapy using foods and some herbs, with many traditional herb-food recipes.

Kushi, Michio. *MACROBIOTIC HOME REMEDIES.* Edited by Marc Van Cauwenberghe, M.D. An excellent practical book on simple home remedies and treatments for a number of health problems.

Kushi, Michio. *THE BOOK OF MACROBIOTICS.* Japan Publ. Presents the basic principles of macrobiotics.

Lu, Henry C. *CHINESE SYSTEM OF FOOD CURES.* Sterling. An outline of the principles of Chinese food therapy.

Ni, Maoshing. *THE TAO OF NUTRITION.* Shrine of the Eternal Breath of Tao, 117 Stonehaven Way, Los Angeles, CA 90049.

Turner, Kristina. *THE SELF HEALING COOKBOOK,* published by Earth Tones, P.O. Box 2341 B, Grass Valley, CA 95945.

ALCHEMY

Albertus, Frater. *ALCHEMIST'S HANDBOOK.* Weiser. Describing how to make spagyric tinctures and other principles of alchemy.

Junius, Manfred. *PRACTICAL HANDBOOK OF PLANT ALCHEMY.* New York, NY: Inner Traditions International Ltd. An excellent and clearly written book on the practical aspects of alchemy. Describes how to maky spagyric tinctures.

Paracelsus. *THE HERMETIC AND ALCHEMICAL WRITINGS OF PARACELSUS.* Shambhala Publications. Edited by Edward Waite. A two volume collection of the fifteenth century giant who layed the foundation for alchemy.

HERBAL CULTIVATION

Foster, Steven. *HERBAL BOUNTY, THE GENTLE ART OF HERB CULTURE.* Salt Lake City, UT: Gibbs M. Smith, Inc. A practical handbook on herbal cultivation with outstanding illustrations by D. D. Dowden.

LIBRARY

The Lloyd's Library and Museum, 917 Plum Street, Cincinnati, OH 45202, ph. (513)721-3707.

SOURCES FOR HERBS AND HERBAL PRODUCTS

The author fully realizes that many of the herbs mentioned in this work are not as yet commonly available through established sources and distributors. However, since it is the personal belief of the author that the Western herbal pharmacopiea has been historically depleted of important therapeutic materials to round off its clinical repertoire, it will eventually be necessary to expand the number of herbs and materials available to at least approximate those described in this work.

Presently the only source for many of these materials is directly from harvesters, wildcrafters, or Chinese herbal pharmacies.

WILDCRAFTERS

Ryan Drum, Waldron, Washington 98297.

Blessed Herbs, Michael Volchok, Rt. 5, Box 191A, Ava, Missouri 85020.

Reevis Mountain School of Survival, 321 E. Northern, Phoenix, Arizona 85020.

Beth Graibeldinger, P.O. Box 1021, Nederland, Colorado 80466.

Mike and Debby Minear, Rt. 1, Box 60, Little Hocking, Ohio 45742.

CHINESE HERB DISTRIBUTORS

Great China Herb Company, 857 Washington St., San Francisco, California 94108.

PLANETARY HERBAL PRODUCTS, a retail mail order company offering Planetary Formulas and other herbal books and products by outstanding herbalists. They also offer a fine selection of quality Western and Chinese herbs. Send for free catalogue, P.O. Box 7145, Santa Cruz, CA 95061 or call 408-479-7074 for information.

May Way Trading Corporation, 622 Broadway, San Francisco, California 94133. Chinese herb distributors with phone numbers and telex throughout the world.

Herbalist and Alchemist Inc., David Winston, P.O. Box 63, Franklin Park, New Jersey 08823.

Tai Sang Trading Chinese Herb Company, 1018 Stockton, San Francisco, California 94108.

AYURVEDIC HERBAL PRODUCTS

Lotus Light (Wholesale), P.O. Box 1008-PH, Silver Lake, WI 53170 800/548-3824; 262-889-8501; fax 262-889-8591

Internatural (Retail), P.O. Box 33719-PH 116th St.
Twin Lakes, WI 53181. 800/643-4221 www.internatural.com

HERB PRODUCTS

Threshold Distributors, P.O. Box 533, Soquel, California 95073, 1-800-438-1700. Distributes Planetary Herb products.

Herb Pharm, Ed Smith, P.O. Box 116, 347 E. Fork Road, Williams, Oregon 97544.

Herbal Home Products, Bob Brucea, 3405 Angel Lane, Placerville, California 95672.

Brion Corporation, Chinese herb formulas and extracts, 12020 Centralia, Hawaiian Gardens, California 90716.

Lotus Light (Wholesale), P.O. Box 1008-PH, Silver Lake, WI 53170 800/548-3824; 262-889-8501; fax 262-889-8591

Internatural (Retail), P.O. Box 33719-PH 116th St.
Twin Lakes, WI 53181. 800/643-4221 www.internatural.com

HERBAL DISTRIBUTORS

Lotus Light (Wholesale), P.O. Box 1008-PH, Silver Lake, WI 53170 800/548-3824; 262-889-8501; fax 262-889-8591

Internatural (Retail), P.O. Box 33719-PH 116th St.
Twin Lakes, WI 53181. 800/643-4221 www.internatural.com
53181.

ORGANIC HERB FARMS

Trout Lake Herb Farm, Rt. 1, Box 355, Trout Lake, Washington 98650.

EAST-WEST HERBAL
CORRESPONDENCE SCHOOL

We offer two home study courses in herbal medicine. The introductory course includes 12 lessons and is most suitable for home and lay herbal practice. The comprehensive Master Course is 36 lessons and forms the basis for a deeper understanding of the principles of traditional herbal medicine, including diet, diagnoses, materia medica and other studies necessary for a professional understanding of herbal medicine. Both of these courses are an integration of Western, Chinese and Ayurvedic herbal medicine and come with projects and lessons that are individually evaluated. There are also optional study materials including audio and visual cassettes which can be obtained separately.

EAST-WEST SCHOOL OF HERBAL STUDIES
Box 712H
Santa Cruz, CA 95061

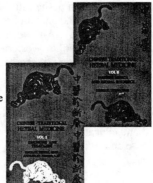

BIOMAGNETIC
and Herbal Therapy
Dr. Michael Tierra

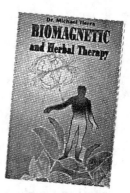

$10.95   96 pp
5 3/8 x 8 1/2 quality trade paper
ISBN 0-914955-33-0

Magnetic energy is the structural force of the universe. In this book the respected herbalist and healer, Dr. Michael Tierra enlightens us on the healing influence of commercially available magnets for many conditions and describes the sometimes miraculous relief from such problems as joint, pain, skin diseases, acidity, blood pressure, tumors, kidney, liver and thyroid problems, and more. Magnetizing herbs, teas, water and their usage in conjunction with direct placement of magnets for synergistic effectiveness is presented in a systematic, succinct and practical manner for the benefit of the professional and lay person alike. Replete with diagrams, and appendices, this is a "how to do" practical handbook for augmenting health and obtaining relief from pain.

The paradigm of health in the future is based on energy flow. This paradigm reaches back to the ancient healing arts of the traditional Chinese, the Ayurvedic and the Native American cultures. It is connected to the work of Hippocrates, the "father" of Western medicine, in ancient Greek culture, and found its way through the herbal and homeopathic science that has flourished in Europe over the last few hundred years.

Dr. Tierra is the author of the all-time best selling herbal *The Way of Herbs* as well as the synthesizing work *Planetary Herbology*. He is a practicing herbalist and educator in the field with a background of studies spanning the Chinese and Ayurvedic, the Native American and the European herbal traditions.

To order your copy, ask your local bookseller or send
$10.95 + 3.00 (s/h) to:
Lotus Press
P O Box 325PH
Twin Lakes, Wi 53181 USA

Request our complete book and alternative health products catalogs
of over 7000 items. Wholesale inquiries welcome.

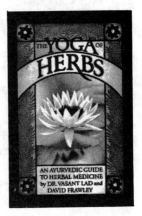

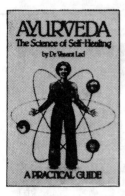

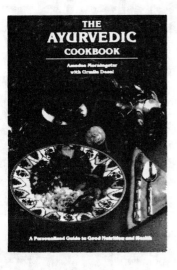

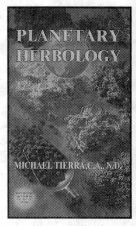